Probiotics in Pediatric Medicine

NUTRITION AND HEALTH SERIES
Adrianne Bendich, PhD, FACN, SERIES EDITOR

For other titles published in this series, go to
www.springer.com/series/7659

Probiotics
in Pediatric Medicine

Editors

Sonia Michail, MD
Department of Gastroenterology and Nutrition, Children's Medical Center,
Wright State Boonshoft School of Medicine, Dayton, OH, USA

Philip M. Sherman, MD, FRCPC
Division of Gastroenterology, Hepatology and Nutrition, The Hospital for Sick
Children, University of Toronto, Toronto, Ontario, Canada

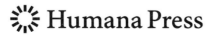 Humana Press

Editors
Sonia Michail, MD
Department of Gastroenterology and Nutrition
Children's Medical Center
Wright State Boonshoft School of Medicine
Dayton, OH
USA

Philip M. Sherman, MD, FRCPC
Division of Gastroenterology, Hepatology
and Nutrition
The Hospital for Sick Children
University of Toronto
Toronto, Ontario
Canada

Series Editor
Adrianne Bendich, PhD, FACN
GlaxoSmithKline Consumer Healthcare
Parsippany, NJ
USA

ISBN: 978-1-60327-288-9   e-ISBN: 978-1-60327-289-6
DOI: 10.1007/978-1-60327-289-6

Library of Congress Control Number: 2008933594

Printed on acid-free paper

springer.com

Biosketch

Sonia K. Michail, MD, FAAP, is an associate professor of pediatrics at Boonshoft School of Medicine, Wright State University and a pediatric gastroenterologist at Dayton Children's Medical Center, in Dayton, Ohio. After receiving her medical degree in 1989, she completed her pediatric residency program at Michigan State University and her pediatric gastroenterology fellowship at the University of Nebraska Medical Center and Creighton University, Omaha, Nebraska. Dr. Michail's research interest is focused on probiotics and gut microflora and has received NIH funding in this pursuit.

Philip M. Sherman, MD, FRCPC, is professor of pediatrics, microbiology, and dentistry at the Hospital for Sick Children, University of Toronto, where he has been on faculty since 1984. Sherman completed medical school at the University of Calgary in 1977 and training in pediatrics at the University of California, San Francisco (1977–1980). He did his training in gastroenterology and conducted his research at the Hospital for Sick Children in Toronto, Canada, and at the Walter Reed Army Institute of Research in Washington, DC (1980–1984), respectively. Sherman is the immediate former president of the North American Society for Pediatric Gastroenterology, Hepatology and Nutrition and a former president of the Canadian Association of Gastroenterology. He is the recipient of a Canada Research Chair (tier 1) in Gastrointestinal Disease (2001–2015). His research program is funded by support currently provided by the Crohn's and Colitis Foundation of Canada and the Canadian Institutes of Health Research. Sherman serves on the Research Advisory Board of Antibe Therapeutics. His research interests focus on epithelial cell signal transduction responses to bacteria and their products.

Series Editor's Introduction

The Nutrition and Health series of books have, as an overriding mission, to provide health professionals with texts that are considered essential because each includes: 1) a synthesis of the state of the science, 2) timely, in-depth reviews by the leading researchers in their respective fields, 3) extensive, up-to-date fully annotated reference lists, 4) a detailed index, 5) relevant tables and figures, 6) identification of paradigm shifts and the consequences, 7) virtually no overlap of information between chapters, but targeted, inter-chapter referrals, 8) suggestions of areas for future research and 9) balanced, data-driven answers to patient/health professionals questions which are based upon the totality of evidence rather than the findings of any single study.

The series volumes are not the outcome of a symposium. Rather, each editor has the potential to examine a chosen area with a broad perspective, both in subject matter as well as in the choice of chapter authors. The international perspective, especially with regard to public health initiatives, is emphasized where appropriate. The editors, whose trainings are both research and practice oriented, have the opportunity to develop a primary objective for their book; define the scope and focus, and then invite the leading authorities from around the world to be part of their initiative. The authors are encouraged to provide an overview of the field, discuss their own research and relate the research findings to potential human health consequences. Because each book is developed de novo, the chapters are coordinated so that the resulting volume imparts greater knowledge than the sum of the information contained in the individual chapters.

Probiotics in Pediatric Medicine, edited by Sonia Michail and Philip M. Sherman is a very welcome addition to the Nutrition and Health Series and fully exemplifies the Series' goals. This volume is especially timely since it stands as the first volume to use an evidence-based approach to examine the clinical role of probiotics in the prevention and treatment of a number of disease conditions in pediatric patients. As one example, there is a growing awareness of the potential for specific probiotics to reduce the risk of serious gastrointestinal conditions such as diarrhea in infants and children. Probiotics that were considered as part of alternative medicine in adults in the recent past are now considered by physicians around the world as well as regulatory agencies to be part of mainstream medical care not only for adults, but also for newborns and toddlers. Probiotics are defined by the World Health Organization as "live microorganisms which, when consumed in adequate amounts as part of food, confer a health benefit". Probiotics are also characterized as non-pathogenic microbes that are normally found in the human gastrointestinal (GI) tract and that are mainly consumed in live form for the benefit of the human host.

The last decade has seen an increased emphasis on the identification and characterization of the human microflora as well as their bioactive, immunomodulatory molecules. At the same time, there has been an increasing awareness of the role of inflammation in the development of GI tract diseases and the potential for probiotics with anti-inflammatory mechanisms of action to help slow disease progression. This text is the first to synthesize the knowledge base concerning gut inflammation, loss of gut integrity and the potential for commensal microbes and/or their products to be factors in the development of autoimmune diseases not only in the GI tract, but throughout the body. This excellent volume will add great value to the practicing health professional as well as those professionals and students who are interest in the latest, up-to-date information on the science behind the probiotics and how these microbes can improve the health throughout the lifespan.

The editors of this benchmark volume are internationally recognized experts in the field of Pediatric Gastroenterology and each has been directly involved in the characterization of the clinical value of probiotics in children. Dr. Michail, M.D. is Associate Professor of Pediatrics and Medicine at the Boonshoft School of Medicine at Wright State University in Dayton Ohio and is NIH funded in the area of probiotics and gut microflora. Dr. Sherman, M.D., FRCPC is Professor of Paediatrics, Microbiology, and Dentistry at the Hospital for Sick Children, University of Toronto in Toronto, Canada and has served as President of the North American Society for Pediatric Gastroenterology, Hepatology and Nutrition and the Canadian Association of Gastroenterology. They have developed an excellent volume that provides the reader with chapters covering the basics of gastrointestinal physiology and the key aspects of the complex area of gut immunity. Importantly, they have included an entire chapter on the microflora within the human gut and include important information about the development of the gut microflora during the first weeks/months of life. The reader learns quickly that the genetic material contained within the gut microbes surpasses that of the human genome by a factor of 140! Another sobering statistic is that there are about 1014 microbes in the adult human gut which is about 10 times the number of cells in the human body. Thus, the introductory chapters provide a comprehensive overview of the functions of the GI tract as well as the resident microbes. Examples of areas covered in these chapters include the importance of maintenance of tight junctions between GI epithelia and the importance of zonulin, discovered by the author of the first chapter, the role of Toll receptors, gut associated lymphoid tissue (GALT), gut peptide hormones and signaling molecules, cytokines and interleukins. Readers are introduced to the links between gut immunity and the microflora and the development of diseases such as irritable bowel disease (IBS), inflammatory bowel disease (IBD) and other systemic conditions including, eczema and allergy. Moreover, the products of the microflora are found in the host's blood, lymph, bile, sweat and urine.

In the chapter entitled Probiotics 101, we learn that the term probiotics was introduced in 1965, however the first commercially available probiotic was produced in 1935. Related terms, such as prebiotic (food for probiotics) and synbiotics (both pre and probiotics in the same product) are discussed in detail. The following chapter describes the multiple functions of probiotics and their mechanisms of action and the next chapter examines the data related to the safety of probiotics including the areas of potential sepsis, enhancement of antibiotic resistance and other potential adverse effects. Importantly, probiotics are considered as generally recognized as safe (GRAS) by the US FDA; well-controlled trials have not documented serious adverse events. The critical caveat is that the data are strain specific as well as population specific and cannot be generalized. Case studies of specific adverse events appear to be mainly in individuals with additional risk factors such as being immunocompromised, having cancer and/or other complicating diseases or conditions.

Several chapters review the development of the GI tract. The development of the fetal gut becomes a more critical factor when the infant is born preterm. Prior to 34 weeks of gestation, the gut has not matured to a point where colonization by the normal gut flora is possible. However, if the infant is born before 34 weeks, it will be exposed to microbes even when the greatest care is given to keep the environment sterile. These factors explain the increased occurrence of necrotizing enterocolitis in the most premature infants. Also, the use of antibiotics in the very preterm infants may adversely affect gut colonization. The chapter on neonatal and infant microflora includes an extensive discussion about the role of the microflora in gut maturation in pre-term and term infants. There is a unique, valuable chapter that describes the maternal/infant path of microbe colonization and reviews the role of vaginal microbes as well as those in breast milk and other sources of the maternal microbiota. Probiotics' role in infant dietetics is clearly reviewed with emphasis on the specific microbes that have been shown to reduce infant gastritis in well-controlled studies.

Specific, in-depth chapters examine the biological rationale and clinical data pointing to the potential for probiotic use in prevention as well as treatment in disease states including necrotizing enterocolitis, irritable bowel syndrome, infectious diarrhea, antibiotic-associated diarrhea, Crohn's disease, ulcerative colitis, pouchitis, Helicobacter pylori infection, allergy, asthma and the immunocompromised host. These chapters contain excellent tables that outline the published clinical studies and also contain helpful figures that indicate the functions of the probiotics in these disease states. The authors of these chapters are experienced clinicians and researchers who provide practical guidelines and assessments of the data to help health professionals determine strategies for their patients based upon the totality of the clinical evidence rather than based upon a single study. Also, the authors identify key areas where data are lacking as well as areas for future research.

The final section of the volume is devoted to examining the sources of probiotics in our food supply, the potential of prebiotic consumption to enhance gut function and the added value of combining pre and probiotics in a synbiotic food or dietary supplement source. Another important chapter reviews the current quality control practices in the US versus what is seen in Europe and Asia. Clear guidance is provided for accessing objective analyses from reputable information sources about products sold in the US. This information will be of great use to health professionals, educators, regulators and students interested in the quality of currently marketed probiotic-containing products. The chapter on the future of probiotics outlines the requirements for further acceptance of probiotics by scientists and physicians and highlights the areas of quality control, appropriate regulation, validated shelf life, and importantly, validated health claims. In the future, there may be a role for dead probiotics and/or their biologically active components (including DNA) and the products of probiotics. Probiotics may be genetically engineered to deliver beneficial immunomodulators or small quantities of allergens to enhance the development of tolerance. Other diseases and conditions outside of the GI tract may be shown to benefit from probiotics including the respiratory tract, the joints and even obesity. Such a future for probiotics further verifies the timeliness of this critically important volume.

This volume's 24 chapters serve a dual purpose of providing an overview of the biology behind the functioning of the GI tract and gut immune function and the role of the gut microflora related to diseases affected by an imbalance between commensal and pathogenic microorganisms. The authors have focused on the state of the science with regard to clinical studies using probiotics for the most commonly seen GI tract conditions in the pediatric population. There is a consistent overriding caution from the chapter authors that clinicians must be advised that results are dependent upon the probiotic products used because specific species have been found to be effective for specific conditions at a defined dosage level for a defined age group. Each chapter includes a review of current clinical findings and puts these into historic perspective as well as pointing the way to future research opportunities.

Drs. Michail and Sherman are excellent communicators and have worked tirelessly to develop a book that is destined to be considered the best in the field because of its extensive, in-depth chapters covering the most important aspects of the complex interactions between the human GI tract and its microbiota, and the effects of consumed microbes on this balance. The introductory chapters provide readers with the basics so that the more clinically-related chapters can be easily understood. The editors have chosen 36 of the most well recognized and respected authors from around the world to contribute the 24 informative chapters in the volume. The chapter authors have integrated the newest research findings so the reader can better understand the complex interactions that can result from the development of gastrointestinal dysfunction in the pediatric population. Hallmarks of all of the chapters include complete definitions of terms with the abbreviations fully defined for the reader and consistent use of terms between chapters. Key features of this comprehensive volume include the informative bulleted summary points and key words that are at the beginning of each chapter, appendices that include a detailed list of related websites, books and Journals. The volume contains more than 30 detailed tables and informative figures, an extensive, detailed index and more than 1600 up-to-date references that provide the reader with excellent sources of worthwhile information about the gastrointestinal system, gut immunity and its role in allergy and autoimmune disease, gut microbes, probiotics, pediatric gastroenterology, pediatric gastric diseases and gut health.

In conclusion, "Probiotics in Pediatric Medicine", edited by Sonia Michail and Philip M. Sherman provides health professionals in many areas of research and practice with the most up-to-date, well-referenced volume on the importance of probiotics for the prevention and treatment of GI tract-related conditions in the pediatric population as well as for the maintenance of their overall health. This volume will serve the reader as the benchmark in this complex area of interrelationships between the GI tract epithelium, gut immune cells, lymphoid tissue, gut micro-organisms, microbiota-generated nutrients, bioactive molecules and regulatory signals, probiotics, prebiotics and related factors. The volume also includes critical detailed descriptions of probiotic product development, regulatory status and the safety assessments currently used for the probiotic substances that we consume. Moreover, these topics are clearly delineated so that students as well as practitioners can better understand the current understanding of probiotics in medicine today. Dr. Michail and Dr. Sherman are applauded for their efforts to develop the most authoritative resource in the field to date and this excellent text is a very welcome addition to the Nutrition and Health Series.

Adrianne Bendich, PhD, FACN,
Series Editor

Preface

The concept of probiotics was conceived hundreds and thousands of years ago but became more tangible at the turn of the century when Metchnikoff documented his intelligent correlation between the health of Bulgarian peasants and the consumption of what would now be considered probiotics. Since then many scientists and investigators have diligently designed and performed experiments and trials to prove or disprove the power of probiotics. A great number of probiotic products in various shapes and forms have become available to the consumer and more than ever clinicians are dealing with children and patients that consider the use of probiotics.

The purpose of this project is to provide clinicians in general and clinicians caring for children more specifically, with a tool to understand the current evidence for the role of probiotics in various pediatric disorders related to the gastrointestinal as well as the extra-intestinal tract. This book will provide evidence-based up-to-date information from experts in the field to help clinicians make decisions regarding the use of probiotics. Currently, the market for probiotics continues to rely heavily on health claims made by manufacturers and retailers and clinicians ultimately have the sole responsibility to understand the various strains and preparations that are commercially available and be able to advise patients accordingly.

We hope that this book will serve as a helpful tool and a critical resource for health professionals to enhance their ability to make the appropriate decisions regarding the use of probiotics.

Contents

Section C. Probiotics and the Gut

Section D. Probiotics Outside the Gut

Section E. Probiotics Products

Section F. Probiotic Future

Contributors

CARLO AGOSTONI • *Department of Paediatrics, San Paolo Hospital, University of Milan, Via A. di Rudinì, 8, I-20143 Milan, Italy*

MARINA ALOI • *Pediatric Gastroenterology and Liver Unit, University of Rome "La Sapienza"*

KINGSLEY C. ANUKAM, PhD, MHPH • *Canadian Research & Development Centre for Probiotics, Lawson Health Research Institute, London, Ontario, Canada*

SHERYL BERMAN, MS, PhD • *Department Chair of Basic Sciences, Bastyr University, Kenmore, WA*

SAMRA SARIGOL BLANCHARD, MD • *Department of Pediatric Gastroenterology, University of Maryland School of Medicine, Baltimore, MD*

ATHOS BOUSVAROS, MD, MPH • *Associate Professor of Pediatrics, Harvard Medical School, Associate Director, Inflammatory Bowel Disease Center, Children''s Hospital, Boston, MA*

MICHAEL D. CABANA, MD, MPH • *Departments of Pediatrics, Epidemiology and Biostatistics, & Institute of Health Policy Studies, University of California, San Francisco, CA*

STEVEN J. CZINN, MD • *Department of Pediatrics, University of Maryland School of Medicine, Baltimore, MD*

SALVATORE CUCCHIARA • *Pediatric Gastroenterology and Liver Unit, University of Rome "La Sapienza"*

ALESSIO FASANO, MD • *Mucosal Biology Research Center and Department of Physiology, University of Maryland School of Medicine*

RICHARD FEDORAK, MD • *Director, Center of Excellence for Gastrointestinal Inflammation and Immunity Research (CEGIIR), Director, Northern Alberta Clinical Trials and Research Center (NACTRC), Professor of Medicine, Division of Gastroenterology, University of Alberta, Edmonton, Alberta, Canada*

R. FÖLSTER-HOLST • *Department of Dermatology, University of Kiel, Kiel, Germany*

GEORGE J. FUCHS, MD • *Department of Pediatrics, University of Arkansas for Medical Sciences and Arkansas Children's Hospital, Little Rock, AR*

PAOLO GIONCHETTI • *Department of Internal Medicine and Gastroenterology University of Bologna, Italy*

STUART S. KAUFMAN MD • *Georgetown University, Children's Medical Center, Washington, DC*

ESI S. N. LAMOUSÉ-SMITH, MD, PHD • *Fellow in Gastroenterology, Children's Hospital, Boston, MA*

ANNE LIZA MCCARTNEY, BSC(HONS), PHD • *Food Microbial Sciences Unit School of Chemistry, University of Reading, Reading UK*

DAVID R. MACK, MD, FRCPC • *Department of Pediatrics, Biochemistry, Microbiology and Immunology Faculty of Medicine, University of Ottawa, and Gastroenterology, Hepatology & Nutrition Department of Pediatrics, Children's Hospital of Eastern Ontario*

SONIA MICHAIL, MD • *Department of Gastroenterology and Nutrition, Children's Medical Center, Wright State University Boonshoft School of Medicine, Dayton, OH*

JOSEF NEU • *College of Medicine, University of Florida, Gainesville, FL*

B. OFFICK • *Institute for Physiology and Biochemistry of Nutrition, Federal Research Centre for Nutrition and Food, Kiel, Germany*

D. BRENT POLK, MD • *Departments of Pediatrics, Division of Gastroenterology, Hepatology & Nutrition, Vanderbilt University School of Medicine, Nashville, TN*

E. PROKSCH • *Department of Dermatology, University of Kiel, Kiel, Germany*

EAMONN M. M. QUIGLEY, MD, FRCP, FACP, FACG, FRCPI • *Alimentary Pharmabiotic Centre, National University of Ireland, Cork, Ireland*

SAMULI RAUTAVA • *Mucosal Immunology Laboratory, Massachusetts General Hospital for Children, Charlestown, MA*

ANUKUM REID, PHD, MBA, ARM, CCM • *Canadian Research & Development Centre for Probiotics, Lawson Health Research Institute and Department of Microbiology and Immunology and Surgery, University of Western Ontario, London, Ontario Canada*

YULIYA REKHTMAN, MD • *Georgetown University, Children's Medical Center, Washington, DC*

LAURE CATHERINE ROGER, BSC(HONS) • *Food Microbial Sciences Unit School of Chemistry, University of Reading, Reading UK*

FILIPPO SALVINI • *Department of Paediatrics, San Paolo Hospital, University of Milan, Via A. di Rudinì, 8, I-20143 Milan, Italy*

SHAFIQUL A. SARKER MD, PHD • *International Centre for Diarrhoeal Diseases Research, Bangladesh*

J. Schrezenmeir, · *Institute for Physiology and Biochemistry of Nutrition, Federal Research Centre for Nutrition and Food, Kiel, Germany*

TEREZ SHEA-DONOHUE, PHD • *Mucosal Biology Research Center and Department of Physiology, University of Maryland School of Medicine*

PHILIP M. SHERMAN, MD, FRCP • *Division of Gastroenterology, Hepatology and Nutrition, The Hospital for Sick Children, University of Toronto, Toronto, Ontario Canada*

HANIA SZAJEWSKA, MD • *The 2nd Department of Paediatrics [II Katedra Pediatrii], The Medical University of Warsaw, Poland*

GERALD W. TANNOCK • *Department of Microbiology and Immunology, University of Otago, Dunedin, New Zealand*

W. WALKER • *Mucosal Immunology Laboratory, Massachusetts General Hospital for Children, Charlestown, MA*

ZWI WEIZMAN • *Pediatric Gastroenterology and Nutrition Unit, Soroka Medical Center Faculty of Health Sciences, Ben-Gurion University, Beer-Sheva, Israel*

FANG YAN, MD., PhD • *Departments of Pediatrics, Division of Gastroenterology, Hepatology & Nutrition, Vanderbilt University School of Medicine, Nashville, TN*

Section A
Probiotics: The Basics

1 Basics of GI Physiology and Mucosal Immunology

Alessio Fasano and Terez Shea-Donohue

Key Points

- The intestine has the largest mucosal surface interfacing with external environment.
- Tight junctions are pivotal in intestinal barrier function.
- Gut associated lymphoid tissue (GALT) serves to prevent harmful antigens from reaching systemic circulation as well as inducing immune tolerance.
- Intestinal microbiota surpasses the human genome by 140-fold and is critical in the development of GALT.
- Loss of intestinal barrier function secondary to a dysfunction of the intercellular tight junctions is one of the key ingredients in the pathogenesis of autoimmune diseases.

Key Words: Intestinal mucosa, gut-associated lymphoid tissue, tight junctions, microbiota, toll like receptors, innate immunity, adaptive immunity, autoimmunity.

INTRODUCTION

The intestinal epithelium is the largest mucosal surface providing an interface between the external environment and the mammalian host. Its exquisite anatomical and functional arrangements and the finely tuned coordination of digestive, absorptive, motility, neuroendocrine, and immunological functions are testimony to the complexity of the gastrointestinal (GI) system. Also pivotal is the regulation of molecular trafficking between the intestinal lumen and the submucosa, leading to either tolerance or immune responses to non-self antigens. Macromolecule trafficking is dictated mainly by intestinal permeability, whose regulation depends on the modulation of intercellular tight junctions (tj). A century ago, tj were conceptualized as a secreted extracellular cement forming an absolute and unregulated barrier within the paracellular space. The contribution of the paracellular pathway of the GI tract to the general economy of molecule trafficking between environment and host, therefore, was judged to be negligible. It is now apparent that tj are extremely dynamic structures involved in developmental, physiological, and pathological circumstances.

From: *Nutrition and Health: Probiotics in Pediatric Medicine*
Edited by: S. Michail and P.M. Sherman © Humana Press, Totowa, NJ

PRINCIPLES OF GI PHYSIOLOGY

Structural Characteristics of the GI Tract

Each region of the gut provides a distinct contribution to the digestion of a meal, which is supported by unique morphology and function. At every level, the wall can be divided into four basic layers: serosa, muscularis externa, submucosa, and mucosa. There are variations in the type and distribution of mucosal cells present along the length of the GI tract that reflect the specialized function of a particular region. The mucosal layer of the small intestine is designed to provide a large surface area for exposure of luminal contents to absorptive cells. Three anatomic factors contribute to the amplification of the absorptive surface beyond that of a simple cylinder. The circular folds of the intestinal mucosa called plicae circulares, valvulae conniventes, or folds of Kerckring increase the surface area by threefold. The mucosal surface is further extended tenfold by the presence of villi and crypts along the surface. The apical aspect of the enterocytes are covered with microvilli further increasing the absorptive surface some 600-fold.

There are several types of epithelial cells lining the villi and crypts of the small intestine and this variety allows the intestine to perform its varied functions. The most common epithelial cells are columnar cells, which can be divided further on the basis on their proliferative activity. Cells in the crypt region have the highest activity while the surface cells are less active. Functionally, crypt cells are thought to be primarily secretory, while enterocytes are primarily absorptive cells with the apical brush border containing hydrolases and other enzymes critical in the terminal digestion of carbohydrates and proteins. Recent studies in the colon challenge this classical compartmentalization of crypt secretion and surface cell absorption by showing that epithelial cells have both secretory and absorptive abilities in this region.[1,2] Goblet cells are present all along the GI tract especially in the terminal jejunum and ileum and the mucus they secrete acts as a lubricant as well as protect the mucosa from irritation.[3]

Two populations of cells in the gut have unique roles: the enteroendocrine (EC) cells and the gut associated lymph tissue (GALT). The gut is the largest endocrine organ in the body and EC cells play a key role in gut sensing by releasing peptide hormones such as secretin and cholescytokinin (CCK) or amines, such as 5-HT, in response to stimuli in the lumen. They comprise about 1% of surface cells and hormones like CCK, glucagons like peptide-1 (GLP-1), peptide YY (PYY) and ghrelin, are important in the regulation of appetite and satiety.[4] The GALT is composed of several specialized cells, including Peyers patches, M cells, and intraepithelial lymphocytes, which play key roles in host defense.[5] It is well-documented that bacterial colonization is required for the structural and functional development of the GALT. One of the most important functions of the GALT is to discriminate between commensal versus pathogenic microorganisms.[6] Microflora derived from the mother at birth initiates microbial-epithelial crosstalk that serves as a defense against enteric pathogens. Epithelial cells become active participants in mucosal immunity through expression of Toll-like receptors (TLR) that induce transcription of immune and inflammatory responses.[7] Processing of these bacterial antigens promote the development of memory T cells that make up most of the T cells in gut lymphoid tissues. The structural arrangement of intestinal epithelial and immune cells just underneath the epithelial mucosa is a testimony to their coordinated complex series of response to microorganisms and macromolecules present in the intestinal lumen.

Functional Features of the GI Tract

Digestive Functions

Digestion is a coordinated activity involving all regions of the GI tract. Secretions from the accessory organs such as salivary glands, pancreas, and liver, provide the bulk of fluid that is presented for absorption as well as specialized components, such as hydrochloric acid or bile salts, that are critical for digestion. These secretions vary in amount based on luminal stimuli that activate both neural and hormonal mechanisms, which ensure that the timing of the secretions along the GI tract is closely linked to the arrival of gut contents. Absorption of nutrients is a primary feature of the small intestine and can be divided arbitrarily into two components, intraluminal digestion followed by brush border digestion and transport of nutrients into absorptive cells. Movement of chyme along the gut is possible because of coordinated contractions of the smooth muscle that are regulated by intersitital cells of Cajal, intrinsic and extrinsic nerves, as well as release of gut hormones.

Absorptive Functions

The small intestine is the major site of fluid, electrolyte and nutrient aborption in the gut. Carbohydrates are a primary energy source for numerous physiological functions and appropriately, comprise 45–65% of total calories in a Western diet. Digestive enzymes secreted by the pancreas in response to neural (vagal) and endocrine (CCK and secretin) stimuli following emptying of a meal from the stomach into the duodenum, are critical for nutrient digestion. Undigested carbohydrates, in the form of resistant starches and dietary fibers (both soluble and insoluble), along with a small amount of dietary carbohydrates that escape digestion and absorption in the small bowel, undergo fermentation by resident colonic anaerobic bacteria giving rise to short-chain fatty acids (SCFA). Butyrate, the preferred fuel for colonocytes,[8] is important for colonic homeostasis and is tranpsorted by the monocarboxylate transporter, MCT-1, with some evidence for a sodium linked transporter, slc5a8 (or SMCT).[9,10] SCFA alter colonic pH, which indirectly influences the bacterial composition of the microbiota. There is also evidence for undigested carbohydates reaching the colon, acting as competitors for epithelial bacterial receptors, making it difficult for adherence of pathogenic bacteria.[11] Changes in pH influence both the quantity and compostion of the colonic microbiota, an important factor in the development of chronic inflammatory bowel diseases.[12,13] Given the role of the microflora in the generation of SCFA, there is a growing interest in the impact of probiotics on colonic fermentation of undigested carbohydrates. This is particularly relevant to the evaluation of the benefical effects of prebiotics, nondigestible foods, such as inulin and fructo-oligosaccharides, which promote gut health by selectively stimulating the growth of specific bacteria in the colon.[14,15]

Water and Electrolyte Transport

One of the most important functions of the GI tract is absorption of water and electrolytes. Fluid absorption is passive and dependent on rate of solute transport and is, therefore, isotonic. The energy dependent $3Na^+–2K^+$ pump in the basolateral plasma membrane provides the energy-requiring step for driving transcellular and paracellular flow of water across the epithelium. Other factors that influence fluid absorption are luminal osmolality and the region of the gut. There is a cephalocaudal increase in transepithelial resistance, which is regulated largely by intercellular tj, along the intestine that underlies the greater paracellular flow of water in the small intestine compared to the colon. Transcellular flow of water is intimately coupled to solute transport, with the greatest flux occuring in the small intestine because of sodium-linked solute transporters.[16] The role of aquaporins (AQP), integral membrane protiens with high water selectivity,[17] must also be considered in transcellular fluid transport. These water channels are located at both the apical and basolateral aspects of the epithelial cell in the small intestine and colon. Shifts in the location of AQP 7 and 8 from the apical to the basolateral membrane of enterocytes in IBD patients suppports a role for these channels in the defective fluid transport in these patients.[14] Nonsolute coupled sodium transport is attributed to neutral NaCl absorption that is predominant during the interdigestive period. The sodium/hydrogen exchangers, NHE-2 and NHE-3, are present in the apical membrane of surface epithelial cells in both the small intestine and colon. Of interest, elevation of cyclic nucleotides induced by either endogenous signals or bacterial toxins such as *Vibrio cholerae*–derived cholera toxin or heat stable enterotoxin elaborated by enteorotoxigenic *Escherichia coli*, inhibit neutral sodium chloride absorption and NHE-3 activity.[16]

While sodium transport provides the driving force for absorption, intestinal secretion is linked to movement of chloride through the cystic fibrosis transmembrane regulator (CFTR) located in the apical plasma membrane. Cyclic nucleotide-dependent phosphorylation increases the conductance of the CFTR channel. Excessive CFTR activity causes secretory diarrhea that occurs in response to the bacterial toxins such as choleragen, which elevates cyclic nucleotide production in the gut. In addition to the CFTR channel, there are also two other classes of Cl⁻ channels in the intestine, the CLC family and a calcium activated chloride channel (CLCA).[18] The CLC gene family are broadly expressed chloride channels, the most prominent in the intestine being CLC-2.[19] These channels can be activated by hyperpolarization, cell swelling and extracellular acidification.[18] The precise physiological function of this channel remains to be elucidated, however, it is proposed to play a role in cholinergic mediated secretion in the colon.[20]

Intestinal Barrier Function

The paracellular route is the dominant pathway for passive solute flow across the intestinal epithelial barrier, and its functional state depends on the regulation of the intercellular tj, also known as the zonula occludens (ZO).[4] The tj is one of the hallmarks of absorptive and secretory epithelia. As a barrier between apical and basolateral compartments, it selectively regulates the passive diffusion of ions and small water-soluble solutes through the paracellular pathway, thereby compensating for any gradients generated by transcellular pathways.[21] Due to the high resistance of the enterocyte plasma membrane, variations in transepithelial conductance have been ascribed to changes in the paracellular pathway.[22] The tj represents the major barrier within this paracellular pathway with electrical resistance of epithelial tissues dependent on the number and complexity of transmembrane protein strands within the tj, as observed by freeze-fracture electron microscopy.[23] Evidence now exists that tj, once regarded as static structures, are in fact dynamic, and readily adapt to a variety of developmental,[24–26] physiological[27–30] and pathological[31–33] circumstances.

To meet the diverse physiological challenges to which the intestinal epithelial barrier is subjected, tj must be capable of rapid and coordinated responses. This requires the presence of a complex regulatory system that orchestrates the state of assembly of the tj multiprotein network. While knowledge about tj ultrastructure and intracellular signaling events has progressed significantly during the past decade, relatively little is known about their pathophysiological regulation secondary to extracellular stimuli. The discovery of zonulin, a molecule that reversibly modulates tj permeability, sheds light on how the intestinal barrier function is regulated in health and disease[34] (Fig. 1.1). The physiological role of the zonulin system remains to be established. However, it is likely that this pathway is involved in several functions, including tj regulation responsible for the movement of fluid, macromolecules, and leukocytes between the bloodstream and the intestinal lumen, and vice versa. Another physiological role of intestinal zonulin is protection against colonization by microorganisms of the proximal intestine (that is innate immunity).[22] Given the complexity of both cell signaling events and intracellular structures involved in the zonulin system, it is not surprising that this pathway is affected when the physiological state of epithelial and endothelial cells is dramatically changed, as it is in many of the autoimmune diseases in which tj dysfunction appears to be the primary defect (see below).

GI MUCOSAL IMMUNOLOGY

The Gut Associated Lymphoid Tissue

Paracellular passage of macromolecules, under either physiological or pathological circumstances, is safeguarded by the GALT. The GALT serves as a containment system preventing potentially harmful intestinal antigens from reaching the systemic circulation and induces systemic tolerance against luminal antigens by a process that involves polymeric IgA secretion and the induction of regulatory T cells. GALT is composed of both inductive (Peyer's patches) and effector sites (intraepithelial cells and lamina propria). Recent studies also include isolated lymphoid follicles (ILF), which are tertiary lymphoid stuctures formed in autoimmune diseases as well as in a number of inflammatory pathologies of the gut.[21] Mature ILF bear a resemblance to Peyer's patches in cellular composition and localization in the distal intestine, as well as a dependence on lymphotoxin β receptor (LTβR) for formation of these structures.[23] Another important factor for the intestinal immunological responsiveness is the major histocompatibility complex (MHC). Human leukocyte antigen (HLA) class I and class II genes are located in the MHC on chromosome 6. These genes code for glycoproteins, which bind peptides, and this HLA-peptide complex is recognized by certain T-cell receptors in the intestinal mucosa.[35,36] Susceptibility to at least 50 diseases is associated with specific HLA class I or class II alleles.

The balance between immunity and tolerance is essential for a healthy intestine, and abnormal or inappropriate immune responses may result in inflammatory pathologies. Antigen- presenting M cells efficiently take up and transport a variety of microorganisms and present antigen[37]; therefore, ILF are proposed to be local sites for lympocytic, antigen and antigen presenting cell interactions. In addition to M cells, dendritic cells also capture antigens present in the intestinal lumen by sending dendrites through tight

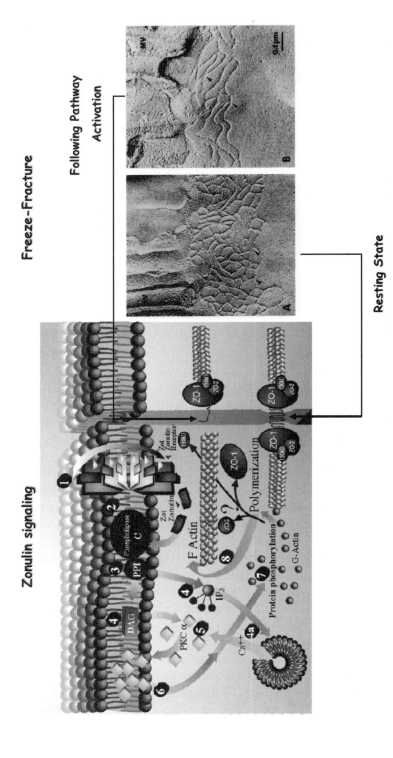

Fig. 1.1. Proposed zonulin intracellular signaling leading to the opening of intestinal TJ Zonulin interacts with a specific surface receptor (1) whose distribution within the intestine varies. The protein then activates phospholipase C (2) that hydrolyzes phosphatidyl inositol (3) to release inositol 1,4,5-*tris* phosphate (PPI-3) and diacylglycerol (DAG) (4). PKCα is then activated (5), either directly (via DAG) (4) or through the release of intracellular Ca^{2+} (via PPI-3) (4a). Membrane-associated, activated PKCα (6) catalyzes the phosphorylation of target protein(s), with subsequent polymerization of soluble G-actin in F-actin (7). This polymerization causes the rearrangement of the filaments of actin and the subsequent displacement of proteins (including ZO-1) from the junctional complex (8). As a result, intestinal TJ become looser (see freeze fracture electron microscopy). Once the zonulin signaling is over, the TJ resume their baseline steady state.

junctions between epithelial cells while maintaining barrier integrity[24,25] and then rapidly migrating to other areas, such as mesenteric lymph nodes.[26] There is evidence that antigen-presenting dendritic cells are educated by memory T cells and subsequently induce naïve T cells,[27] thereby supporting the role for dendritic cells in coupling innate and adaptive immune responses that affect intestinal permeability.

Innate and Adaptive Immunity and Their Interactions

Recognition of antigens by dendritic cells triggers a family of pattern recognition receptors, TLR, which change dendritic cell phenotype and function. TLR are the major receptors involved in the discrimination between self and non-self based on the recognition of conserved bacterial molecular patterns (Fig. 1.2). In intestinal epithelial cells (IECs), TLR play a role in normal mucosal homeostasis and are particularly important in the interaction between the mucosa and the luminal flora.[29] There are a number of TLRs, all of which are present in the gut and respond to different stimuli resulting in different adaptive immune responses.[28,30,32] There is now evidence for a differential response to stimuli arising from TLRs located at the basolateral versus the apical surface.[38]

TLR direct immune responses by activating signaling events leading to elevated expression of factors, such as cytokines and chemokines that recruit and regulate the immune and inflammatory cells, which then either initiate or enhance host immune responses.[39] The peripheral memory T cell response is a critical outcome of adaptive immunity and TLR likely are required for the generation and maintenance of memory T cells.[33] TLR are implicated in chronic diseases such as enteric inflammation and may have both proinflammatory and protective roles. Of interest, commensal flora acting through TLR4 positively influence the susceptibility to food antigens[31] and implicate

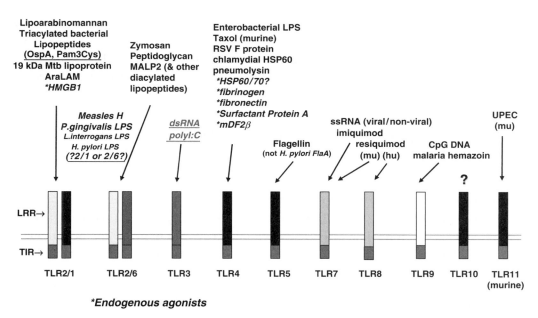

Fig. 1.2. Toll-like receptors and their ligands.

TLR in the regulation of intestinal permeability. This concept is supported by recent in vitro studies using IEC cultures, which show that TLR-2 enhances epithelial integrity by a rearrangement of the tight junction protein, ZO-1.[28] In addition, TLR signaling is important in the anti-inflammatory effects of probiotics.[40] These data show the critical role of bacteria in shaping the immune response and underscore the current interest in probiotic effects on permeability[41–43] that may act to limit polarization to Th1 or Th2 responses and, thereby, maintain intestinal barrier function.

Intestinal Microbiota

The human gut is host to a large and diverse population of microbiota that are known to play a critical role in the development of the GALT. The collective bacterial genome of the human microbiota encodes an estimated 2–4 million genes, surpassing the human genome by a staggering 140-fold.[44] Intestinal bacteria carry thousands of enzymatic reactions not catalyzed by the mammalian host and, thus, act as an "organ within an organ." Therefore, acquisition of the intestinal microbiota at birth from the mother's microbiota can be considered as the inheritance of a parallel genome. One of most important functions of the mucosal epithelium is the ability to discern commensal from pathogenic bacteria to maintain tolerance. The epithelium recognizes specific microbiota and responds with increased production of chemokine and cytokines that serve to promote an antigen-specific immune response.[45] The mechanisms that govern this recognition of bacterial species are of interest, particularly with respect to the mechanisms of the beneficial effect of probiotics on autoimmune diseases that are associated with an impaired mucosal barrier function such as type 1 diabetes.[46] The nucleotide oligomerization domain (NOD) proteins are another set of recognition receptors that function in the innate immune response. Genetic polymorphisms in NOD-2 are linked to an increased susceptibility to Crohn's disease in certain populations.[47,48] Recent studies show that DNA derived from the combination probiotic VSL3 improved inflammation in IL-10 deficient mice,[49] suggesting a novel mechanism by which bacteria are recognized by epithelial cells. Recent studies showed increased expression of surface TLR9 expression on cell cultures in response to pathogenic bacteria,[50] evidence that can negate inflammatory signals initiated by activation of basolateral TLR.[38]

COORDINATION OF PHYSIOLOGICAL AND IMMUNOLOGICAL FUNCTIONS OF THE GI TRACT IN HANDLING NON-SELF ANTIGENS IN HEALTH AND DISEASE

The Intestinal Neuro-Endocrine Network

Intestinal homeostasis is coordinated by responses of different cell types, including both immune and nonimmune cells. The interaction between immune and nonimmune cells is amplified by the influx of inflammatory and immune cells, increasing the exposure of nonimmune cells to soluble mediators, such as cytokines, that are released from immune cells. Macrophages, leukocytes and mucosal mast cells (MMC) all elaborate a number of mediators that alter gut function. Of interest, MMC appear to play a role in both Th1 and Th2 driven adaptive immune responses, release a number of preformed mediators (such as histamine and serotonin), as well as newly synthesized mediators, including leukotrienes, prostaglandins, platelet activating factor, as well as IL-4 and TNF-α, many of which have an effect on epithelial permeability.[51–55] This may explain, at least in part, the increased permeability that is a feature of both Th1- and Th2-driven pathologies.

CLASSICAL AND NEW THEORIES IN THE PATHOGENESIS OF AUTOIMMUNE DISEASES

Classical Theories

Autoimmune diseases are the third most common category of diseases in the United States after cancer and heart disease, affecting up to 8% of the population or 14–22 million persons.[56] They can affect virtually every site in the body, including the GI tract. At least 15 diseases are the direct result of an autoimmune response, while circumstantial evidence links >80 conditions with autoimmunity.[57]

Soon after autoimmune diseases were first recognized more than a century ago, researchers began to associate them with viral and bacterial infections. A mechanism often called on to explain the association of infection with autoimmune disease is "molecular mimicry," where antigens (or, more properly, epitopes) of the microorganism are postulated to closely resemble self-antigens.[58] The induction of an immune response to the microbial antigen then results in a cross-reaction with self-antigens and the induction of autoimmunity. Once the process is activated, the autoimmune response becomes independent of continuous exposure to the environmental trigger and, therefore, the process is self-perpetuating and irreversible. Epitope-specific cross-reactivity between microbes and self-tissues has been shown in some animal models.[59] Conversely, molecular mimicry in most human autoimmune diseases seems to be a factor in the progression of a pre-existing sub-clinical autoimmune response, rather than in the initiation of autoimmunity by breaking tolerance.[60]

Another theory suggests that microorganisms expose self-antigens to the immune system by directly damaging tissues during active infection. This mechanism has been referred to as the "bystander effect" and occurs when the new antigen is presented with the originally fed antigen.[61] Whether pathogens mimic self-antigens, release sequestered self-antigens, or both, remains to be elucidated.

Recently, increased hygiene and a lack of exposure to various microorganisms has been proposed to be responsible for the "epidemic" of autoimmune diseases that has occurred over the past 30–40 years in industrialized countries, including the US[62] The essence of the "hygiene hypothesis," argues that rising incidence of immune-mediated (including autoimmune) diseases is due, at least in part, to lifestyle and environmental changes that have made us too "clean." This hypothesis is supported by immunological data showing that the response to microbial antigens induces Th1 cyokine expression that offsets the T-helper 2-polarized cytokine production in neonates. In the absence of microbes, the gut may be conducive to an exaggerated IgE production, atopy and atopic diseases. Alternately, the absence of helminth infections eliminates the normal up-regulation of Th2 in childhood, culminating in a more Th1 prone immune environment that is characteristic of autoimmune and inflammatory diseases.[63] Regardless of whether autoimmune diseases are due to too much, or too little, exposure to microorganisms, it is now generally considered that adaptive immunity and imbalance among Th1, Th2,

Th17, and T regulatory cells responses are key elements of the pathogenesis of the autoimmune process.[64]

New Theories

A common denominator of autoimmune diseases is the presence of several preexisting conditions leading to an autoimmune process. The first is a genetic susceptibility for the host immune system to recognize, and potentially misinterpret, an environmental antigen presented within the GI tract. Second, the host must be exposed to the antigen. Finally, the antigen must be presented to the GI mucosal immune system following its paracellular passage (normally prevented by the tj competency) from the intestinal lumen to the gut submucosa.[65] In many cases, increased permeability appears to precede disease and causes an abnormality in antigen delivery that triggers the multiorgan process leading to the autoimmune response.[66]

Therefore, the following hypothesis can be formulated to explain the pathogenesis of autoimmune diseases that encompasses the following three key points:

1. Autoimmune diseases involve a miscommunication between innate and adaptive immunity.
2. Molecular mimicry or bystander effects alone may not explain entirely the complex events involved in the pathogenesis of autoimmune diseases. Rather, continuous stimulation by nonself antigens (environmental triggers) appears necessary to perpetuate the process. This concept implies that the autoimmune response can be theoretically stopped and, perhaps, reversed if the interplay between autoimmune predisposing genes and trigger(s) is either prevented or eliminated.
3. In addition to genetic predisposition and the exposure to the triggering nonself antigen, the third key element necessary to develop autoimmunity is the loss of the protective function of mucosal barriers (mainly the GI and lung mucosa) that interface with the environment.

CONCLUSIONS

The GI tract has been extensively studied for its digestive and absorptive functions. A more attentive analysis of its anatomo-functional characteristics, however, clearly indicates that its functions go well beyond the handling of nutrients and electrolytes. The exquisite regional-specific anatomical arrangements of cell subtypes and the finely regulated cross talk between epithelial, neuroendocrine and immune cells highlights other less-studied, yet extremely important functions of the GI tract. Of particular interest is the regulation of antigen trafficking and intestinal mucosa-microbiota interactions. These functions dictate the switch from tolerance to immunity, and are likely integral mechanisms involved in the pathogenesis of GI inflammatory processes.

The classical paradigm of autoimmune pathogenesis involving specific genetic makeup and exposure to environmental triggers has been challenged recently by the addition of a third element, the loss of intestinal barrier function. Genetic predisposition, miscommunication between innate and adaptive immunity, exposure to environmental triggers, and loss of intestinal barrier function secondary to a dysfunction of the intercellular tj, all seem to be key ingredients involved in the pathogenesis of autoimmune diseases. This new theory implies that once the autoimmune process is activated, it is not auto-perpetuating. Rather, it can be modulated or even reversed by preventing the continuous interplay between genes and the environment. Since tj dysfunction allows such interactions, new therapeutic strategies aimed at re-establishing the intestinal barrier function offer innovative and hitherto unexplored approaches for the management of these devastating chronic diseases.

REFERENCES

1. Binder HJ, Rajendran V, Sadasivan V, Geibel JP. Bicarbonate secretion: a neglected aspect of colonic ion transport. *J Clin Gastroenterol* 2005;39:S53–S58.
2. Geibel JP. Secretion and absorption by colonic crypts. *Annu Rev Physiol* 2005;67:471–490.
3. Allen A, Flemstrom G. Gastroduodenal mucus bicarbonate barrier: protection against acid and pepsin. *Am J Physiol Cell Physiol* 2005;288:C1–19.
4. Naslund E, Hellstrom PM. Appetite signaling: from gut peptides and enteric nerves to brain. *Physiol Behav* 2007;92:256–262.
5. Nagler-Anderson C. Man the barrier! Strategic defences in the intestinal mucosa. *Nat Rev Immunol* 2001;1:59–67.
6. Lanning DK, Rhee KJ, Knight KL. Intestinal bacteria and development of the B-lymphocyte repertoire. *Trends Immunol* 2005;26:419–425.
7. Cobrin GM, Abreu MT. Defects in mucosal immunity leading to Crohn's disease. *Immunol Rev* 2005;206:277–295.
8. Cummings JH. Colonic absorption: the importance of short chain fatty acids in man. *Scand J Gastroenterol Suppl* 1984;93:89–99.
9. Coady MJ, Chang MH, Charron FM, Plata C, Wallendorff B, Sah JF, Markowitz SD, Romero MF, Lapointe JY. The human tumour suppressor gene SLC5A8 expresses a Na+-monocarboxylate cotransporter. *J Physiol* 2004;557:719–731.
10. Cuff MA, Lambert DW, Shirazi-Beechey SP. Substrate-induced regulation of the human colonic monocarboxylate transporter, *MCT1. J Physiol* 2002;539:361–371.
11. Gassull MA. Review article: the intestinal lumen as a therapeutic target in inflammatory bowel disease. *Alimentary Pharmacol Therapeutics* 2006;24:90–95.
12. Macfarlane S, Furrie E, Cummings JH, Macfarlane GT. Chemotaxonomic analysis of bacterial populations colonizing the rectal mucosa in patients with ulcerative colitis. *Clin Infect Dis* 2004;38:1690–1699.
13. Prindiville T, Cantrell M, Wilson KH. Ribosomal DNA sequence analysis of mucosa-associated bacteria in Crohn's disease. *Inflamm Bowel Dis* 2004;10:824–833.
14. Hardin JA, Wallace LE, Wong JFK, OΓÇÖLoughlin EV, Urbanski SJ, Gall DG, MacNaughton WK, Beck PL. Aquaporin expression is downregulated in a murine model of colitis and in patients with ulcerative colitis, CrohnΓÇÖs disease and infectious colitis. *Cell Tissue Res* 2004;318:313–323.
15. Langlands SJ, Hopkins MJ, Coleman N, Cummings JH. Prebiotic carbohydrates modify the mucosa associated microflora of the human large bowel. *Gut* 2004;53:1610–1616.
16. Rao MC. Oral rehydration therapy: new explanations for an old remedy. *Annu Rev Physiol* 2004; 66:385–417.
17. Matsuzaki T, Tajika Y, Ablimit A, Aoki T, Hagiwara H, Takata K. Aquaporins in the digestive system. *Med Electron Microsc* 2004;37:71–80.
18. Jentsch TJ, Stein V, Weinreich F, Zdebik AA. Molecular structure and physiological function of chloride channels. *Physiol Rev* 2002;82:503–568.
19. Lipecka J, Bali M, Thomas A, Fanen P, Edelman A, Fritsch J. Distribution of ClC-2 chloride channel in rat and human epithelial tissues. *Am J Physiol Cell Physiol* 2002;282:C805–C816.
20. Schultheiss G, Siefjediers A, Diener M. Muscarinic receptor stimulation activates a Ca(2+)-dependent Cl(-) conductance in rat distal colon. *J Membr Biol* 2005;204:117–127.
21. Lorenz RG, Newberry RD. Isolated lymphoid follicles can function as sites for induction of mucosal immune responses. *Ann NY Acad Sci* 2004;1029:44–57.

22. El Asmar R, Panigrahi P, Bamford P, Berti I, Not T, Coppa GV, Catassi C, Fasano A. Host-dependent zonulin secretion causes the impairment of the small intestine barrier function after bacterial exposure. *Gastroenterology* 2002;123:1607–1615.

23. Lorenz RG, Chaplin DD, McDonald KG, McDonough JS, Newberry RD. Isolated lymphoid follicle formation is inducible and dependent upon lymphotoxin-sufficient B lymphocytes, lymphotoxin {beta} receptor, and TNF receptor I function. *J Immunol* 2003;170:5475–5482.

24. Bilsborough J, Viney JL. Gastrointestinal dendritic cells play a role in immunity, tolerance, and disease. *Gastroenterology* 2004;127:300–309.

25. Hayday A, Viney JL. The ins and outs of body surface immunology. *Science* 2000;290:97–100.

26. Mellman I, Steinman RM. Dendritic cells: specialized and regulated antigen processing machines. *Cell* 2001;106:255–258.

27. Alpan O, Bachelder E, Isil E, Arnheiter H, Matzinger P. 'Educated' dendritic cells act as messengers from memory to naive T helper cells. *Nat Immunol* 2004;5:615–622.

28. Cario E, Gerken G, Podolsky DK. Toll-like receptor 2 enhances ZO-1-associated intestinal epithelial barrier integrity via protein kinase C. *Gastroenterology* 2004;127:224–238.

29. Rakoff-Nahoum S, Paglino J, Eslami-Varzaneh F, Edberg S, Medzhitov R. Recognition of commensal microflora by toll-like receptors is required for intestinal homeostasis. *Cell* 2004;118:229–241.

30. Rumio C, Besusso D, Palazzo M, Selleri S, Sfondrini L, Dubini F, Menard S, Balsari A. Degranulation of Paneth cells via toll-kike receptor 9. *Am J Pathol* 2004;165:373–381.

31. Bashir ME, Louie S, Shi HN, Nagler-Anderson C. Toll-like receptor 4 signaling by intestinal microbes influences susceptibility to food allergy. *J Immunol* 2004;172:6978–6987.

32. Otte JM, Cario E, Podolsky DK. Mechanisms of cross hyporesponsiveness to toll-like receptor bacterial ligands in intestinal epithelial cells. *Gastroenterology* 2004;126:1054–1070.

33. Pasare C, Medzhitov R. Toll-dependent control mechanisms of CD4 T cell activation. *Immunity* 2004;21:733–741.

34. Wang W, Uzzau S, Goldblum SE, Fasano A. Human zonulin, a potential modulator of intestinal tight junctions. *J Cell Sci* 2000;113:4435–4440.

35. Bjorkman PJ, Saper MA, Samraoui B, Bennett WS, Strominger JL, Wiley DC. Structure of the human class-I histocompatibility antigen, *Hla-A2*. *Nature* 1987;329:506–512.

36. Cuvelier C, Barbatis C, Mielants H, Devos M, Roels H, Veys E. Histopathology of intestinal inflammation related to reactive arthritis. *Gut* 1987;28:394–401.

37. Jang MH, Kweon MN, Iwatani K, Yamamoto M, Terahara K, Sasakawa C, Suzuki T, Nochi T, Yokota Y, Rennert PD, Hiroi T, Tamagawa H, Iijima H, Kunisawa J, Yuki Y, Kiyono H. Intestinal villous M cells: an antigen entry site in the mucosal epithelium. *PNAS* 2004;101:6110–6115.

38. Lee J, Mo JH, Katakura K, Alkalay I, Rucker AN, Liu YT, Lee HK, Shen C, Cojocaru G, Shenouda S, Kagnoff M, Eckmann L, Ben-Neriah Y, Raz E. Maintenance of colonic homeostasis by distinctive apical TLR9 signalling in intestinal epithelial cells. *Nat Cell Biol* 2006;8:1327–1336.

39. Akira S, Takeda K. Toll-like receptor signalling. *Nat Rev Immunol* 2004;4:499–511.

40. Rachmilewitz D, Katakura K, Karmeli F, Hayashi T, Reinus C, Rudensky B, Akira S, Takeda K, Lee J, Takabayashi K, Raz E. Toll-like receptor 9 signaling mediates the anti-inflammatory effects of probiotics in murine experimental colitis. *Gastroenterology* 2004;126:520–528.

41. Montalto M, Maggiano N, Ricci R, Curigliano V, Santoro L, Di Nicuolo F, Vecchio FM, Gasbarrini A, Gasbarrini G. Lactobacillus acidophilus protects tight junctions from aspirin damage in HT-29 cells. *Digestion* 2004;69:225–228.

42. Rosenfeldt V, Benfeldt E, Valerius NH, rregaard A, Michaelsen KF. Effect of probiotics on gastrointestinal symptoms and small intestinal permeability in children with atopic dermatitis. *J Pediatrics* 2004;145:612–616.

43. Seehofer D, Rayes N, Schiller R, Stockmann M, Muller AR, Schirmeier A, Schaeper F, Tullius SG, Bengmark S, Neuhaus P Probiotics partly reverse increased bacterial translocation after simultaneous liver resection and colon ic anastomosis in rats. *J Surg Res* 2004;117:262–271.

44. Hao WL, Lee YK. Microflora of the gastrointestinal tract: a review. *Methods Mol Biol* 2004; 268:491–502.

45. Xavier RJ, Podolsky DK. Unravelling the pathogenesis of inflammatory bowel disease. *Nature* 2007;448:427–434.

46. Yadav H, Jain S, Sinha PR. Antidiabetic effect of probiotic dahi containing Lactobacillus acidophilus and Lactobacillus casei in high fructose fed rats. *Nutrition* 2007;23:62–68.

47. Hugot JP, Chamaillard M, Zouali H, Lesage S, Cezard JP, Belaiche J, Almer S, Tysk C, O'Morain CA, Gassull M, Binder V, Finkel Y, Cortot A, Modigliani R, Laurent-Puig P, Gower-Rousseau C, Macry J, Colombel JF, Sahbatou M, Thomas G. Association of NOD2 leucine-rich repeat variants with susceptibility to Crohn's disease. *Nature* 2001;411:599–603.

48. Ogura Y, Bonen DK, Inohara N, Nicolae DL, Chen FF, Ramos R, Britton H, Moran T, Karaliuskas R, Duerr RH, Achkar JP, Brant SR, Bayless TM, Kirschner BS, Hanauer SB, Nunez G, Cho JH. A frameshift mutation in NOD2 associated with susceptibility to Crohn's disease. *Nature* 2001; 411:603–606.

49. Jijon H, Backer J, Diaz H, Yeung H, Thiel D, McKaigney C, De Simone C, Madsen K. DNA from probiotic bacteria modulates murine and human epithelial and immune function. *Gastroenterology* 2004;126:1358–1373.

50. Ewaschuk JB, Backer JL, Churchill TA, Obermeier F, Krause DO, Madsen KL. Surface expression of toll-like receptor 9 is upregulated on intestinal epithelial cells in response to pathogenic bacterial DNA. *Infect Immun* 2007;75:2572–2579.

51. Madden KB, Yeung KA, Zhao A, Gause WC, Finkelman FD, Katona IM, Urban JF Jr., Shea-Donohue T. Enteric nematodes induce stereotypic STAT6-dependent alterations in intestinal epithelial cell function. *J Immunol* 2004;172:5616–5621.

52. Madden KB, Whitman L, Sullivan C, Gause WC, Urban JF Jr., Katona IM, Finkelman FD, Shea-Donohue T. Role of STAT6 and mast cells in IL-4- and IL-13-induced alterations in murine intestinal epithelial cell function. *J Immunol* 2002;169:4417–4422.

53. Shea-Donohue T, Sullivan C, Finkelman FD, Madden KB, Morris SC, Goldhill J, Pineiro-Carrero V, Urban Jr.JF The role of IL-4 in *Heligmosomoides polygyrus*-induced alterations in murine intestinal epithelial cell function. *J Immunol* 2001;167:2234–2239.

54. Ma TY, Boivin MA, Ye D, Pedram A, Said HM. Mechanism of TNF-{alpha} modulation of Caco-2 intestinal epithelial tight junction barrier: role of myosin light-chain kinase protein expression. *Am J Physiol Gastrointest Liver Physiol* 2005;288:G422–G430.

55. Wang F, Graham WV, Wang Y, Witkowski ED, Schwarz BT, Turner JR. Interferon-γ and tumor necrosis factor-α synergize to induce intestinal epithelial barrier dysfunction by up-regulating myosin light chain kinase expression. *Am J Pathol* 2005;166:409–419.

56. Cooper GS, Stroehla BC. The epidemiology of autoimmune diseases. *Autoimmunity Reviews* 2003; 2:119–125.

57. Fasano A, Shea-Donohue T. Mechanisms of disease: the role of intestinal barrier function in the pathogenesis of gastrointestinal autoimmune diseases. *Nature Clinical Practice Gastroenterol Hepatol* 2005;2:416–422.

58. Perl A. Pathogenesis and spectrum of autoimmunity. *Methods Mol Med* 2004;102:1–8.

59. Ercolini AM, Miller SD. Molecular mimics can induce novel self peptide-reactive CD4 + T cell clonotypes in autoimmune disease. *J Immunol* 2007;179:6604–6612.

60. Christen U, von Herrath MG. Induction, acceleration or prevention of autoimmunity by molecular mimicry. *Molecular Immunol* 2004;40:1113–1120.

61. Fujinami RS, von Herrath MG, Christen U, Whitton JL. Molecular mimicry, bystander activation, or viral persistence: infections and autoimmune disease. *Clin Microbiol Rev* 2006;19:80–94.

62. Rook GA, Brunet LR. Microbes, immunoregulation, and the gut. *Gut* 2005;54:317–320.

63. Korzenik JR. Past and current theories of etiology of IBD: toothpaste, worms, and refrigerators. *J Clin Gastroenterol* 2005;39:S59–S65.

64. Korzenik JR, Podolsky DK. Evolving knowledge and therapy of inflammatory bowel disease. *Nat Rev Drug Discov* 2006;5:197–209.

65. Picco P, Gattorno M, Marchese N, Vignola S, Sormani MP, Barabino A, Buoncompagni A. Increased gut permeability in juvenile chronic arthritides. A multivariate analysis of the diagnostic parameters. *Clin Exp Rheumatol* 2000;18:773–778.

66. Watts T, Berti I, Sapone A, Gerarduzzi T, Not T, Zielke R, Fasano A. Role of the intestinal tight junction modulator zonulin in the pathogenesis of type I diabetes in BB diabetic-prone rats. *PNAS* 2005;102:2916–2921.

2

What Pediatricians Need to Know about the Analysis of the Gut Microbiota

Gerald W. Tannock

Key Points

- The biodiverse, individualistic bowel microbiota of humans is acquired by a sequential process that produces a characteristic biological succession.
- Bifidobacteria predominate in the infant gut and may have a long-lasting impact on the physiology of the child (biological Freudianism).
- The mechanisms that regulate the composition and activities of the bowel community likely involve competitive exclusion and efficient regulation of microbial physiology.
- Nucleic acid-based methods of analysis are widely used to determine and monitor the composition of the bowel microbiota. This is because, currently, a large proportion of the members of the bacterial community cannot be cultured under laboratory conditions by traditional bacteriological methods.

Key Words: Microbiota, bowel, bifidobacteria, molecular analysis, infants.

Over evolutionary time, humans have developed an equilibrium with the microbial world, which consists of cloaking the body inside and out with microorganisms that are likelier to be friends than enemies. (Abigail Salyers and Dixie Whitt [microbiologists])

INTRODUCTION

Fabrication of the metaphorical cloak of microbes begins within hours of birth when bacteria from the environment, the mother and other humans who interact intimately with the baby inoculate the sterile skin and accessible body cavities of the infant. The baby is exposed to a diversity of microbial life during the ensuing days, weeks and months yet only certain bacterial types find the body to be "fertile soil" that provides their required carbon and energy sources and other physicochemical factors conducive to their life. It is easy to imagine that the infant body is assailed from every direction by microbes, and studies of the temporal acquisition of the gut microbiota, for example,

From: *Nutrition and Health: Probiotics in Pediatric Medicine*
Edited by: S. Michail and P.M. Sherman © Humana Press, Totowa, NJ

show that the composition of the microbial community of the bowel, essentially composed in modern times of bacteria, progresses in the form of a characteristic biological succession [1–8]. The first heterogeneous collection of bacterial species quickly simplifies and facultative anaerobes (*Escherichia coli* and enterococci) assume numerical dominance. Obligately, anaerobic bacteria belonging to the genus *Bifidobacterium* are also numerous and, by the age of three months, are the predominant members of the bowel microbiota, even in formula-fed babies [1,6,9–11]. To all intents and purposes, the neonate during the first few months of life is almost, in gnotobiotic terms, a monoassociated animal, such is the simplicity in composition of the microbiota and the numerical predominance of bifidobacteria.

Gnotobiotic mouse experiments have demonstrated that, at least in the short term, the presence of bacteria in the bowel influences the physiology of the animal host. Particularly striking have been the reports of the effects on murine gene expression in relation to the epithelial barrier and the induction of angiogenesis in the ileum, and the accumulation of body fat [12–15]. If these reported effects on mice are applicable to humans, then the biological successions occurring in early life become pivotal in the development of the child. Colonization of the bowel by certain bacterial species may have lifelong consequences. Dubos et al. [16] aptly referred to this enduring influence of early microbial associations as "biological Freudianism." Microbial influences replace, in this view, environmental and social factors that mould the "unconscious." We are not conscious of the impact of early microbial associations, but their long-lasting influences shape our adult physiology – the microbiological past is alive in the physiological present.

Immune deviation, the process in which the bias toward a Th2 response by the immune system of the infant is removed, may be an important consequence of exposures to microbes in early life [17,18]. Many affluent countries have experienced an increase in the prevalence of allergic diseases in recent decades, including atopic dermatitis, asthma, and atopic rhinitis [19]. With reference to "biological Freudianism," colonization of the infant bowel by specific species of bacteria might be important in the initial regulation of the developing immune system. Modern lifestyles and environments may alter qualitative exposure of infants to bowel commensals and this might influence the risk of atopic diseases [20,21]. Members of the genus *Bifidobacterium* are likely to be important bacteria in this respect because, as indicated above, they form a major portion of the bowel community in early life.

The rules and regulations that govern the bacterial community resident in the bowel must be legislated anew each time a neonate is colonized. This is because the bacterial collection is not the same in every human [22,23]. Probably fundamental to the homeostasis of ecosystems associated with the human body is the phenomenon of "competitive exclusion," which is particularly well known in the case of the bowel community [24]. Long ago demonstrated in gnotobiotic experiments, the presence of the microbiota enhances nonspecific resistance to infection. For example, germfree mice can be infected by the oral route by a dose of *Salmonella typhimurium* as small as ten cells; the infectious dose for conventional mice is about 10^9 cells. The self-regulated, homeostatic community already established in the conventional bowel provides a hurdle that only large numbers (a high dose) of pathogenic cells can surmount [25]. We are not exactly sure how competitive exclusion is mediated mechanistically but may best be summarized in the "niche exclusion principle": two species cannot simultaneously occupy the same ecological niche [26]. Only the better adapted will be successful. This can easily be envisaged in the case of nutritional competition because the species/strain that best binds and transports a source of energy and carbon into its cells will out-compete a biochemically less capable organism. Not to be forgotten, moreover, is the production of antimicrobial molecules that could give a competitive edge by altering the chemical environment, making it unsuitable for growth of other species. Short chain fatty acids can be invoked in this respect, as can hydrogen sulfide, and perhaps "bacteriocins" [25,27]. Multiple mechanisms must participate synergistically in the control of populations within complex communities. It is extremely difficult, however, to define competitive mechanisms even using experimental animal models. The order in which bacterial strains are introduced into the experimental system can ordain which of the two organisms eventually dominates the ecosystem numerically [28]. The diet fed to experimental animals can also influence the outcome of competition experiments [29,30]. By changing the diet, the number and types of available ecological niches are changed. The bowel community is composed of hundreds of species, which in turn implies that this is the number of ecological niches in the ecosystem – the more niches, the more biodiversity. The diversity of bacterial types in the human bowel reflects, therefore, the intensely competitive nature of this ecosystem in which mutations and horizontal gene transfer have permitted adaptation of bacteria to perform diverse functions in the bowel community.

Clearly, investigations of the impacts of commensal bacteria on the infant in early life require analytical procedures that can be used in the laboratory to monitor the composition and activities of the bacterial community of the bowel. Much of the bacteriological information of the bowel community has been generated through the application of nucleic acid-based methodologies, most of which rely on the nucleotide base sequence of small ribosomal subunit RNA (16S rRNA in the case of bacteria) which provides a cornerstone of microbial taxonomy. Nucleic acid-based methods of detection suggest that about 50% of the bacterial cells seen microscopically in feces of adults cannot yet be cultured in the laboratory, even when accounting for the fact that some of the bacteria are dead [31]. This phenomenon, also manifested even more dramatically in terrestrial and aquatic ecosystems was, based on traditional bacteriological experience, totally unexpected and has been called "the great plate count anomaly" [32]. Operational taxonomic units (OTU; molecular species) never encountered in culture-based bacteriology are detectable by the molecular methods, revealing a new world remaining to be investigated by bacteriologists of the future. Although, in the case of infants, the microbiota is dominated in early life by the bifidobacteria, which are relatively easily cultured under laboratory conditions, nucleic acid-based analytical methods provide evidence of the increasing complexity of community composition as babies grow and develop.

The starting point for nucleic acid-based, analytical methods is the extraction of bacterial DNA or RNA directly from the fecal or other sample of interest, avoiding the need to cultivate any members of the bacterial community. 16S rRNA or the gene that encodes it has become a cornerstone of bacterial classification because it contains regions of nucleotide base sequence that are highly conserved across the bacterial world and that are interspersed with variable regions (V regions). These variable regions contain the "signatures" of phylogenetic groups and even species [33]. For this reason, variable regions of 16S rRNA (or 16S rRNA gene sequences) are the basis of the analytical methods. Bacterial DNA or RNA extracted from the samples (in theory nucleic acid from all of the bacterial types in the sample will be represented in the extracts) and polymerase chain reaction (PCR) amplification (reverse transcription-PCR in the case of RNA extracts) of the 16S rRNA gene in part or complete, is carried out. Clone libraries of the 16S rRNA genes can be made and sequenced, or emulsion-based high-throughput PCR sequencing can be carried out, producing a catalog of the bacterial constituents of the ecosystem [23,35–37]. It is unfortunate that as much as 5% of the 16S rRNA gene sequences in databanks are inaccurate. This is because the results of high-throughput sequencing projects have polluted the DNA databanks with unreliable 16S rRNA gene sequences making meaningful analysis of catalogs of bacterial inhabitants difficult to achieve [38,39].

Nevertheless, from this sequence information, DNA probes can be designed. DNA (oligonucleotide) probes that target specific rRNA sequences (16S or 23S) within ribosomes, to which they hybridize, are used in this method [40–45]. The probes are 5′ labeled with a fluorescent dye, which permits both detection and quantification of specific bacterial populations (fluorescence in situ hybridization [FISH]). Bacterial cells within which hybridization with a probe has occurred fluoresce and hence can be detected and counted. Permeablization of the bacterial cells is required in order to standardize intracellular access of DNA probes to their targets [46]. Within the cell, the secondary structure of rRNA molecules and their molecular interactions within the ribosome may hinder the access of the probes to their target sites. In situ accessibility influences the amount of fluorescence generated from the probe [47]. A high degree of in situ accessibility would facilitate the binding of the probe to its target site and therefore permit the probe to emit a bright fluorescence signal. The determination of the brightness of fluorescence (probe relative fluorescence) conferred by a probe is a means of evaluating its in situ accessibility [46,47]. Modeling of the secondary structure of 16S rRNA molecules allows in silico investigation of the in situ accessibility of the entire molecule [47–49] and the target site can be assessed in terms of accessibility. If the target region is located in a poor or nonaccessible site, helper probes (unlabeled oligonucleotides) can be derived that are complementary to regions adjacent to the probe's target site, promoting the binding of the probe and therefore amplifying the fluorescence signal [49–51]. Other important technical considerations include (i) the physiological state of the bacterial cells because the number of ribosomes per bacterial cell is greater the higher their metabolic activity. Therefore, bacterial cells in a quiescent state have weak fluorescence and may not be detected. (ii) the degree of hybridization stringency, which depends on three factors: temperature, salt concentration, and formamide concentration of the hybridization solution. The manipulation of these factors influences the specificity of hybridisation and hence detection and quantification. (iii) a 16S rRNA gene database that is rapidly increasing is size. More than 600,000 16S rRNA sequences are available from the Ribosomal Database (http://rdp.cme.msu.edu), permitting the in silico development and validation of a large panel of probes targeting different phylotypes resident in the human bowel. Several of the currently used probes were designed and tested using older versions of the Ribosomal Database so continual reassessment of specificity and coverage of these probes is essential in order to update and confirm their continuing reliability. (iv) epifluoresence microscopic detection and quantification of bacterial populations was used originally to enumerate fluorescent cells but, because of the laborious and time-consuming nature of this work, automated systems have been developed [52], culminating in the use of flow cytometry to count the fluorescent cells. Rapid and easy to set up, flow cytometry combines quantitative and multifactor analysis (size, internal granularity, fluorescence signal).

Deriving a catalog of bowel inhabitants, or enumerating groups of bacteria using DNA probes for every sample that needs to be investigated is a daunting task. A relatively simple, semiquantitative screening method to compare the bacterial composition of multiple samples is provided by PCR combined with denaturing gradient gel electrophoresis (DGGE) or temporal temperature gradient gel electrophoresis (TTGE). This approach, which provides comparative "snapshots" of microbiota compositions, has been demonstrated to have enormous utility in a number of bowel microbiota studies [53–56]. DNA or RNA is extracted directly from intestinal or faecal samples. Then a variable 16S rRNA gene sequence is amplified using PCR primers that anneal with conserved sequences that span the selected V region. One of the PCR primers has a GC-rich 5′ end (GC clamp) to prevent complete denaturation of the DNA fragments during gradient gel electrophoresis. To separate the 16S fragments amplified from different types of bacteria and present in the PCR product, a polyacrylamide gel is used. The double-stranded 16S fragments migrate through a polyacrylamide gel containing a chemical or thermal gradient until they are partially denatured by the chemical or temperature conditions. The fragments do not completely denature because of the GC clamp, and migration is radically slowed when partial denaturation occurs. Because of the variation in the 16S sequences of different bacterial species, chemical and thermal stability is also different; therefore different 16S "species" can be differentiated by this electrophoretic method. 16S rRNA gene fragments from different bacteria have different migration distances in the electrophoretic gel and a profile of the numerically predominant members of the microbiota is thereby generated [57,58]. Individual fragments of DNA can be cut from electrophoretic gels, further amplified and cloned, then sequenced. The sequence can be compared to those in gene databanks in order to obtain identification of the bacterium from which the 16S sequence originated. In a further development of this methodology, PCR primers specific for bacterial groups can be derived. These primers generate an electrophoretic profile of the species comprising a specific bacterial genus, for example bifidobacterial species, within the bacterial community [59–61].

Specific strains of bacteria can be differentiated by producing their DNA fingerprint, much as is done in human forensics. Chromosomal DNA is extracted from pure cultures of bacteria. The DNA is digested by a restriction endonuclease chosen on the basis of the mol % G + C content of the DNA of the bacterial species and on the recognition sequence of the enzyme. An endonuclease that will cut the DNA rarely is desired so that a relatively small number of DNA fragments result from the digestion and a relatively simple pattern will be generated in the electrophoretic gel. The digestion generates large fragments of DNA that would not separate by the usual agarose gel electrophoresis that is based on molecular sieving. Therefore, pulsed field gel electrophoresis (PFGE) is used in which the mixture of fragments in the DNA digest are exposed to alternating electrical fields that force the fragments to change orientation rather than to migrate through the agarose gel immediately after the electrical field is changed from one direction to another. The rate of reorientation is size dependent, so larger molecules change direction more slowly than smaller ones. The pulse time (the time spent in a field of particular direction) is varied and this dictates the DNA class size that spends most of the time reorientating rather than migrating. The DNA fragments are thus separated by the retardation of net movement rather than by sieving. The pattern of fragments generated in the gel represents the genetic fingerprint of the bacterial culture and is characteristic of that strain of bacteria [62]. A particularly useful application of PFGE of DNA digests is to provide a means by which a probiotic bacterial strain can be tracked during the course of a probiotic study. The bacterial group of interest can be selectively cultured and colonies are randomly picked to obtain pure cultures. The genetic fingerprint of these isolates is then determined by PFGE of DNA digests, and compared with that of the probiotic bacterial strain. The presence or absence of the probiotic strain in fecal samples can be determined by this method. The advantage of PFGE of DNA digests is that a specific strain can be tracked during studies aimed at determining the persistence of the probiotic strain in the gut. Disadvantages include the requirement for bacteriological culture and the immense logistical effort required to genetically fingerprint hundreds or thousands of bacterial isolates.

An example of the use of genetic fingerprinting in a probiotic study is provided by the work of Tannock et al. [63] who analyzed the composition of the *Lactobacillus* populations present in the feces. The composition of the fecal bacterial community of ten human subjects was monitored before (control period of six months), during (test period of six months) and after (posttest period of three months) the administration of a milk product containing *Lactobacillus rhamnosus* DR20 (daily dose of 1.6×10^9 lactobacilli). The composition of the *Lactobacillus* population of each subject was analyzed by PFGE of bacterial DNA digests in order to differentiate between DR20 and other strains present in the fecal samples. Consumption of the probiotic transiently altered the composition of the *Lactobacillus* populations of the subjects, but to varying degrees. The detection of DR20 among the numerically predominant strains was related to the presence or absence of a stable autochthonous population of lactobacilli during the control period. The probiotic strain did not predominate in samples collected from subjects with *Lactobacillus* populations of stable composition.

What predicates which bacterial species or strain will establish in the infant bowel? The short answer is probably: only bacteria that can utilize the substrates provided by the diet and the particular human host. Bifidobacteria, *E. coli* and enterococci can utilize a wide range of monosaccharides and oligosaccharides, which would be provided by the diet. Genomic analysis of bifidobacterial species shows that these bacteria are indeed endowed well with enzymic capacity to hydrolyze and ferment oligosaccharides [64,65]. After weaning, however, the range of fermentable substrates available to the bacteria changes from monosaccharides and oligosaccharides to complex plant polymers (dietary fiber) that pass undigested through the small bowel and hence become one of the principle sources of carbon and energy for bowel bacteria [66]. The other major source of complex carbohydrates is provided by the mucins (constituents of mucus) that are continually secreted into the bowel from goblet cells present in the mucosal lining [67]. Assessment of obligately anaerobic inhabitants of the adult bowel through analysis of a few representative fully sequenced genomes, as well as by studies of community genetics [68–70] show that they are superbly adapted to digesting complex polysaccharides. The bacteria produce numerous hydrolytic enzymes and can regulate their use according to the kinds of substrates that they sense in their environment. Strict regulation of catabolic pathways must be an extremely important attribute in a habitat where the nutritional profile will vary from day to day according to the omnivorous and varied dietary preferences of the human host, and helps to explain the remarkable consistency in biochemistry and biodiversity of the human bowel [71].

Increasingly, it becomes clear that, because of the individualistic compositions of the microbiota, phylogenetic analysis of the bowel community of infants may not offer useful information, beyond that which has already been accumulated [6]. New methodologies are required to explore the impact of the maturing bowel microbiota of the developing child. "Who is there?" needs to be replaced by "What are they doing, and how are they doing it?" We need to define the molecular webs that interconnect bacteria-bowel milieu-infant mucosa. In this view, the identity of the phylogenetic entities inhabiting the bowel is minimized and their biochemistry is emphasized. Because much of the microbiota has not yet been cultivated, new culture-independent methodologies must be invented and applied to investigations of the bowel.

Metagenomics is a facet of microbial ecology in which a microbial community is studied in terms of its collective genomes (community genetics), rather than focusing on the diversity of species and their individual genomes [32]. For functional studies, the metagenomic approach traditionally entails the cloning of large fragments of community genomic DNA that have been extracted directly from the ecosystem of choice. The cloned DNA fragments are large enough to encode operons and therefore might result in the expression, by a surrogate bacterial host, of several enzymes that could catalyze a relatively complex metabolic process, including the synthesis of secondary metabolites. Metagenomic libraries derived from microbial community genomes can be screened for heterologous phenotypic traits that include enzymes and other proteins that are essential to the functioning of the ecosystem. Hence they provide a means of accessing and assessing details of community biochemistry through its underpinning genetics.

Measurement of the impact of bacteria on the transcriptome of the bowel mucosa of the child, such has been achieved with experimental animals, would be ethically and technically difficult to achieve. A new approach to determine the impact of the microbiota on the infant's tissues is therefore required. Metabolomics is the nontargeted, holistic, quantitative analysis of changes in the complete set of metabolites in the cell (the metabolome) in response to environmental or cellular changes [72]. Metabolites are low-molecular weight organic compounds (<1000 Da) that participate in general metabolic reactions, or, are required for maintenance, growth, and normal functioning of a cell. Changes in cellular physiology are amplified through transcription of genes and translation to proteins but, due to regulatory mechanisms and/or substrate availability, a tenfold increase in concentration of a transcript or enzyme is not necessarily reflected in a tenfold increase in a particular cell activity. Alterations in transcriptome or proteome do, however, have large effects on the concentrations of intermediary metabolites in the cell because they reflect the activities of metabolic pathways. Of particular importance is the ability of metabolomics to penetrate the mechanisms of intracellular signaling in which both concentrations of metabolites and their associated dynamics are important. Whereas knowledge of the intracellular metabolites (metabolic fingerprint, the endometabolome) is essential in this work, changes in the physiology of the bowel ecosystem could be more easily revealed by investigation of the exometabolome (metabolic footprint) represented by the extracellular milieu which contains metabolites secreted or consumed by bacteria in the bowel [73]. The metabolic footprint of the bowel bacteria is reflected in the metabolome of the animal host because bacterial metabolites are absorbed from the gut lumen into the lymph and blood circulations. Hence, the body fluids (blood, lymph, bile, sweat, urine) of the host contain numerous bacterial products that may provide biomarkers of food–microbe–host interrelationships and possible indicators of health or disease. The host metabolome is the sum of the interacting metabolomes of the whole organism and thus represents the end product of genetic, environmental, and host–bacterial relationships. The study of microbiota and host metabolomes might therefore contribute to a full systems biology approach to understanding and maintaining bowel health of the infant [74]. Preparation of the blueprint of the interactive bowel networks will require a systems biology investigation encompassing a diversity of scientists from different disciplines. The primary aim of the research will be to understand how all of the heterogeneous parts (dietary components, bacterial consortia, host physiology, and development) are integrated in early life, with a supplementary aim of identifying biomarkers of health or disease. A fusing of biological and computational expertise will be required for success.

> *From all points of view, the child is truly the father of the man, and for this reason we need to develop an experimental science that might be called biological Freudianism. Socially and individually the response of human beings to the conditions of the present is always conditioned by the biological remembrance of things past.* (Rene Dubos, Dwayne Savage, and Russell Schaedler [microbiologists])

SUMMARY AND CONCLUSION

The infant bowel becomes colonized by a biodiverse collection of bacteria soon after birth. A regulated process (succession) can be recognized in which the proportions of different bacterial groups comprising the microbiota change during the first few years of life. The physiological impact of this bacterial succession may have long-lasting, physiological consequences. Much of the microbiota is uncultivable by traditional bacteriological methods, therefore nucleic acid-based analytical methods are widely used to appraise the state of the microbiota. The highly individualistic compositions of individual bowel communities, even in infants, confound comparisons of dietary and other environmental influences. Increased understanding in the future of bacteria–host interactions will probably result from the application of advanced chemical analyses.

REFERENCES

1. Cooperstock MS, Zedd AJ. Intestinal flora of infants. In: Hentges DJ, ed., Human intestinal microflora in health and disease. New York: Academic Press, 1983:79–99.
2. Tannock GW, Fuller R, Smith SL, Hall MA. Plasmid profiling of members of the family *Enterobacteriaceae*, lactobacilli, and bifidobacteria to study the transmission of bacteria from mother to infant. *J Clin Microbiol* 1990;28:1225–1228.
3. Zoetendal EG, Akkermans ADL, Akkermans-van Viliet WM, de Visser JAGM, de Vos WM. The host genotype affects the bacterial community in the human gastrointestinal tract. *Microb Ecol Health Dis* 2001;13:129–134.
4. Martin R, Langa S, Revriego C, Jiminez E, Marin ML, Xaus J, Fernandez L, Rodriguez JM. Human milk is a source of lactic acid bacteria for the infant gut. *J Pediatr* 2003;143:754–758.
5. Martin R, Heilig HGHJ, Zoetnedal EG, Jiminez E, Fernandez L, Smidt H, Rodriguez JM. Cultivation-independent assessment of the bacterial diversity of breast milk among healthy women. *Res Microbiol* 2007;158:31–37.

6. Mah KW, Chin VIL, Wong WS, Lay C, Tannock GW, Shek LP, Aw M, Chua KY, Wong HB, Panchalingham A, Lee BW. Analysis of the fecal microbiota of infants at risk of atopic diseases shows a distinctive colonization pattern regardless of probiotic administration. *Pediatr Res* 2007;62:674–679.

7. Tannock GW. Normal microflora. An introduction to microbes inhabiting the human body. London: Chapman & Hall, 1995.

8. Rawls JF, Mahowald MA, Ley RE, Gordon JI. Reciprocal gut microbiota transplants from zebrafish and mice to germfree recipients reveal host habitat selection. *Cell* 2006;127:423–433.

9. Norin KE, Gustafsson BE, Lindblad BS, Midtvedt T. The establishment of some microflora associated biochemical characteristics in feces from children during the first years of life. *Acta Paediatr Scand* 1985;74:207–212.

10. Tannock GW, Cook G. Enterococci as members of the intestinal microflora of humans. In: Gilmore MS, Clewell DB, Courvalin P, Dunny GM, Murray BE, Rice LB ed., The Enterococci: pathogenesis, molecular biology, and antibiotic resistance. Washington, DC: ASM Press, 2002:101–132.

11. Harmsen HJM, Wildeboer ACM, Raangs GC, Wagendorp AA, Klijn N, Bindels JG, Welling GW. Analysis of intestinal flora development in breast-fed and formula-fed infants by using molecular identification and detection methods. *J Pediatr Gastroenterol Nutr* 2000;30:61–67.

12. Hooper LV, Wong MH, Thelin A, Hansson L, Falk PG, Gordon JI. Molecular analysis of commensal host–microbial relationships in the intestine. *Science* 2001;291:881–884.

13. Hooper LV, Xu J, Falk PG, Midtvedt T, Gordon JI. A molecular sensor that allows a gut commensal to control its nutrient foundation in a competitive ecosystem. *Proc Natl Acad Sci USA* 1999;96: 9833–9838.

14. Stappenbeck TS, Hooper LV, Gordon JI. Developmental regulation of intestinal angiogenesis by indigenous microbes via Paneth cells. *Proc Natl Acad Sci USA* 2002;99:15451–15455.

15. Backhed F, Ding H, Wang T, Hooper LV, Koh GY, Nagy A, Semenkovich CF, Gordon JI. The gut microbiota as an environmental factor that regulates fat storage. *Proc Natl Acad Sci USA* 2004;101: 15718–15723.

16. Dubos R, Savage D, Schaedler R. Biological freudianism: lasting effects of early environmental influences. *Pediatrics* 1996;38:789–800.

17. Yabuhara A, Macaubas C, Prescott SL, Venaille TJ, Holt BJ, Habre W, Sly PD, Holt PG. Th2-polarized immunological memory to inhalant allergens in atopics is established during infancy and early childhood. *Clin Exp Allergy* 1997;27:1237–1239.

18. Prescott SL, Macaubus C, Holt BJ, Smallacombe TB, Loh R, Sly PD, Holt PG. Transplacental priming of the human immune system to environmental allergens: universal skewing of initial T cell responses toward the Th2 cytokine profile. *J Immunol* 1998;160:4730–4737.

19. Hopkin JM. Mechanisms of enhanced prevalence of asthma and atopy in developed countries. *Curr Opin Immunol* 1997;9:788–792.

20. Murray CS, Woodcock A. Gut microflora and atopic disease. In: Tannock GW, ed., Probiotics and prebiotics: where are we going? Wymondham, UK: Caister Academic Press, 2002:239–261.

21. Gore C, Munro K, Lay C, Bibiloni R, Morris J, Woodcock A, Custovic A, Tannock GW. *Bifidobacterium pseudocatenulatum* is associated with atopic eczema – a nested case-control study investigating the fecal microbiota of infants. *J Allergy Clin Immunol* 2008;121:135–140.

22. Zoetendal EG, Akkermans ADL, de Vos WM. Temperature gradient gel electrophoresis analysis of 16S rRNA from human faecal samples reveals stable and host-specific communities of active bacteria. *Appl Environ Microbiol* 1998;64:3854–3859.

23. Eckburg PB, Bik EM, Bernstein CN, Purdom E, Dethlefsen L, Sargent M, Gill SR, Nelson KE, Relman DA. Diversity of the human intestinal microbial flora. *Science* 2005;308:1635–1638.

24. Van der Waaij D, Berghuis de Vries JM, Lekkerkerk JEC. Colonisation resistance of the digestive tract in conventional and antibiotic-treated mice. *J Hyg* 1971;69:405–411.

25. Tannock GW. Control of gastrointestinal pathogens by normal flora. In: Klug MJ, Reddy CA, ed., Perspectives in microbial ecology. Washington, DC: American Society for Microbiology, 1984:374–382.

26. Hardin G. The competitive exclusion principle. *Science* 1960;131:1292–1297.

27. Corr SC, Yin L, Riedel CU, O'Toole PW, Hill C, Gahan CGM. Bacteriocin production as a mechanism for the anti-infective activity of *Lactobacillus salivarius* UCC118. *Proc Natl Acad Sci USA* 2007;104:7617–7621.

28. Hentges DJ, Freter R. In vivo and in vitro antagonism of intestinal bacteria against *Shigella flexneri*. I. Correlation between various tests. *J Infect Dis* 1962;110:30–37.

29. Freter R, Abrams GD, Aranki A. Patterns of interaction in gnotobiotic mice among bacteria of a synthetic "normal" intestinal flora. In: Heneghan JB, ed., *Germfree Research*, New York: Academic Press, 1973:429–433.

30. Ducluzeau R, Raibaud P. Ecologie microbienne du tube digestif. Paris: Masson, 1979.

31. Ben-Amor K, Heilig H, Smidt H, Vaughan EE, Abee T, de Vos, WM. Genetic diversity of viable, injured, and dead faecal bacteria assessed by fluorescence-activated cell sorting and 16S rRNA gene analysis. *Appl Environ Microbiol* 2005;71:4679–4689.

32. Handelsman J. Metagenomics: application of genomics to uncultured microorganisms. *Microbiol Mol Biol Res* 2004;68:669–685.

33. Woese CR. Bacterial evolution. *Microbiol Rev* 1987;51:221–271.

34. Wilson KH, Blitchington RB. Human colonic biota studied by ribosomal DNA sequence analysis. *Appl Environ Microbiol* 1996;62:2273–2278.

35. Suau A, Bonnet R, Sutren M, Godon JJ, Gibson GR, Collins MD, Doré J. Direct analysis of genes encoding 16S rRNA from complex communities reveals many novel molecular species within the human gut. *Appl Environ Microbiol* 1999;65:4799–4807.

36. Hayashi H, Takahashi R, Nishi T, Sakamoto M, Benno Y. Molecular analysis of jejunal, ileal, caecal and recto-sigmoidal human colonic microbiota using 16S rRNA gene libraries and terminal restriction fragment length polymorphism. *J Med Microbiol* 2005;54:1093–1101.

37. Wang M, Ahrne S, Jeppsson B, Molin G. Comparison of bacterial diversity along the human intestinal tract by direct cloning and sequencing of 16S rRNA genes. *FEMS Microbiol Ecol* 2005;54:219–231.

38. Ashelford KE, Chuzhanova NA, Fry JC, Jones AJ, Weightman AJ. At least 1 in 20 16S rRNA sequence records currently held in public repositories is estimated to contain substantial anomalies. *Appl Environ Microbiol* 2005;71:7724–7736.

39. Ashelford KE, Chuzhanova NA, Fry JC, Jones AJ, Weightman AJ. New screening software shows that most recent large 16S rRNA gene clone libraries contain chimeras. *Appl Environ Microbiol* 2006;72:5734–5741.

40. Amann RI, Ludwig W, Schleifer KH. Phylogenetic identification and in situ detection of individual microbial cells without cultivation. *Microbiol Rev* 1995;59:143–169.

41. Harmsen HJM, Raangs GC, He T, Degener JE, Welling GW. Extensive set of 16S rRNA-based probes for detection of bacteria in human faeces. *Appl Environ Microbiol* 2002;68:2982–2990.

42. Franks A, Harmsen HJM, Raangs GC, Jansen GJ, Schut F, Welling GW. Variations of bacterial population in human faeces measured by fluorescent in situ hybridization with group-specific 16S rRNA-targeted oligonucleotide probes. *Appl Environ Microbiol* 1988;64:3336–3345.

43. Langendijk P, Schut F, Jansen GJ, Raangs GC, KamphuisGR, Wilkinson MHF, Welling GW. Quantitative fluorescence in situ hybridization of *Bifidobacterium* spp. with genus-specific 16S rRNA-targeted probes and its application in faecal samples. *Appl Environ Microbiol* 1995;61:3069–3075.

44. Sghir A, Gramet G, Suau A, Rochet V, Pochart P, Dore J. Quantification of bacterial groups within the human faecal flora by oligonucleotide probe hybridisation. *Appl Environ Microbiol* 2000;66:2263–2266.

45. Lay C, Rigottier-Gois L, Holmstrom K, Rajilic M, Vaughan EE, de Vos WM, Collins MD, Thiel R, Namsolleck P, Blaut M, Dore J. Colonic microbiota signatures across five northern European countries. *Appl Environ Microbiol* 2005;71:4153–4155.

46. Lay C, Sutren M, Rochet V, Saunier K, Dore J, Rigottier-Gois L. Design and validation of 16S rRNA probes to enumerate members of the *Clostridium leptum* subgroup in human faecal microbiota. *Environ Microbiol* 2005;7:933–946.

47. Fuchs BM, Wallner G, Beisker W, Schwippl I, Ludwig W, Amann R. Flow cytometric analysis of the in situ accessibility of *Escherichia coli* 16S rRNA for fluorescently labeled oligonucleotide probes. *Appl Environ Microbiol* 1998;64:4973–4982.

48. Kumar Y, Westram R, Behrens S, Fuchs B, Glockner FO, Amann R, Meier H, Ludwig W. Graphical representation of ribosomal RNA probe accessibility data using ARB software package. *BMC Bioinformatics* 2005;6:61.

49. Saunier K, Rouge C, Lay C, Rigottier-Gois L, Dore J. Enumeration of bacteria from the *Clostridium leptum* subgroup in human faecal microbiota using Clep1156 16S rRNA probe in combination with helper and competitor oligonucleotides. *Syst Appl Microbiol* 2005;28:454–464.

50. Fuchs BM, Glockner FO, Wulf, Amann R. Unlabeled helper oligonucleotides increase the in situ accessibility to 16S rRNA of fluorescently labeled oligonucleotide probes. *Appl Environ Microbiol* 2000;66:3603–3607.

51. Dinoto A, Suksomcheep A, Ishizuka S, Kimura H, Hanada S, Kamagata Y, Asano K, Tomita F, Yokota A. Modulation of rat cecal microbiota by administration of raffinose and encapsulated *Bifidobacterium breve*. *Appl Environ Microbiol* 2006;72:784–792.

52. Jansen GJ, Wildeboer-Veloo AC, Tonk RH, Franks AH, and Welling GW. Development and validation of an automated, microscopy-based method for enumeration of groups of intestinal bacteria. *J Microbiol Meth* 1999;37:215–221.

53. Knarreborg A, Simon MA, Engberg RM, Jensen BB, Tannock GW. Effects of dietary fat source and subtherapeutic levels of antibiotic on the bacterial community in the ileum of broiler chickens at various ages. *Appl Environ Microbiol* 2002;68:5918–5924.

54. Tannock GW, Munro K, Bibiloni R, Simon MA, Hargreaves P, Gopal P, Harmsen H, Welling G. Impact of consumption of oligosaccharide-containing biscuits on the fecal microbiota of humans. *Appl Environ Microbiol* 2004;70:2129–2136.

55. Bibiloni R, Mangold M, Madsen KL, Fedorak RN, Tannock GW. The bacteriology of biopsies differs between newly diagnosed, untreated, Crohn's disease and ulcerative colitis patients. *J Med Microbiol* 2006;55:1141–1149.

56. Snart J, Bibiloni R, Grayson T, Lay C, Zhang H, Allison GE, Laverdiere JK, Temelli F, Vasanthan T, Bell R, Tannock GW. Supplementation of the diet with high-viscosity beta-glucan results in enrichment for lactobacilli in the rat cecum. *Appl Environ Microbiol* 2006;72:1925–1931.

57. Felske A, Rheims H, Wolerink A, Stackebrandt E, Akkermans ADL. Ribosome analysis reveals prominent activity of an uncultured member of the class Actinobacteria in grassland soils. *Microbiology* 1997;143:2983–2989.

58. Muyzer G, Smalla K. Application of denaturing gradient gel electrophoresis (DGGE) and temperature gradient gel electrophoresis (TGGE) in microbial ecology. *Antonie van Leewenhoek* 1998; 73,127–141.

59. Satokari RM, Vaughan EE, Akkermans ADL, Saarela M, de Vos WM. Bifidobacterial diversity in human faeces detected by genus-specific PCR and denaturing gradient gel electrophoresis. *Appl Environ Microbiol* 2001;67:504–513.

60. Requena T, Burton J, Matsuki T, Munro K, Simon MA, Tanaka R, Watanabe K, Tannock GW. Identification, detection, and enumeration of human *Bifidobacterium* species by PCR targeting the transaldolase gene. *Appl Environ Microbiol* 2002;68:2420–2427.

61. Walter J, Hertel C, Tannock GW, Lis CM, Munro K, Hammes WP. Detection of *Lactobacillus, Pediococcus, Leuconostoc,* and *Weissella* species in human faeces by using group-specific PCR primers and denaturing gradient gel electrophoresis. *Appl Environ Microbiol* 2001;67:2578–2585.

62. Gardiner K. Pulsed field gel electrophoresis. *Anal Chem* 1991;63:658–665.

63. Tannock GW, Munro K, Harmsen HJM, Welling GW, Smart J, Gopal PK. Analysis of the faecal microflora of human subjects consuming a probiotic product containing *Lactobacillus rhamnosus* DR20. *Appl Environ Microbiol* 2000;66:2578–2588.

64. Ward RE, Ninonuevo M, Mills DA, Lebrilla CB, German JB. In vitro fermentation of breast milk oligosaccharides by *Bifidbacterium infantis* and *Lactobacillus gasseri*. *Appl Environ Microbiol* 2006;72:4497–4499.

65. Schell MA, Karamirantzou M, Snel B, Vilanova D, Berger B, Pessi G, Zwahlen MC, Desiere F, Bork P, Delby M, Pridmore RD. The genome sequence of *Bifidobacterium longum* reflects its adaptation to the human gastrointestinal tract. *Proc Natl Acad Sci USA.* 2002;99:14422–14427.

66. Cummings JH, Macfarlane GT. The control and consequences of bacterial fermentation in the human colon. *J Appl Bacteriol* 1991;70:443–459.

67. Roberton AM, Corfield AP. Mucin degradation and its significance in inflammatory conditions of the gastrointestinal tract. In: GW Tannock, ed., Medical importance of the normal microflora. Dordrecht, the Netherlands: Kluwer Academic, 1999:222–261.

68. Xu J, Bjursell MK, Himrod J, Deng S, Carmichael LK, Chiang HC, Hooper LV, Gordon JI. A genomic view of the human-*Bacteroides thetaiotaomicron* symbiosis. *Science* 2003; 299:2074–2076.

69. Gill SR, Pop M, DeBoy RT, Eckburg PB, Turnbaugh PJ, Samuel BS, Gordon JI, Relman DA, Fraser-Liggett CM, Nelson KE. Metagenomic analysis of the human distal gut microbiome. *Science* 2006;312:1355–1359.

70. Flint HJ, Duncan SH, Scott KP, Louis P. Interactions and competition within the microbial community of the human colon: links between diet and health. *Environ Microbiol* 2007;9:1101–1111.

71. Tannock GW. The intestinal microflora. In: Fuller R, Perdigon G, ed., Gut Flora. Nutrition, immunity and health. Oxford: Blackwell Press, 2003:1–23.

72. Werf van der MJ, Jellema RH, Hankemeier T. Microbial metabolomics: replacing trial-and-error by the unbiased selection and ranking of targets. *J Indust Microbiol Biotechnol* 2005;32:234–252.

73. Kell DB, Brown M, Davey HM, Dunn WB, Spasic I, Oliver SG. Metabolic footprinting and systems biology: the medium is the message. *Nature Rev* 2005;3:557–565.

74. Nicholson JK, Holmes E, Lindon JC, Wilson ID. The challenges of modeling mammalian biocomplexity. *Nature Biotechnol* 2004;22:1268–1274.

3   Role of Microflora in Disease

Salvatore Cucchiara and Marina Aloi

Key Points

- Gut microflora normally live in a symbiotic relationship with the host.
- The relationship between indigenous gut microbes and their hosts can shift from commensalism toward pathogenicity in certain diseases.
- In the animal models there is no intestinal inflammation or it is extremely attenuated in axenic animals.
- Several observations implicate intestinal bacteria in the pathogenesis of inflammatory bowel disease (IBD).
- Recent evidence suggests that altered bacterial–neuromotor interactions could play a role in irritable bowel syndrome (IBS).
- Infants with food allergies have been reported to have a disturbed balance between beneficial and potentially harmful bacteria in the intestine.

Key Words: Gut, microflora, overgrowth, inflammatory bowel disease, irritable bowel syndrome.

INTRODUCTION

The gut microflora, which is mainly anaerobic and localized in the colon, comprises about 10^{14} microorganisms, corresponding to more than ten times the number of the body's own cells. This inner biomass accounts for >1000 bacterial species [1,2], living in terms of symbiotic, commensal, and pathogenic relationship with the host. The former refers to a relationship between two different species where at least one partner benefits without harming the other. The term "commensal" comes from the Latin "commensalis," meaning "at table together" and generally refers to partners that coexist without detriment but without obvious benefit. Finally, a pathogenic relationship results in damage to the host.

This complex bacterial community includes native species, mainly acquired during the first year of life, that permanently colonize the tract, and a variable set of living microorganisms that transit temporarily through the gastrointestinal tract and are continuously ingested from the external environment (food, drinks, etc.) [3]. The composition

From: *Nutrition and Health: Probiotics in Pediatric Medicine*
Edited by: S. Michail and P.M. Sherman © Humana Press, Totowa, NJ

of the enteric microbiota varies along the length of the gut with a concentration increasing from the stomach to the colon and, after the first years of life, is individual but stable in humans.

Symbiotic relationship between gut bacteria and host is established during the first 2–3 years of life, with human babies being sterile before birth. Primary colonization is orderly, aerobic species predominating first, followed by anaerobic species, with the timing and composition of the microbial successions being influenced both by the mother (vaginal vs caesarean delivery, breast vs bottle fed, and genetic factors) and the environment (hygiene).

Commensal bacteria exerts several metabolic functions leading to saving of energy and absorbable nutrients, trophic effects on the intestinal epithelia, promotion of gut maturation and integrity, maintenance of intestinal immune homeostasis and defence against pathogenic bacteria [4]. In particular, in this context, microflora plays a crucial role in postnatal development of the immune system. During the early postnatal period, intestinal gut bacteria stimulates the development of both local and systemic immunity; later on, these components evoke, on the contrary, regulatory (inhibitory) mechanisms intended to keep both mucosal and systemic immunity in balance [5,6].

Alterations in normal intestinal microflora and its activities are now thought to be critical factors contributing to many chronic gastrointestinal and extraintestinal diseases. Indeed inflammatory bowel disease (IBD), irritable bowel syndrome (IBS), atopic dermatitis, rheumatoid arthritis, and ankylosing spondylitis have been linked to alterations of gut microbiota.

Aim of this chapter is to review the current evidences about the role of gut microflora in the pathophysiology of these diseases, focusing on IBD, IBS, and atopic dermatitis.

IBD, which includes ulcerative colitis and Crohn's disease, has an incidence in pediatric subjects in Western countries of approximately 10 new cases per 100,000 people per year. Although the etiology of IBD is unclear, the most widely held hypothesis about the pathogenesis is that these diseases are the outcome of four essential interactive cofactors: host susceptibility, enteric microflora, mucosal immunity, and environmental factors. The mucosal immune system is required to sense and interpret the local microenvironment, recognize and avoid reacting to commensal flora (tolerance), yet retain the capacity to respond to episodic challenge from pathogens [7]. In IBD, in a susceptible individual, an "inappropriate" activation of the mucosal immune system occurs. This abnormal activation has been linked to a loss of tolerance to gut commensals [8,9].

Several observations implicate intestinal bacteria in the pathogenesis of ulcerative colitis and Crohn's disease [10]. First, the incidence of inflammation in the case of these disorders is greatest in the area with the highest concentrations of luminal bacteria. Second, the continuity of the fecal stream has been implicated in disease activity, and interruption of this stream is associated with disease improvement in the distal areas. Third, intestinal inflammation and mucosal ulceration can be induced by direct instillation of fecal contents from an inflamed gut into a noninflamed gut of susceptible individuals [11]. The most compelling evidence about the importance of gut microbiota in the IBD pathogenesis is derived from animal models. Despite a great diversity in genetic defects and immunopathology, a consistent feature is the dependency on the presence of normal enteric flora for a full expression of disease. Most animal models of colitis depend on the presence of the bacterial microflora in the gut lumen [12]. A "hyperreactivity" to normal gut microflora has been observed in several animal models with different underlying genetic defects (IL-2, IL-10, or Gia1 deficiency) that led to abnormal responses of T-cell effector or Treg [13]. Intriguingly, gut inflammation did not occur if the mouse was maintained in a strictly germ-free milieu. Hence, it was apparent that normal gut commensals could drive mucosal inflammation in these mouse models and, to the extent that these models mimic human IBD, they also drive mucosal inflammation in human disease. What is not clear is whether the inflammatory process in IBD is elicited in response to a specific subset of intestinal bacteria. To date, no specific bacterial agent has been identified as potential factor triggering intestinal inflammation, although the involvement of pathogenic bacteria cannot be excluded.

An altered balance of beneficial versus aggressive microbial species (dysbiosis) could lead to a pro inflammatory luminal environment that drives chronic intestinal inflammation in a susceptible host. Numerous studies have implicated several commensal organisms, such as *Escherichia coli*, *Bacteroides*, *Enterococcus*, and *Klebsiella* species, in the pathogenesis of experimental intestinal inflammation and human IBD [14]. By contrast, various *Lactobacillus* and *Bifidobacterium* species have been thought to have protective effects and have been used therapeutically as probiotics [15].

Many studies have shown that bacterial flora differ between patients with IBD and healthy people [16–20]. Patients with IBD have higher amounts of bacteria attached to their intestinal epithelial surface, even in the noninflamed mucosa, than healthy controls [21,22]. Using conventional culture techniques, Swidsinski et al. demonstrated thick layers of adherent mucosal-associated bacteria in biopsy specimens obtained from patients with IBD, in comparison with specimens from healthy controls. Higher bacterial concentrations were found in Crohn's disease subjects [21]. However, noninflamed areas were associated with a higher amount of adherent bacteria than was inflamed mucosa, contradicting the hypothesis that microbial pathogens are directly responsible for local lesions in IBD. In another study, Darfeuille-Michaud et al. reported increased numbers of mucosa-associated bacteria in IBD [23]: in this study, a pathogen-like invasive *E. coli* (as defined by in vitro studies) was associated with the mucosa of 20–40% of ileal biopsy specimens from Crohn's disease patients as compared with the mucosa of 6% of specimens derived from controls.

Recently, Conte et al. demonstrated a higher number of mucosa-associated aerobic and facultative-anaerobic bacteria in biopsy specimen of children with IBD than in controls. Moreover, the authors found an overall decrease in some bacterial species belonging to the normal anaerobic intestinal microflora; in particular, occurrence of *Bacteroides vulgatus* was markedly lower in Crohn's disease, ulcerative colitis, and indeterminate colitis than in healthy controls, suggesting that *B. vulgatus* may have a protective role [24].

Experimental evidence indicates that loss of tolerance to commensal bacteria can be underlined by different factors, such as abnormal mucosal T-cell effector population that overreacts to usual microbial antigens or, alternatively, by a defective mucosal Treg cell population such that even normal effector T-cells are not properly modulated, and by an excessive stimulation of mucosal dendritic cells and changes in the receptor pattern (the role of the NOD2/CARD15 Crohn's disease susceptibility gene in bacterial peptidoglycan recognition strengthens the links between gut bacteria and mucosal inflammation) [25,26].

Previous studies in IBD patients demonstrated that cells derived from inflamed intestinal IBD tissue showed strong stimulation when cultured with sonicates of autologous or heterologous gut microflora, whereas cells from normal subjects responded only to sonicates of heterologous microflora [8]. These data suggested that IBD patients lack tolerance to antigens of autologous microflora. However, these observations might be the result of an altered epithelium leading to increased exposure to autologous microflora and hence increased reactivity.

The hygiene hypothesis [27] offers an alternative explanation for the increased incidence of IBD, asthma, and autoimmune disorders such as rheumatoid arthritis and type I diabetes in Western society. This theory suggests that increases in chronic inflammatory disorders in developed countries are partly attributable to diminishing exposure to organisms that are part of the mammalian evolutionary history. This decreased exposure was traditionally thought to promote an exaggerated immunological response based on a prevailing Th2 profile. However, this would not account for the reported increased incidence of Th1 immunomediated disorders in the same countries. The recently described "old friend" hypothesis [28] suggests that crucial organisms, including helminths and saprophytic mycobacteria, are viewed by the innate immune system as harmless or as organisms, that once established must be tolerated. This recognition then triggers development of Treg or dendritic cells that drive regulatory T cell responses to the "old friends" themselves and to simultaneously "forbidden" antigens of the chronic inflammatory disorders.

In normal conditions, gut microbiota exert a key role on the development of gut neuromotor function. The relationship bacteria-motility is bidirectional, since gut motor function controls the growth of intestinal microflora by the physiological removal of exceeding microorganisms. There is evidence suggesting that altered bacterial–neuromotor interactions could play a role in motor and sensory gastrointestinal disorders, including IBS [29].

Physiological studies showed that germ-free animals exhibit profound altered motility patterns that are normalized upon reconstitution with normal flora [30]. Interestingly, the influence of the intestinal microbiota on small intestine myoelectric activity was species dependent [31]. In vivo functional recordings in animals have shown that intestinal microbiota promotes distal propagation [32,33] and cyclic recurrence of interdigestive motor complexes (MMCs) [34]. In particular, the effect of *Lactobacillus acidophilus* and *Bifidobacterium bifidum* in the promotion and aboral migration of MMCs along with acceleration of small intestinal transit has been established [33]. On the other hand, *Micrococcus luteus* and *E. coli* showed an inhibitory action.

The precise mechanism through which the intestinal microbiota modulates this variety of gastrointestinal functions remains unknown. Under normal conditions, bacteria interact with the gastrointestinal tract through receptors on the epithelial cells such as toll-like and NOD receptors, and bacterial passage of viable bacteria to mesenteric lymph nodes (translocation) or other organs is minimal [35]. However, secreted products of bacteria normally gain access to the submucosa to stimulate the mucosal immune system. Moreover, even in healthy subjects, passage of bacteria to the submucosa occurs periodically without consequences for the individual, because bactericidal mechanisms are in place [36]. Though, this penetration may be sufficient to induce changes in intestinal immunity and physiology that are independent of bacterial interaction with the epithelial cell. *B. thethaiotaomicron*, a common gut commensal in mice and humans, was recently found to alter expression of genes involved in smooth-muscle function and neurotransmission [35]. To what extent this altered gene expression can affect intestinal function, and its precise pathway, remains unclear.

Several observations have direct attention toward the gastrointestinal microflora in patients with IBS, although the influence of gut bacteria in the IBS pathophysiology has not been clearly elucidated. IBS is a common gastrointestinal disorder. Typical symptoms reported are abdominal pain, flatulence, and irregular bowel movements. Studies indicate that 10–20% of the general population have these symptoms [37], corresponding to about 25–50% of all patients who visit a gastroenterologist's clinic [38]. Despite the frequency of the condition, the etiology is largely unknown. Etiological considerations range from psychosomatic factors, altered gastrointestinal motility, visceral hypersensitivity, or even abnormal illness behavior [39]. Recently, attention has been directed to the supposed role of low grade mucosal inflammation, on the basis of evidence showing that some patients with IBS have an increased number of inflammatory cells in the colonic and ileal mucosa [40]. Previous episodes of infectious enteritis, undiagnosed food allergies, and changes in enteric microflora may all play a role in promoting and perpetuating this low grade inflammatory process.

Common risk factors associated with the onset of symptoms of IBS include a recent course of antibiotics [41,42] and a previous episode of gastroenteritis [43]. Prospective studies of cohorts with proven bacterial gastroenteritis have demonstrated the persistence of gastrointestinal symptoms in 25–30% of patients 6–12 months following the initial infection [43,44], a 12-fold relative risk in comparison to those without such a history [45]. Both antibiotics and gastrointestinal infections have the potential to alter the gut flora [46]. Data on intestinal microbiota abnormalities have been obtained by comparing the fecal bacterial population of IBS patients and healthy controls [47] and by the analysis of bowel fermentation patterns [48,49]. It has been suggested that differences in the intestinal microflora between healthy subjects and patients with IBS may underlie symptom generation by promoting abnormal colonic fermentation [50]. The gut flora in IBS appears to differ from that in asymptomatic individuals, with an increase in anaerobes, *E. coli* and *Bacteroides* in the colonic mucosa of IBS patients in comparison to healthy individuals and a reduction in *Bifidobacterium* spp. [51]. Long-term follow-up of the flora in IBS patients suggests that the flora is unstable, with alteration in the rank order of species in contrast to healthy subjects [52]. Many IBS patients report exacerbation of symptoms by specific foods, and restrictive diets avoiding such foods may lead to improvement of their symptoms [53,54]. Exposure to intolerant foods results in changes in the gut flora and an increase in bacterial metabolic activity as demonstrated by increased production of short-chain fatty acids [54].

Recent studies suggest that small intestinal bacterial overgrowth (SIBO) may be an underlying factor in a subgroup of patients with IBS [55]. Pimentel et al. using a lactulose hydrogen breath test (LHBT) to detect indirectly quantitative changes in intestinal microbiota, found that 78% of the 202 community-referred IBS patients had a positive LHBT suggestive of SIBO [56]. Furthermore, qualitative changes in intestinal gas production were associated with different IBS symptom presentation. Methane production during LHBT was consistently associated with the predominant constipation subgroup of IBS patients [57], and this subgroup of patients showed decreased postprandial serotonin levels in comparison to patients with a predominant hydrogen production [58].

Some studies have been conducted targeting changes in intestinal microflora using different medical approaches, like probiotics and antibiotics. Randomized, placebo-controlled trials assessing the role of probiotics in IBS have produced controversial results [59–66]. Some of these studies showed beneficial effects, including improvement in global symptom scores [59,61,65] or in single symptoms such as abdominal pain [61,62], flatulence [62], and bloating [60]. Although encouraging, these results should be considered with caution given the small number of patients treated and the contradictory results found.

Recent studies have suggested that enteric flora may play a role in the initiation and perpetuation of allergic inflammation. Infants with food allergies have been reported to have a disturbed balance between beneficial and potentially harmful bacteria in the large intestine [67,68]. Differences in intestinal microbiota composition have been shown between infants in countries with high (Sweden) and low (Estonia) allergy prevalence and also between allergic and healthy infants [67]. Most reports were based on small populations and although the majority of observational studies found an association between the gut microbiota and allergy, no protective or potentially harmful bacteria have yet been identified [69]. Indeed, data suggest that an aberrant microbial composition in the gut such as inadequate bifidobacterial biota may deprive the developing immune system from counter-regulatory signals against T helper 2 mediated allergic responses [70,71] Conversely, by triggering inflammatory responses or by toxin formation, some bacteria may increase gut permeability and thus exposure to potential allergens [72,73]. Of the predominant bacterial groups in infancy, some strains of *E. coli*, *Bacteroides*, and clostridia seem to have such properties [74,75].

Bifidobacterial supplementation alleviates atopic eczema [76]. A similar effect may also contribute to the protective effect of exclusive breast in infants at high risk for allergic disease [77]; the gut flora of breast-fed neonates is essentially dominated by *Bifidobacteria*, while formula fed infants exhibit a more complex flora with relatively high numbers of *Bacteroides* and *E. coli* [78].

A prospective clinical study demonstrated that differences in neonatal gut microflora preceded the development of skin prick test reactivity to dietary and environmental antigens. Neonates who later developed skin prick test reactivity had higher counts of clostridia and lower counts of bifidobacteria in their fecal samples as analyzed by fluorescence in-situ hybridization [70]. These data suggest that an imbalance in the gut flora and differences in the indigenous intestinal flora might affect the development and priming of the immune system in early childhood. This in turn could affect the risk for allergy. The fact that differences in the endogenous microflora are present before any clinically manifest disease [79] seems to indicate that they are not secondary phenomena. In two recent prospective studies, less bifidobacteria were detected during the first weeks of life in babies who developed allergy during infancy [69,78]. Furthermore, colonization intensity during the first week of life was lower in babies who developed allergy during the first year of life [79]. A randomised placebo-controlled trial in 159 high-risk children demonstrated that perinatal administration of intestinal probiotic bacteria *Lactobacillus* GG halved the later development of atopic eczema during the first 2 years of life [80]. Moreover, specific probiotic strains have successfully been used in the treatment of infants suffering from atopic eczema and cow's milk allergy [81,82].

Penders et al. found an association between *C. difficile* and *E. coli* and atopic manifestations (83). The consistent findings of a positive association between *C. difficile* and atopic features strengthen the probability of a causal relationship between gut microbiota and atopy, and support the potential role of probiotics in the prevention and therapy of these disease.

In conclusion, there is a delicate balance in which intestinal microbiota interact with host tissues to determine intestinal and extraintestinal physiological functions in normal conditions. Factors that perturb this equilibrium can promote abnormal dysfunction and are likely to be involved in symptom generation in IBD, IBS, and allergy. Although quantitative differences in the intestinal microbiota are demonstrated in these diseases as compared to healthy subjects, it is still unclear whether a causal relationship exists. The hypothesis that a disruption of the intestinal microbiota may be involved in these disorders suggests that a restoration of this equilibrium (pharmacobiotics) may be of therapeutic benefit.

SUMMARY AND CONCLUSION

The gut microflora includes native species, that permanently colonise the tract, and a variable set of living microorganisms that transit temporarily through the gastrointestinal tract. Alterations in normal microbiota and its activities are now thought to be critical factors contributing to many chronic gastrointestinal and extraintestinal diseases, for instance IBD, IBS, and atopic dermatitis. Most animal models of colitis depend on the presence of the bacterial microflora in the gut lumen. An altered balance of beneficial versus aggressive microbial species (dysbiosis) could lead to a pro inflammatory luminal environment that drives chronic intestinal inflammation in a susceptible host. Numerous studies have implicated several commensal organisms, such as *E. coli*, *Bacteroides*, *Enterococcus*, and *Klebsiella* species, in the pathogenesis of IBD. Altered bacterial–neuromotor interactions could play a role in motor and sensory gastrointestinal disorders, including IBS. The gut flora in IBS appears to differ from that in asymptomatic individuals, with an increase in anaerobes, *E. coli* and *Bacteroides* in the colonic mucosa of IBS patients and a reduction in *Bifidobacterium* spp. Infants with food allergies have been reported to have a disturbed balance between beneficial and potentially harmful bacteria in the large intestine. An imbalance in the gut flora and differences in the indigenous intestinal flora might affect the development and priming of the immune system in early childhood. This in turn could affect the risk for allergy. The hypothesis that a disruption of the intestinal microbiota may be involved in these disorders suggests that a restoration of this equilibrium may be of therapeutic benefit.

REFERENCES

1. Sonnemburg JL, Angenent LT, Gordon JI. Getting a grip on things: How do communities of bacterial symbionts become established in our intestine? *Nat Immunol* 2004;5:569–73.
2. Xu J, Gordon JI. Inaugural article: honor thy symbionts. *Prod Natl Acad Sci USA* 2003;100:1042–9.
3. Guarner F. Enteric flora in health and disease. *Digestion* 2006;73(Suppl. 1):5–12.
4. Hooper LV, Gordon JI. Commensal host–bacterial relationships in the gut. *Science* 2001;292:1115–18.

5. Tlaskalova-Hogenova H, Tuckova L, Lodinova-Zadnikova R, Stepankova R, Cukrowska B, Funda DP, Striz I, Kozakova H, Trebichavsky I, Sokol D, Rehakova Z, Sinkora J, Fundova P, Horakova D, Jelinkova L, Sanchez D. Mucosal immunity: its role in defense and allergy. *Int Arch Allergy Immunol* 2002;128(2):77–89.

6. Tlaskalova-Hogenova H, Stepankova R, Hudcovic T, Tuckova L, Cukrowska B, Lodinova-Zadnikova R, Kozakova H, Rossmann P, Bartova J, Sokol D, Funda DP, Borovska D, Rehakova Z, Sinkora J, Hofman J, Drastich P, Kokesova A. Commensal bacteria (normal microflora), mucosal immunity and chronic inflammatory and autoimmune diseases. *Immunol Lett* 2004;93(2–3):97–108.

7. Shanahan F. Inflammatory bowel disease: immunodiagnostics, immunotherapeutics, and ecotherapeutics. *Gastroenterology* 2001;120(3):622–35.

8. Duchmann R, Kaiser I, Hermann E, Mayet W, Ewe K, Meyer zum Buschenfelde KH. Tolerance exists towards resident intestinal flora but is broken in active inflammatory bowel disease (IBD). *Clin Exp Immunol* 1995;102(3):448–55.

9. MacPherson A, Khoo UY, Forgacs I, Philpott-Howard J, Bjarnason I. Mucosal antibodies in inflammatory bowel disease are directed against intestinal bacteria. *Gut* 1996;38(3):365–75.

10. Shanahan F. Probiotics in inflamatory bowel disease. *Gut* 2001;48(5):609.

11. Fedorak RN, Madsen KL, Probiotics and the management of inflammatory bowel disease. *Inflamm Bowel Dis* 2004;10(3):286–99.

12. Balfour Sartor R. Mechanism of disease: pathogenesis of Crohn's disease and ulcerative colitis. *Nat Clin Pract Gastroenterol Hepatol* 2006 July;3(7):390–407.

13. Strober W, Fuss IJ, Blumberg RS. The immunology of mucosal models of inflammation. *Ann Rev Immunol* 2002;20:495–549.

14. French N, Pettersson S. Microbe-host interactions in the alimentary tract: the gateway to understanding inflammatory bowel disease. *Gut* 2000;47:162–163.

15. Sartor RB. Microbial influences in inflammatory bowel disease: Role in pathogenesis and clinical implications. In: Kirsner's Inflammatory Bowel Diseases. Eds. Sartor RB and Sandborn WJ. Philadelphia: Elsevier, 2004:138–162.

16. Shanahan F. The host-microbe interface within the gut. *Best Pract Res Clin Gastroenterol* 2002;16:915–31.

17. Guarner F, Malagelada JR. Gut flora in health and disease. *Lancet* 2003;361:512–19.

18. Marteau P, Lepage P, Mangin I, et al. Gut flora and inflammatory bowel disease. *Aliment Pharmacol Ther* 2004;20:18–23.

19. Boudeau J, Glasser AL, Masseret E, et al. Invasive ability of an *Escherichia coli* strain isolated from the ileal mucosa of a patient with Crohn's disease. *Infect Immun* 1999;67:4499–509.

20. Boudeau J, Barnich N, Darfeuille-Michaud A. Type 1 pili-mediated adherence of *Escherichia coli* strain LF82 isolated from Crohn's disease is involved in bacterial invasion of intestinal epithelial cells. *Mol Microbiol* 2001;39:1272–8.

21. Swidsinski A, Ladhoff A, Pernthaler A, et al. Mucosal flora in inflammatory bowel disease. *Gastroenterology* 2002;122:44–54.

22. Schultz C, Van Den Berg FM, Ten Kate FW, et al. The intestinal mucus layer from patients with inflammatory bowel disease harbours high numbers of bacteria compared with controls. *Gastroenterology* 1999;117:1089–97.

23. Darfeuille-Michaud A, Neut C, Barnich N, Lederman E, Di Martino P, Desreumaux P, Gambiez L, Joly B, Cortot A, Colombel JF. Presence of adherent *Escherichia coli* strains in ileal mucosa of patients with Crohn's disease. *Gastroenterology* 1998;115:1405–1413.

24. Conte MP, Schippa S, Zamboni I, Penta M, Chiarini F, Seganti L, Osborn J, Falconieri P, Borrelli O, Cucchiara S. Gut-associated bacterial microbiota in paediatric patients with inflammatory bowel disease. *Gut* 2006;55(12):1760–7.

25. Furrie E, Macfarlane S, Cummings JH, et al. Systemic antibodies towards mucosal bacteria in ulcerative colitis and Crohn's disease differentially activate the innate immune response. *Gut* 2004;53:91–8.

26. Tamboli CP, Neut C, Desreumaux P, Colombel JF. Dysbiosis in inflammatory bowel disease. *Gut* 2004;53(1):1–4.

27. Strachan DP. Hay fever, hygiene, and household size. *BMJ* 1989;299:1259–60.

28. Rook GA, Brunet LR. Microbes, immunoregulation, and the gut. *Gut* 2005;54(3):317–20.

29. Barbara G, Stanghellini V, Brandi G, Cremon C, Di Nardo G, De Giorgio R, Corinaldesi R. Interactions between commensal bacteria and gut sensorimotor function in health and disease. *Am J Gastroenterol* 2005;100:2560–8.

30. Caenepeel P, Janssens J, Vantrappen G et al. Interdigestive myoelectric complex in germ-free rats. *Dig Dis Sci* 1989;34:1180–1184.

31. Husebye E, Hellstrom PM, Sundler F et al. Influence of microbial species on small intestinal myoelectric activity and transit in germ-free rats. *Am J Physiol Gastrointest Liver Physiol* 2001;280:G368–80.

32. Husebye E, Hellstrom PM, Midtvedt T. Introduction of conventional microbial flora to germfree rats increases the frequency of migrating myoelectric complexes. *J Gastrointest Mot* 1992;4:39–45.

33. Husebye E, Hellstrom PM, Midtvedt T. Intestinal microflora stimulates myoelectric activity of rat small intestine by promoting cyclic initiation and aboral propagation of migrating myoelectric complex. *Dig Dis Sci* 1994;39:946–56.

34. Caenepeel P, Janssens J, Vantrappen G, et al. Interdigestive myoelectric complex in germ-free rats. *Dig Dis Sci* 1989;34:1180–4.

35. Berg RD. Bacterial translocation from the gastrointestinal tract. *Adv Experi Med Biol* 1999; 473:11–30.

36. McPherson AJ. Immune regulation of the normal intestinal bacterial flora. The host response to the normal intestinal flora. In: Gut ecology, Uhr T, Ed., 2002.

37. Talley NJ, Zinsmeister AR, Van Dyke C, et al. Epidemiology of colonic symptoms and the irritable bowel syndrome. *Gastroenterology* 1991;101:927–34.

38. Everhart JE, Renault PF. Irritable bowel syndrome in office-based practice in the United States. *Gastroenterology* 1991;100:998–1005.

39. Quigley EMM. Current concepts of the irritable bowel syndrome. *Scand J Gastroenterol* 2003;38(Suppl. 237):1–8.

40. Jones J, Boorman J, Cann P, et al. British Society of Gastroenterology guidelines for the management of the irritable bowel syndrome. *Gut* 2000; 47(Suppl. 2):1–19.

41. Jones AV, Wilson AJ, Hunter JO, Robinson RE. The aetiological role of antibiotic prophylaxis with hysterectomy in irritable bowel syndrome. *J Obstet Gynaecol* 1984;5:522–523.

42. Maxwell PR, Rink E, Kumar D, Mendall MA. Antibiotics increase functional abdominal symptoms. *Am J Gastro* 2002;97:104–108.

43. McKendrick MW, Read NW. Irritable bowel syndrome: post *Salmonella* infection. *J Infect* 1994;29:1–3.

44. Neal KR, Hebden J, Spiller R. Prevalence of gastrointestinal symptoms six months after bacterial gastroenteritis and risk factors for development of the irritable bowel syndrome: postal survey of patients. *BMJ* 1997;314:779–782.

45. Garcya C, Rodryguez LA, Ruigomez A. Increased risk of irritable bowel syndrome after bacterial gastroenteritis: cohort study. *BMJ* 1999;318:565–66.

46. Dear KL, Elia M, Hunter JO. *Do interventions which reduce colonic bacterial fermentation improve symptoms of irritable bowel syndrome? Dig Dis Sci* 2005;50(4):758–66.

47. Balsari A, Ceccareli A, Dubini F, et al. The fecal microbial population in the irritable bowel syndrome. *Microbiologica* 1982;5:185–94.

48. King TS, Elia M, Hunter JO. Abnormal colonic fermentation in the irritable bowel syndrome. *Lancet* 1998;352:1187–9.

49. Treem W, Ahsan N, Kastoff G, et al. Fecal short-chain fatty acids in patients with diarrhea-predominant irritable bowel syndrome: in vitro studies of carbohydrate fermentation. *J Ped Gastroent Nutr* 1996;23:280–6.

50. Drossman DA, Sandler RS, McKee DC, Lovitz AJ. Bowel patterns among subjects not seeking health care: use of a questionnaire to identify a population with bowel dysfunction. *Gastroenterology* 1982;83:529–34.

51. Swidsinski A, Khilkin M, Ortner M, et al. Alteration of bacterial concentration in colonic biopsies from patients with irritable bowel syndrome (IBS). *Gastroenterology* 1999;116:A1.

52. Bradley HK, Wyatt GM, Bayliss CE, Hunter JO. Instability of the faecal flora of a patient suffering from food-related irritable bowel syndrome. *J Med Microbiol* 1987;23:29–32.

53. Nanda R, James R, Smith H, Dudley CRK, Jewell DP. Food intolerance and the irritable bowel syndrome. *Gut* 1989;30:1099–1104.

54. Wyatt GM, Bayliss CE, Lakey AF, Bradley HK, Hunter JO, Alun-Jones V. The faecal flora of two patients with food intolerant irritable bowel syndrome during challenge with symptom-provoking foods. *J Med Micobiol* 26:295–299.

55. Lin HC. Small intestinal bacterial overgrowth: a frame-work for understanding irritable bowel syndrome. *JAMA* 2004;292:852–8.

56. Pimentel M, Chow EJ, Lin HC. Eradication of small intestinal bacterial overgrowth reduces symptoms of irritable bowel syndrome. *Am J Gastroenterol* 2000;95:3503–6.

57. Pimentel M, Mayer AG, Park S, et al. Methane production during lactulose breath test is associated with gastrointestinal disease presentation. *Dig Dis Sci* 2003;48:86–92.

58. Pimentel M, Kong Y, Park S. IBS subjects with methane on lactulose breath test have lower postprandial serotonin levels than subjects with hydrogen. *Dig Dis Sci* 2004;49:84–7.

59. Halpern GM, Prindiville T, Blankenburg M, et al. Treatment of irritable bowel syndrome with Lacteol Fort: a randomized, double-blind, cross-over trial. *Am J Gastroenterol* 1996;91:1579–85.

60. Kim HJ, Camilleri M, McKinzie S, et al. A randomized controlled trial of a probiotic, VSL#3, on gut transit and symptoms in diarrhoea-predominant irritable bowel syndrome. *Aliment Pharmacol Ther* 2003;17:895–904.

61. Niedzielin K, Kordecki H, Birkenfeld B. A controlled, double-blind, randomized study on the efficacy of *Lactobacillus plantarum* 299V in patients with irritable bowel syndrome. *Eur J Gastroenterol Hepatol* 2001;13:1143–7.

62. Nobaek S, Johansson ML, Molin G, et al. Alteration of intestinal microflora is associated with reduction in abdominal bloating and pain in patients with irritable bowel syndrome. *Am J Gastroenterol* 2000;95:1231–8.

63. O'Sullivan MA, O'Morain CA. Bacterial supplementation in the irritable bowel syndrome. A randomised double blind placebo-controlled crossover study. *Dig Liver Dis* 2000;32:294–301.

64. Sen S, Mullan MM, Parker TJ, et al. Effect of *Lactobacillus plantarum* 299v on colonic fermentation and symptoms of irritable bowel syndrome. *Dig Dis Sci* 2002;47:2615–20.

65. O'Mahony L, McCarthy J, Kelly P, et al. *Lactobacillus* and *bifidobacterium* in irritable bowel syndrome: symptom responses and relationship to cytokine profiles. *Gastroenterology* 2005;128:541–51.

66. Bjorksten B, Naaber P, Sepp E, et al. The intestinal microflora in allergic Estonian and Swedish 2-year-old children. *Clin Exp Allergy* 1999;29:342–6.

67. Kalliomäki M, Kirjavainen P, Eerola E, et al. Distinct patterns of neonatal gut microflora in infants developing or not developing atopy. *J Allergy Clin Immunol* 2001;107:129–34.

68. Bjorksten B. Effects of intestinal microflora and the environment on the development of asthma and allergy. *Springer Semin Immunopathol* 2004;25:257–70.

69. Kalliomäki M, Kirjavainen P, Eerola E, et al. Distinct patterns of neonatal gut microflora in infants developing or not developing atopy. *J Allergy Clin Immunol* 2001;107:129–34.

70. Kirjavainen PV, Apostolou E, Arvola T, et al. Characterizing the composition of intestinal microflora as a prospective treatment target in inflant allergic disease. *FEMS Immunol Med Microbiol* 2001;32:1–7.

71. Sudo N, Sawamura S, Tanaka K, et al. The requirement of intestinal bacterial flora for the development of an IgE production system fully susceptible to oral tolerance induction. *J Immunol* 1997;159:1739–45.

72. Hessle C, Andersson B, Wold AE. Gram-positive bacteria are potent inducers of monocytic interleukin-12 (IL-12) while gram-negative bacteria preferentially stimulate IL-10 production. *Infect Immun* 2000;68:3581–6.

73. Deitch EA, Specian RD, Berg RD. Endotoxin-induced bacterial translocation and mucosal permeability: role of xanthine oxidase, complement activation, and macrophage products. *Crit Care Med* 1991;19:785–91.

74. Obiso RJJr, Lyerly DM, Van Tassell RL, et al. Proteolytic activity of the *Bacteroides fragilis* enterotoxin causes fluid secretion and intestinal damage in vivo. *Infect Immun* 1995;63:3820–6.

75. Isolauri E, Arvola T, Sütas Y, et al. Probiotics in the management of atopic eczema. *Clin Exp Allergy* 2000;30:1604–10.

76. Committee on Nutrition. Hypoallergenic infant formulas. *Pediatrics* 2000;106:346–9.

77. Harmsen HJM, Wildeboer-Veloo ACM, Raangs GC, et al. Analysis of intestinal flora development in breast-fed and formula-fed infants by using molecular identification and detection methods. *J Pediatr Gastr Nutr* 2000;30:61–7.

78. Bjorksten B, Sepp E, Julge K, Voor T, Mikelsaar M. Allergy development and the intestinal microflora during the first year of life. *J Allergy Clin Immunol* 2001;108:516.

79. Kalliomaki M, Salminen S, Arvilommi H, et al. Probiotics in the primary prevention of atopic disease: a randomised placebo-controlled trial. *Lancet* 2001;357:1076–79.

80. Majamaa H, Isolauri E. Probiotics: a novel approach in the management of food allergy. *J Allergy Clin Immunol* 1997; 99:179–185.

81. Isolauri E, Arvola T, Sutas Y, et al. Probiotics in the management of atopic eczema. *Clin Exp Allergy* 2000;30:1604–10.

82. Penders J, Thijs C, van der Brandt PA, et al. Gut microbiota composition and development of atopic manifestations in infancy: the KOALA Birth Cohort Study. *Gut* 2007;56:661–7.

4 Probiotics 101

Samuli Rautava and W. Allan Walker

Key Points

- Consumption of probiotics has a long history characterized by wide use, nonspecific claims for therapeutic potential and anecdotal evidence.
- Solid scientific data in reducing the risk or treatment of human disease by specific probiotics has emerged during past decades.
- Our understanding of the mechanisms of specific probiotic effects is expanding.
- Intestinal microbes can be a source of maturational signals to the developing intestine.
- Probiotic bacteria have been observed to have remarkable immunomodulatory functions.

Key Words: Atopic disease, diarrhea, immunology, infant, necrotizing enterocolitis, prevention, probiotics.

INTRODUCTION

Probiotics are live specific microbial cultures which, when consumed in adequate amounts, confer documented health benefits in the form of either reducing the risk or treatment of disease [1,2]. In most countries, probiotics as therapeutic agents are not controlled by legislation comparable to that pertaining to pharmaceuticals. Hence the use of probiotics has become widespread in many countries despite the fact that, with the exception of infectious diarrhea, solid scientific evidence for the use of probiotic interventions in pediatric practice is only emerging. Probiotics are often lamentably considered to fall into the category of "alternative" therapies without clearly defined indications for use or therapeutic effects. All of this notwithstanding, advances in scientific research in the past decade may be considered to have provided proof of concept for specific probiotic interventions in the field of pediatrics and new avenues for probiotic use are likely to emerge as a result of research efforts elucidating the role of indigenous intestinal microbes in health and disease.

Early evidence suggesting efficacy of probiotic interventions to prevent or treat human disease originated from anecdotal accounts of success and pioneering studies

From: *Nutrition and Health: Probiotics in Pediatric Medicine*
Edited by: S. Michail and P.M. Sherman © Humana Press, Totowa, NJ

based on sparse theoretical background. Subsequently, a growing number of rigorously designed and conducted clinical trials have documented the potential of probiotic interventions in prevention and treatment of a variety of disorders afflicting infants and children, including infectious disease (particularly of the gastrointestinal tract), allergic and atopic disorders, and intestinal inflammatory conditions such as neonatal necrotizing enterocolitis (NEC) and inflammatory bowel disease (IBD) [3,4] (Table 4.1). The complexity of the intestinal microbiota and its role in human health and disease have gradually become fully appreciated. Experimental studies using animals devoid of intestinal microbes (germ-free) have revealed the truly symbiotic relationship between these organisms and the mammalian host. In particular, recent research advances highlight the crucial role of microbial stimuli in normal gut development and maturation in infancy but intestinal microbes provide the intestinal immune system with stimuli necessary for maintenance of immune homeostasis also later in life. Epidemiological studies linking gut microbiota composition and certain disorders demonstrate the clinical relevance of this host–microbe crosstalk to human health and disease [4]. The exact mechanisms of host–microbe crosstalk and probiotic effects are gradually being

Table 4.1
Pediatric conditions which potentially may be alleviated or prevented by probiotics

Condition	Currently available evidence
Acute infectious diarrhea	Efficacy in treatment established by several independent meta-analyses of clinical trials; several different strains appear to be beneficial
	A number of studies suggest benefit in prevention of nosocomial spread of infection
Antibiotic-associated diarrhea	Meta-analyses of clinical trials suggest efficacy in prevention; optimal strains not established
NEC	Slightly discrepant data from clinical trials using different probiotic strains and protocols; meta-analysis suggests efficacy
Atopic disease	Three clinical trials with different strains and protocols suggest that probiotic supplementation in early infancy might reduce the risk of atopic eczema in high-risk infants; further studies needed
	Several species appear to have potential to alleviate symptoms of atopic eczema and/or cow's milk allergy in infancy; optimal intervention yet to be determined
IBD	Clinical trials with relatively small numbers of patients suggest benefit in maintaining remission in adults; recent meta-analysis found no evidence of benefit
Viral infections of the respiratory tract	One clinical trial suggesting mild reduction in infections in children in daycare; another trial using different probiotics and protocol found probiotics ineffective in reducing infectious episodes
Dental caries	One clinical trial suggests long-term consumption of probiotic-supplemented milk to reduce caries in children

elucidated by research in microbiology and molecular biology laboratories [5]. The purpose of this chapter is to briefly overview the historical origins and current status of the three pillars (role of intestinal microbes in health and disease, molecular mechanisms of probiotic effects and clinical evidence) of the rationale for the use of probiotics to prevent and treat disease in infants and children.

A BRIEF HISTORY OF PROBIOTICS – FROM ANECDOTES TO SCIENTIFIC EVIDENCE

Louis Pasteur's revolutionary notion that microbes are important causative agents in human disease brought about a celebrated paradigm shift in prevention and treatment of infectious disorders in the form of antiseptic practices, vaccines and later antimicrobial drugs. Pasteur's junior colleague and coworker Elie Metchnikoff later proposed that, in addition to causing disease, certain lactic acid-producing bacteria found in fermented milk products might have health-promoting effects [6]. Inspired by Metchnikoff's theory, the Japanese microbiologist Minoru Shirota was able to isolate and identify a lactic acid-producing microbe, which was capable of surviving in the human digestive tract. A fermented milk drink containing the bacterium, named *Lactobacillus casei* strain s*hirota*, was the first probiotic product to become commercially available in 1935. Specific strains of lactic acid-producing bacteria including lactobacilli and bifidobacteria are the most commonly used and thoroughly investigated probiotic bacteria today (Table 4.2).

According to an anecdote told by Murch [7], Adolf Hitler was one of the first people reported to have benefited from probiotic intervention: Hitler's eczema and irritable bowel symptoms were interpreted to result from imbalance in intestinal microbes and apparently improved as a result of consuming the probiotic *Escherichia coli* Nissle 1917. A few decades later, another probiotic strain of *E. coli* was used in a pioneer clinical trial conducted in Prague [8]. Altogether 640 newborn infants born in a four-month period were administered *E. coli* O83:K24:H31 during the first week of life. The control group consisted of 640 infants born during another four-month period in the same hospital who were not administered probiotics. Based on data obtained from questionnaires filled when the subjects were 10 and 20 years of age, neonatal probiotic intervention reduced the risk of both repeated infections and allergic disease. By present standards, the study design has obvious and severe flaws including lack of randomization and retrospective data collection, but it is to our knowledge the first trial to assess long-term clinical effects of early probiotic supplementation. Interestingly, similar effects, albeit with different probiotic strains and administration protocols, have recently been observed in more rigorously designed prospective clinical trials [9,10].

The term "probiotic" was introduced in 1965 to refer to any organism or substance produced by a microbe, which has a positive effect on intestinal microbial balance [11]. This definition reflects the conception, explicit or implicit, that probiotics exert their health effects via modulating gut microecology. Accumulating data indicate, however, that whilst probiotic supplementation may induce transient changes in the composition of gut microbes, probiotic microbes also have a wide array of direct strain-specific effects on host physiology. Consistently with the demands of evidence-based medicine, the current definition of probiotics has no reference to gut microbes but emphasizes scientifically proven health-promoting effects instead [1,2]. The term "prebiotics" has

Table 4.2
Examples of current probiotics and their potential uses

Probiotic	Potential use
L. rhamnosus GG	Treatment of acute diarrheal disease
	Prevention of antibiotic-associated diarrhea
	Prevention and treatment of atopic eczema
	Prevention of viral respiratory tract infections
	Prevention of dental caries
L. acidophilus	Treatment of acute diarrheal disease
	Prevention of necrotizing enterocolitis
B. lactis	Prevention of acute diarrheal disease
	Prevention of antibiotic-associated diarrhea
	Treatment of atopic eczema
B. infantis	Treatment of acute diarrheal disease
	Prevention of necrotizing enterocolitis
E. coli Nissle 1917	Maintenance of remission in ulcerative colitis
S. boulardii	Treatment of acute diarrheal disease
	Prevention of antibiotic-associated diarrhea
VSL#3	Treatment of IBD
Combination of	Prevention and treatment of pouchitis
L. casei	Alleviation of irritable bowel symptoms
L. plantarum	
L. acidophilus	
L. delbrueckii subsp. bulgaricus	
B. longum	
B. breve	
B. infantis	
Streptococcus salivarius subsp. thermophilus	

been reserved for factors, which selectively promote the growth of intestinal bacteria and thereby may elicit health benefits [12]. The concept of prebiotics originates from breast milk factors such as oligosaccharides, which are known to favor the growth of bifidobacteria in the infant gut. Consequently, typical prebiotics used today are nondigestable food ingredients such as fructo-oligosaccharides, galacto-oligosaccharides or lactulose. When pre- and probiotics are administered in combination, the term synbiotics may be used [13].

INTESTINAL MICROBIOTA IN HEALTH AND DISEASE – PROBIOTICS AS MODULATORS OF GUT MICROECOLOGY

One of the founding principles underlying the concept of probiotic interventions is the notion that disturbances in gut microecology, sometimes referred to as "dysbiosis," might play a causal role in human disease. Initially, human gut microbiota composition was investigated using culture-based methods, but recently advances in molecular biology have widened our perspective through the use of culture-independent techniques [14]. Our current knowledge of intestinal microbiota composition is far from comprehensive but it is clear that the human gut harbors an immensely complex ecosystem with hundreds of bacterial species, a large portion of which are hitherto not identified [15]. Moreover, the composition and quantity of bacteria varies greatly between different parts of the gastrointestinal tract as a function of pH, presence of antimicrobial or digestive molecules and transit time. It has also become evident that whilst the intestinal microbiota in a given individual tends to remain relatively stable after infancy, gut microbiota composition between individuals varies by as much as 70% [16]. Human gut microbiota as a clearly defined entity therefore hardly exists [14] and it is difficult to identify features of healthy intestinal microbial balance disruptions of which might be corrected with probiotics. Nonetheless, exogenous factors such as antimicrobial therapy to treat bacterial infections are known to severely affect gut microecology, e.g., by allowing overgrowth of *Clostridium difficile* or other potentially pathogenic microbes, and result in diarrheal disease. Probiotics such as lactobacilli or *Saccharomyces boulardii* have successfully been used to treat antibiotic-associated diarrhea and, according to a recent meta-analysis, probiotic therapy to manage the condition is efficacious [17,18]. However, it is not clear whether amelioration of symptoms of antibiotic-associated diarrhea by probiotics is achieved chiefly by "balancing gut microecology" or by other, more specific means (e.g., *S. boulardii* reducing responsiveness to *C. difficile* toxin [19]). It is also of note that the therapeutic efficacy of probiotics in pediatric practice is most convincingly demonstrated in prevention and treatment of acute infectious diarrhea and particularly in rotaviral gastroenteritis [20–22], which do not result from "dysbiosis." The mechanisms by which probiotics, such as *Lactobacillus* GG, exert their effects in treating acute diarrheal disease may include enhancement of intestinal mucosal barrier function [23] or inducing mucosal rotavirus-specific IgA-production [24]. Similar mechanisms affecting the mucosal immune system may also explain the observed effects of probiotics in reducing the risk of nosocomial rotavirus infections [25] and even viral infections of the respiratory tract [10], which certainly have little to do with gut microbiota. Retrospectively, it is interesting to note that the first clinical trials assessing the efficacy of probiotics in treatment of acute diarrhea were based on sparse data on mechanisms of action but more on anecdotal evidence of benefit.

Despite the difficulties in defining healthy intestinal microbiota discussed above, there are epidemiological studies indicating differences in gut microbiota composition between individuals with certain intestinal or immune-mediated disorders, such as allergic disease, and healthy controls [26–28]. However, the direction of causality between intestinal microbiota composition and development of disease remains open in these case-control studies. More convincing evidence for the notion that gut microbiota composition plays a causal role in the development of atopic disease is derived from prospective epidemiological studies according to which differences in fecal microbes in infancy precede the development of atopic sensitization or atopic eczema [29,30]. According to these reports, large amounts of clostridia and low numbers of enterococci and bifidobacteria in feces in infancy are associated with subsequent development of atopic disorders. This connection has lead to the hypothesis that interventions aiming to modulate early microbial contacts might prevent the development of atopic disease and, indeed, administration of probiotic lactobacilli in early infancy has shown promising results in reducing the risk of atopic eczema in high-risk infants [31–33]. It is by no means clear, however, that the reduction in morbidity observed in these studies is solely or even predominantly the consequence of altered gut microbiota composition even though there are data indicating that the occurrence of atopic eczema in infancy may also be reduced by prebiotic oligosaccharides which promote the growth of intestinal bifidobacteria [34] and that *Lactobacillus* GG, the probiotic strain used in one of the studies, has bifidogenic effects [35].

INTESTINAL MICROBES AS A SOURCE OF MATURATIONAL SIGNALS TO THE DEVELOPING INTESTINE – A WINDOW OF OPPORTUNITY FOR PROBIOTIC INTERVENTION

In addition to affecting gut microbiota composition, probiotics may have direct effects on infant gut. It is well established that the neonatal intestine and the intestinal immune system in particular are dependent on external stimuli to become fully developed. The establishment of indigenous intestinal microbiota coincides with this maturational process and accumulating experimental data demonstrate that, in addition to breast milk, intestinal microbes provide the developing gut with maturational stimuli. It is therefore plausible that these developmental processes may be susceptible to manipulation by probiotics administered in the postnatal period [4].

Colonization of the sterile neonatal gastrointestinal tract begins with first contact of the extrauterine environment. It is well established that a number of environmental factors, including mode of delivery [36], feeding practices (breast milk versus formula [37]) and treatment with antibiotics and/or in a neonatal intensive care unit [38] may have an impact on early microbial colonization. Moreover, there are data indicating that the differences in intestinal microbiota composition between infants delivered vaginally or by caesarian section are still detectable at one year of age [36]. Disruptions in early colonization have been suggested to play a role in the pathogenesis of NEC in preterm infants [39] and the health benefits of breastfeeding have been partially attributed to the bifidogenic properties of breast milk [40]. As alluded to above, early aberrations in gut colonization have been shown to be associated with subsequent development of atopic eczema [29,30]. Given the immunological basis of the pathogenesis of atopic disease, this may be interpreted to imply a significant link between early colonizers and healthy immune development. Consequently, a hypothesis according to which changes in early microbial exposure resulting from lifestyle in the developed world, such as increasing caesarian sections and antibiotic use in infancy, changing pattern of infectious diseases, decreased importance of fermenting as a means to preserve food etc., may underlie the increase of immune-mediated disorders including atopic and autoimmune diseases has been proposed [14]. This "hygiene hypothesis" was originally devised based on epidemiological findings linking decreased occurrence of infectious diseases in early childhood with increased risk of allergic disease [41,42]. However, this view has subsequently been revised to emphasize the role of gut microbiota in healthy immune maturation [14].

The immunological processes resulting in gut immune maturation and establishment of tolerance toward indigenous microbes are not fully understood but both innate immune recognition mechanisms and adaptive immune responses orchestrated by dendritic cells and T lymphocytes are involved. Studies conducted using experimental animal models suggest that toll-like receptors (TLRs), an evolutionarily conserved family of molecules, which recognize microbe-associated molecular patterns, are involved in recognizing and responding to initial pioneer colonizing bacteria. Initially, TLRs have been implicated in innate immune defense against pathogens, but it appears that they may also have developmental and homeostatic functions. Germ-free rats colonized solely with *Bifidobacterium lactis*, a predominant component of gut microbiota in breastfed infants, have been observed to exhibit a transient and self-limiting TLR2-mediated inflammatory gene expression response in intestinal epithelial cells without evidence of inflammatory tissue damage [43]. In a similar fashion, other TLR ligands present on colonizing bacteria have been observed to initially activate inflammatory responses but subsequent challenges fail to induce inflammation, i.e., tolerance is achieved [44,45]. Interestingly, after initial colonization, TLR ligands present on potential pathogens still induce an inflammatory reaction to prevent and control infection but stimulation by similar ligands on indigenous microbes results in apparent nonresponsiveness. These observations are consistent with the fact that the host is tolerant to its indigenous microbes. Moreover, TLR-stimulation by indigenous microbiota appears to be necessary for maintenance of gut immune homeostasis, as lack of TLR-signaling increases mortality in a murine model of IBD [46].

Given the great variability in gut microbes between individuals alluded to above, it is likely that there is significant redundancy with regard to species and strains of bacteria which provide the host with crucial maturational signals. It is therefore somewhat difficult to conceive how introduction of a probiotic strain might influence the maturational process. Nonetheless, intriguing data from animal models demonstrate that defective morphological and immunological maturation in germ-free animals may be salvaged by colonization by a single bacterial strain. Mice reared in germ-free conditions exhibit impaired ability to establish immune tolerance but colonization with bifidobacteria, a predominant component of gut microbiota in breastfed infants, leads to the establishment of tolerance [47]. It has subsequently been demonstrated that indigenous microbes are involved in tolerance formation via TLR-mediated mechanisms [48]. Germ-free mice colonized with the indigenous microbe *Bacteroides thetaiotaomicron* display an array of changes in the expression of genes involved in intestinal maturation and function [49]. In an elegant series of experiments, Mazmanian et al. showed that monocolonization of germ-free mice with another *Bacteroides* species, *B. fragilis*, is sufficient to restore the defects in immune maturation associated with lack of microbial stimulation and these effects were also achieved by administration of only one specific surface polysaccharide of the bacterium [50]. Even taken into account the caveats in extrapolating data from highly controlled experiments using germ-free animals to human subjects exposed to variable environments, these data showing a wide spectrum of significant effects elicited by specific microbes render the results from clinical trials suggesting clinical benefit of neonatal probiotic interventions in reducing the risk of disorders as diverse as NEC, various infections or atopic disease (reviewed in 4, 51) more intelligible. Proper assessment of intestinal immune maturation in neonates and infants would require invasive methods, which for obvious ethical reasons are generally not acceptable. Clinical investigators are therefore often forced to rely on less-sophisticated immune parameters to assess probiotic effects. Nonetheless, some indications of the probiotic effect, enhancing, e.g., mucosal IgA-production or innate immunity, have been observed [52], whereas other studies have been unable to detect probiotic effects on immune maturation [53].

IMMUNOMODULATORY EFFECTS OF PROBIOTICS – TOWARD SPECIFIC THERAPEUTICS

It is of note that there is no data indicating that probiotics permanently colonize the intestine, even when administered in the neonatal period when gut microbiota is first established. Indeed, administration of *Lactobacillus* GG to neonates induces slight but detectable changes in gut microbiota composition [54] but the probiotic strain itself is not detectable in feces after supplementation is discontinued [55]. It may therefore be argued that perhaps probiotic bacteria are recognized as foreign or exogenous stimuli by the intestinal immune system and thus provoke a more pronounced immune response. This notion would explain the perplexing fact that probiotics induce detectable and significant changes in local and systemic immune parameters when typically administered in daily doses not exceeding the total quantity of microbes in just 1 g of colonic content (10^{10}–10^{11} bacteria/g [15]). An impressive body of scientific evidence for the probiotic effects on various immune functions in vivo and in vitro has emerged during the past decade. In children, probiotics have been observed to stimulate antigen-specific IgA production [53,56] and enhance intestinal mucosal barrier function compromised by atopic predisposition [57]. In addition, administration of probiotics to infants and children has been shown to induce changes in immune parameters such as cytokine secretion patterns (reviewed in 4), which are more difficult to correlate with clinical disorders. These effects may partially explain the beneficial effects observed in clinical trials assessing probiotics in treating pediatric disorders such as food allergy, atopic eczema/dermatitis (Chapter 18), IBD (Chapters 12–14) and acute diarrheal disease (reviewed in detail in Chapters 11–13, and 18).

In experimental studies conducted using animal models or in vitro, probiotic bacteria have been observed to have a remarkable array of immunomodulatory functions such as induction of regulatory T cells involved in induction and maintenance of oral tolerance [58,59] and regulating the function of dendritic cells [60], macrophages [61], lymphocytes [58], and intestinal epithelial cells [63]. In addition, probiotic bacteria may directly inhibit the growth and adherence of certain pathogens [63, 64]. It is paramount to understand that these effects are specific to the strain of probiotics used in the studies and extrapolating to other strains, even closely related, is not appropriate. Indeed, different probiotic strains have been observed to elicit distinct epithelial cell responses [65] and probiotic bacteria with similar properties in vitro may elicit different effects in vivo [66].

These observations have a number of consequences for clinical probiotic research. Firstly, it is important to recognize the limits of experimental studies in recapitulating the complex intestinal ecosystem with host–microbe and microbe–microbe interactions. Secondly, it is highly unlikely that, contrary to what is suggested by some advocates of alternative medicine, one probiotic strain or combination of strains should be ideal for a large number of clinical conditions. Thirdly, one should be cautious in interpreting or devising meta-analyses of clinical trials using different probiotic strains. These challenges highlight the importance of basic research into the mechanisms of strain-specific probiotic effects, which will guide future clinical trials with clearly defined interventions and outcomes.

SUMMARY

A century after the notion that intestinal bacteria might elicit beneficial health effects was introduced, probiotics are emerging as a mainstream therapeutic approach in pediatrics. Reflecting the perplexing complexity of the indigenous intestinal microbiota and its crosstalk with the host, probiotics have an impressive array of strain-specific effects, which may be exploited to therapeutic ends. In early infancy, certain probiotics appear to have the potential to enhance immune maturation and thus prevent the development of immune-mediated diseases. Later in life, probiotics may contribute to maintenance of immune homeostasis and thus be of value to treat disease such as IBD. In addition, some probiotic bacteria have effects on host immunophysiology and direct antipathogenic effects, which may contribute to protection against infectious disease.

Currently, meta-analyses of clinical trials have demonstrated the efficacy of probiotic interventions in management of acute diarrheal disease [20,21] and antibiotic-associated diarrhea [17,18] as well as in prevention of NEC [51]. An accumulating body of evidence indicates potential benefits in reducing the risk and treatment of atopic disease [4]. A number of other immune-mediated disorders ranging from IBD to type I diabetes may also be amenable to probiotic interventions. It is to be hoped that concrete guidelines for probiotic use to prevent and treat specific disorders will be drafted in the near future. Before this can be achieved, however, a number of issues including selecting the optimal probiotic strain (or combination of strains), dose and duration of treatment as well as criteria for patients who are likely to benefit from probiotic intervention and safety issues need to be clarified (Table 4.3). Ideally, multicenter clinical trials using clearly defined specific probiotic intervention protocols based on solid scientific data on molecular mechanisms should be carried out.

Table 4.3
Properties of an ideal probiotic

Preclinical criteria
Adequate microbiological characterization
Ability to remain viable in the gastrointestinal tract
Good adherence properties
Well-characterized specific effects on host physiology in vitro and in vivo
Clinical efficacy
Several high-quality clinical trials suggesting efficacy and/or meta-analysis of trials using same Probiotic
Protocol
Clearly described and clinically significant endpoints
Safety
Supplementation does not result in permanent colonization
Low pathogenicity
Not extensively resistant to commonly used antimicrobial agents
Safety data from clinical trials and/or a long history of use in foods
Guidelines for use
Clearly defined clinical conditions the probiotic is used to treat or prevent
Optimal dose defined
Unambiguous criteria describing subjects who are likely to benefit from probiotic intervention
Timing and duration of intervention well-established

REFERENCES

1. Isolauri E, Rautava S, Kalliomaki M, Kirjavainen P, Salminen S. Role of probiotics in food hypersensitivity. *Curr Opin Allergy Clin Immunol* 2002;2:263–71.

2. Reid G, Sanders ME, Gaskins HR, et al. New scientific paradigms for probiotics and prebiotics. *J Clin Gastroenterol* 2003;37:105–18.

3. Chen CC, Walker WA. Probiotics and prebiotics: role in clinical disease states. *Adv Pediatr* 2005;52:77–113.

4. Rautava S. Potential uses of probiotics in the neonate. *Semin Fetal Neonatal Med* 2007;12:45–53.

5. Kalliomäki MA, Walker WA. Physiologic and pathologic interactions of bacteria with gastrointestinal epithelium. *Gastroenterol Clin North Am* 2005;34:383–99.

6. Metchnikoff E. The prolongation of life: optimistic studies. London: William Heinemann 1907.

7. Murch SH. Probiotics as mainstream allergy therapy? *Arch Dis Child* 2005;90(9):881–2.

8. Lodinova-Zadnikova R, Cukrowska B, Tlaskalova-Hogenova H. Oral administration of probiotic *Escherichia coli* after birth reduces frequency of allergies and repeated infections later in life (after 10 and 20 years). *Int Arch Allergy Immunol* 2003;131:209–11.

9. Kalliomäki M, Salminen S, Poussa T, Isolauri E. Probiotics during the first 7 years of life: a cumulative risk reduction of eczema in a randomized, placebo-controlled trial. *J Allergy Clin Immunol* 2007;119:1019–21.

10. Hatakka K, Savilahti E, Ponka A, et al. Effect of long term consumption of probiotic milk on infections in children attending day care centres: double blind, randomised trial. *BMJ* 2001;322:1327.

11. Lilly DM, Stillwell RH. Probiotics: growth-promoting factors produced by micro-organisms. *Science* 1965;47:747–8.

12. Gibson GR, Roberfroid MB. Dietary modulation of the human colonic microbiota: introducing the concept of prebiotics. *J Nutr* 1995;125:1401–12.

13. Salminen S, Bouley C, Boutron-Ruault MC, Cummings JH, franck A, Gibson GR, Isolauri E, Moreau MC, Roberfroid M, Rowland I. Functional food science and gastrointestinal physiology and function. *Br J Nutr* 1998;80:S147–71.

14. Rautava S, Ruuskanen O, Ouwehand A, Salminen S, Isolauri E. The hygiene hypothesis of atopic disease – an extended version. *J Pediatr Gastroenterol Nutr* 2004;38:378–88.

15. Tannock GW. What immunologists should know about bacterial communities of the human bowel. Semin Immunol 2006.

16. Ley RE, Turnbaugh PJ, Klein S, Gordon JI. Microbial ecology: human gut microbes associated with obesity. *Nature* 2006;444:1022–3.

17. Szajewska H, Ruszczynski M, Radzikowski A. Probiotics in the prevention of antibiotic-associated diarrhea in children: a meta-analysis of randomized controlled trials. *J Pediatr* 2006;149:367–72.

18. McFarland LV. Meta-analysis of probiotics for the prevention of antibiotic associated diarrhea and the treatment of *Clostridium difficile* disease. *Am J Gastroenterol* 2006;101:812–22.

19. Chen X, Kokkotou EG, Mustafa N, Bhaskar KR, Sougioultzis S, O'Brien M, Pothoulakis C, Kelly CP. *Saccharomyces boulardii* inhibits ERK1/2 mitogen-activated protein kinase activation both in vitro and in vivo and protects against *Clostridium difficile* toxin A-induced enteritis. *J Biol Chem* 2006;281:24449–54.

20. Szajewska H, Mrukowicz JZ. Probiotics in the treatment and prevention of acute infectious diarrhea in infants and children: a systematic review of published randomized, double-blind, placebo-controlled trials. *J Pediatr Gastroenterol Nutr* 2001;33:S17–25.

21. Van Niel CW, Feudtne C, Garrison MM, Christakis DA. *Lactobacillus* therapy for acute infectious diarrhea in children: a meta-analysis. *Pediatrics* 2002;109:678–84.

22. Sazawal S, Hiremath G, Dhingra U, Malik P, Deb S, Black RE. Efficacy of probiotics in prevention of acute diarrhoea: a meta-analysis of masked, randomised, placebo-controlled trials. *Lancet Infect Dis* 2006;6:374–82.

23. Isolauri E, Kaila M, Arvola T, Majamaa H, Rantala I, Virtanen E, Arvilommi H. Diet during rotavirus enteritis affects jejunal permeability to macromolecules in suckling rats. *Pediatr Res* 1993;33:548–53.

24. Majamaa H, Isolauri E, Saxelin M, Vesikari T. Lactic acid bacteria in the treatment of acute rotavirus gastroenteritis. *J Pediatr Gastroenterol Nutr* 1995;20:333–9.

25. Szajewska H, Kotowska M, Mrukowicz JZ, Armanska M, Mikolajczyk W. Efficacy of *Lactobacillus* GG in prevention of nosocomial diarrhea in infants. *J Pediatr* 2001;138:361–5.

26. Björkstén B, Naaber P, Sepp E, Mikelsaar M. The intestinal microflora in allergic Estonian and Swedish 2-year-old children. *Clin Exp Allergy* 1999;29:342–6.

27. Ouwehand AC, Isolauri E, He F, Hashimoto H, Benno Y, Salminen S. Differences in *Bifidobacterium flora* composition in allergic and healthy infants. *J Allergy Clin Immunol* 2001;108:144–5.

28. Mah KW, Björkstén B, Lee BW, et al. Distinct pattern of commensal gut microbiota in toddlers with eczema. *Int Arch Allergy Immunol* 2006;140:157–63.

29. Kalliomäki M, Kirjavainen P, Eerola E, Kero P, Salminen S, Isolauri E. Distinct patterns of neonatal gut microflora in infants in whom atopy was and was not developing. *J Allergy Clin Immunol* 2001;107:129–34.

30. Björkstén B, Sepp E, Julge K, Voor T, Mikelsaar M. Allergy development and the intestinal microflora during the first year of life. *J Allergy Clin Immunol* 2001;108:516–20.

31. Kalliomäki M, Salminen S, Arvilommi H, Kero P, Koskinen P, Isolauri E. Probiotics in primary prevention of atopic disease: a randomised placebo-controlled trial. *Lancet* 2001;357:1076–9.

32. Kukkonen K, Savilahti E, Haahtela T, et al. Probiotics and prebiotic galacto-oligosaccharides in the prevention of allergic diseases: a randomized, double-blind, placebo-controlled trial. *J Allergy Clin Immunol* 2007;119:192–8.

33. Abrahamsson TR, Jakobsson T, Bottcher MF, et al. Probiotics in prevention of IgE-associated eczema: a double-blind, randomized, placebo-controlled trial. *J Allergy Clin Immunol* 2007;119:1174–80.

34. Moro G, Arslanoglu S, Stahl B, Jelinek J, Wahn U, Boehm G. A mixture of prebiotic oligosaccharides reduces the incidence of atopic dermatitis during the first six months of age. *Arch Dis Child* 2006;91:814–9.

35. Apostolou E, Pelto L, Kirjavainen PV, Isolauri E, Salminen SJ, Gibson GR. Differences in the gut bacterial flora of healthy and milk-hypersensitive adults, as measured by fluorescence in situ hybridization. *FEMS Immunol Med Microbiol* 2001;30:217–21.

36. Grönlund MM, Lehtonen OP, Eerola E, Kero P. Fecal microflora in healthy infants born by different methods of delivery: permanent changes in intestinal flora after cesarean delivery. *J Pediatr Gastroenterol Nutr* 1999;28:19–25.

37. Harmsen HJ, Wildeboer-Veloo AC, Raangs GC, et al. Analysis of intestinal flora development in breast-fed and formula-fed infants by using molecular identification and detection methods. *J Pediatr Gastroenterol Nutr* 2000;30:61–7.

38. Bennet R, Eriksson M, Nord CE, Zetterstrom R. Fecal bacterial microflora of newborn infants during intensive care management and treatment with five antibiotic regimens. *Pediatr Infect Dis* 1986;5:533–9.

39. Claud EC, Walker WA. Hypothesis: inappropriate colonization of the premature intestine can cause neonatal necrotizing enterocolitis. *FASEB J* 2001;15:1398–403.

40. Newburg DS, Walker WA. Protection of the neonate by the innate immune system of developing gut and of human milk. *Pediatr Res* 2007;61:2–8.

41. Gerrard JW, Geddes CA, Reggin PL, Gerrard CD, Horne S. Serum IgE levels in white and metis communities in Saskatchewan. *Ann Allergy* 1976;37:91–100.

42. Strachan DP. Hay fever, hygiene, and household size. *BMJ* 1989;299:1259–60.

43. Ruiz PA, Hoffmann M, Szcesny S, Blaut M, Haller D. Innate mechanisms for *Bifidobacterium lactis* to activate transient pro-inflammatory host responses in intestinal epithelial cells after the colonization of germ-free rats. *Immunology* 2005;115:441–50.

44. Otte JM, Cario E, Podolsky DK. Mechanisms of cross hyporesponsiveness to toll-like receptor bacterial ligands in intestinal epithelial cells. *Gastroenterology* 2004;126:1054–70.

45. Lee J, Mo JH, Katakura K, et al. Maintenance of colonic homeostasis by distinctive apical TLR9 signalling in intestinal epithelial cells. *Nat Cell Biol* 2006;8:1327–36.

46. Rakoff-Nahoum S, Paglino J, Eslami-Varzaneh F, Edberg S, Medzhitov R. Recognition of commensal microflora by toll-like receptors is required for intestinal homeostasis. *Cell* 2004;118:229–41.

47. Sudo N, Sawamura S, Tanaka K, Aiba Y, Kubo C, Koga Y. The requirement of intestinal bacterial flora for the development of an IgE production system fully susceptible to oral tolerance induction. *J Immunol* 1997;159:1739–45.

48. Bashir ME, Louie S, Shi HN, Nagler-Anderson C. Toll-like receptor 4 signaling by intestinal microbes influences susceptibility to food allergy. *J Immunol* 2004;172:6978–87.

49. Hooper LV, Wong MH, Thelin A, Hansson L, Falk PG, Gordon JI. Molecular analysis of commensal host-microbial relationships in the intestine. *Science* 2001;291:881–4.

50. Mazmanian SK, Liu CH, Tzianabos AO, Kasper DL. An immunomodulatory molecule of symbiotic bacteria directs maturation of the host immune system. *Cell* 2005;122:107–18.

51. Deshpande G, Rao S, Patole S. Probiotics for prevention of necrotising enterocolitis in preterm neonates with very low birthweight: a systematic review of randomised controlled trials. *Lancet* 2007;369:1614–20.

52. Rautava S, Arvilommi H, Isolauri E. Specific probiotics in enhancing maturation of IgA responses in formula-fed infants. *Pediatr Res* 2006;60:221–4.

53. Taylor AL, Hale J, Wiltschut J, Lehmann H, Dunstan JA, Prescott SL. Effects of probiotic supplementation for the first 6 months of life on allergen- and vaccine-specific immune responses. *Clin Exp Allergy* 2006;36:1227–35.

54. Rinne M, Kalliomaki M, Salminen S, Isolauri E. Probiotic intervention in the first months of life: short-term effects on gastrointestinal symptoms and long-term effects on gut microbiota. *J Pediatr Gastroenterol Nutr* 2006;43(2):200–5.

55. Gueimonde M, Kalliomaki M, Isolauri E, Salminen S. *Probiotic intervention in neonates – will permanent colonization ensue? J Pediatr Gastroenterol Nutr* 2006;42(5):604–6.

56. Kaila M, Isolauri E, Soppi E, Virtanen E, Laine S, Arvilommi H. Enhancement of the circulating antibody secreting cell response in human diarrhea by a human *Lactobacillus* strain. *Pediatr Res* 1992;32:141–4.

57. Rosenfeldt V, Benfeldt E, Valerius NH, Paerregaard A, Michaelsen KF. Effect of probiotics on gastrointestinal symptoms and small intestinal permeability in children with atopic dermatitis. *J Pediatr* 2004;145:612–6.

58. von der Weid T, Bulliard C, Schiffrin EJ. Induction by a lactic acid bacterium of a population of CD4(+) T cells with low proliferative capacity that produce transforming growth factor beta and interleukin-10. *Clin Diagn Lab Immunol* 2001;8:695–701.

59. Di Giacinto C, Marinaro M, Sanchez M, Strober W, Boirivant M. Probiotics ameliorate recurrent Th1-mediated murine colitis by inducing IL-10 and IL-10-dependent TGF-beta-bearing regulatory cells. *J Immunol* 2005;174:3237–46.

60. Christensen HR, Frokiaer H, Pestka JJ. Lactobacilli differentially modulate expression of cytokines and maturation surface markers in murine dendritic cells. *J Immunol* 2002;168:171–8.

61. He F, Morita H, Ouwehand AC, Hosoda M, Hiramatsu M, Kurisaki J, Isolauri E, Benno Y, Salminen S. Stimulation of the secretion of pro-inflammatory cytokines by *Bifidobacterium* strains. *Microbiol Immunol* 2002;46:781–5.

62. Broekaert IJ, Nanthakumar NN, Walker WA. Secreted probiotic factors ameliorate enteropathogenic infection in zinc-deficient human Caco-2 and T84 cell lines. *Pediatr Res* 2007;62:139–44.

63. Boudeau J, Glasser AL, Julien S, Colombel JF, Darfeuille-Michaud A. Inhibitory effect of probiotic *Escherichia coli* strain Nissle 1917 on adhesion to and invasion of intestinal epithelial cells by adherent-invasive *E. coli* strains isolated from patients with Crohn's disease. *Aliment Pharmacol Ther* 2003;18:45–56.

64. Resta-Lenert S, Barrett KE. Live probiotics protect intestinal epithelial cells from the effects of infection with enteroinvasive *Escherichia coli* (EIEC). *Gut* 2003;52:988–97.

65. Wallace TD, Bradley S, Buckley ND, Green-Johnson JM. Interactions of lactic acid bacteria with human intestinal epithelial cells: effects on cytokine production. *J Food Prot* 2003;66:466–72.

66. Ibnou-Zekri N, Blum S, Schiffrin EJ, von der Weid T. Divergent patterns of colonization and immune response elicited from two intestinal *Lactobacillus* strains that display similar properties in vitro. *Infect Immun* 2003;71:428–36.

5   Mechanisms of Probiotic Regulation of Host Homeostasis

Fang Yan and D. Brent Polk

Key Points

Probiotics regulate host homeostasis by
- Maintaining the intestinal microenvironment through producing antibacterial substances and competing with pathogens for binding.
- Promoting intestinal epithelial cell survival, barrier function, and cytoprotective responses.
- Defining the balance between necessary and excessive immune defense functions to prevent inflammation.
- Activating signaling pathways in intestinal epithelial and immune cells.

Key Words: Antimicrobial, apoptosis, cytokine, immune responses, intestinal epithelium, mechanism, probiotics, signaling pathway, barrier function, toll-like receptor.

INTRODUCTION

Probiotics were first described as selective nonpathogenic living microorganisms, including commensal bacterial flora, which have beneficial effects on host health and disease prevention and/or treatment.[1] Currently, the Food and Agriculture Organization of the United Nations and World Health Organization define probiotics as "live microorganisms which, when consumed in adequate amounts as part of food, confer a health benefit on the host." Probiotic research is beginning to support the potential value for this approach to human health and disease prevention and/or treatment. Clinical efficacy of probiotics in adults, children, and infants has recently been shown for diseases associated with the gastrointestinal tract including inflammatory bowel diseases, diarrhea, irritable bowel syndrome, gluten intolerance, gastroenteritis, *Helicobacter pylori* infection, colon cancer, urogenital tract disorders, and allergy (reviewed in[2, 4]).

One significant question raised regarding clinical use of probiotics is the mechanism underlying the wide range of actions ascribed to various organisms. Recent studies suggest that probiotics can exert beneficial effects on the host through distinct cellular and

From: *Nutrition and Health: Probiotics in Pediatric Medicine*
Edited by: S. Michail and P.M. Sherman © Humana Press, Totowa, NJ

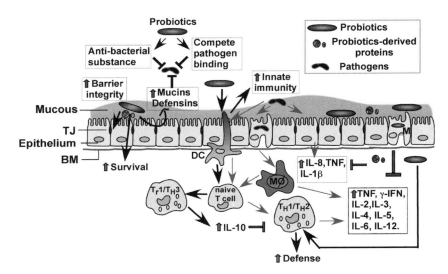

Fig. 5.1. Regulation of host homeostasis by probiotics. Probiotics induce several beneficial host responses. These include producing antibacterial substances, competing with pathogens for binding to epithelial cells, maintaining the intestinal microbial balance, promoting intestinal epithelial cell survival, barrier function, and cytoprotective responses, defining the balance between necessary and excessive defense immunity by increasing innate immunity, up-regulating anti-inflammatory cytokine production, and inhibiting pro-inflammatory cytokine production. BM: basement membrane; DC: dendritic cell; IL: interleukin; M: M-cell; TJ: tight junction.

molecular pathways. These mechanisms of action may vary from one probiotic to another for the same biological response, and may be regulated by a combination of several events, thus making study of the underlying basis of probiotic action a very difficult and complex research area. However, experimental results from basic research including in vitro cell culture experiments and in vivo animal models show that probiotics produce specific enzymes and metabolites that directly regulate host nutritional status and the intestinal microbial environment, and they modulate intestinal epithelial cell or immune cell responses (Fig. 5.1).

This chapter focuses on reviewing significant research findings relevant to the mechanisms by which probiotics promote host homeostasis. Fundamental knowledge of the mechanisms of probiotic action will lead to new hypothesis-driven studies to improve the clinical efficacy of probiotics as alternative treatments for diseases. Furthermore, this chapter will provide clinicians background for conceptualizing a mechanistic-based selection of probiotics for clinical trials.

PROBIOTICS BENEFIT HOST NUTRITION

Probiotic bacteria are widely used as nutritional supplements to improve the digestibility and uptake of some dietary nutrients by some host intestinal cells. For example, bacterial lactase is a well-known enzyme produced by probiotic bacteria, which degrades lactose in the intestine and stomach and prevents symptoms of lactose intolerance. With the development of genomic microarray approaches for transcriptional analysis, many of the molecular and cellular mechanisms whereby bacteria provide metabolic benefits for the host have been revealed. The molecular basis of symbiosis between *Bacteroides thetaiotaomicron* and the host is complex but likely enhanced by the relatively large number of bacterial genes encoding enzymes involved in polysaccharide uptake and degradation and capsular polysaccharide biosynthesis. Interestingly, most of these enzymes capable of breaking down unabsorbed and indigestible dietary and host-derived carbohydrates localize close to the surface layer of the bacterial wall, suggesting this bacterium may use these enzymes for meeting its own energy needs and for regulating the intestinal microenvironment by providing fermentable carbohydrates.[5] This activity represents another layer of complexity to the host–bacterial partnership as it provides an additional source of nutrients for the host and other commensal organisms.

The nutritional benefits that the probiotic bacteria confer on the host extend beyond carbohydrate metabolism. Microarray studies have identified a number of bacteria-regulated genes in intestinal epithelial cells. *B. thetaiotaomicron* colonization increases ileal Na^+/glucose cotransporter, colipase, and apolipoprotein expression.[6] These molecules mediate nutrient absorption and processing in intestinal epithelial cells. Therefore, the molecular mechanisms underlying the nutritional effects of probiotics include both directly metabolizing dietary and host-derived carbohydrates and up-regulating host absorptive capacity.

PROBIOTICS MAINTAIN THE MICROBIAL BALANCE IN THE INTESTINAL TRACT

Establishing normal microbial–host interactions is important for host health. Interruption of these interactions by impaired microbial balance in the gastrointestinal tract may lead to several pathological conditions, such as bacterial overgrowth and increase in the relative numbers of pathogenic bacteria. Probiotics have been proven to exert activity against several pathogens, including pathogenic strains of *Escherichia coli*, *Salmonella*, *Listeria monocytogenes*, *H. pylori*, and rotavirus.[4] At least two mechanisms of action mediate probiotic-induced maintenance of the gastrointestinal microbial balance: production of antibacterial substances and competitive inhibition of pathogen and toxin adherence to the intestinal epithelium.

Probiotic-Derived Antibacterial Substances

Probiotics exert direct antibacterial effects on pathogens through production of anti-bacterial substances, including bacteriocins, acid, and hydrogen peroxide (reviewed in[7]). Studies indicate that these probiotic-derived antibacterial substances exert their effects both alone and synergistically to inhibit the growth of pathogens.

Bacteriocin

Bacteriocins are small antimicrobial peptides produced by *Lactobacilli*. Analysis of the known genomic sequences of *Lactobacillus* strains including *L. plantarum*, *L. acidophilus* NCFM, *L. johnsonii* NCC 533, and *L. sakei* predicts a broad group of bacteriocins with highly divergent sequences.[8, 9, 10, 11] Despite the sequence variation, these peptides have a relatively narrow spectrum of activity and are mostly toxic to Gram-positive bacteria, including *Lactococcus, Streptococcus, Staphylococcus, Listeria,* and *Mycobacteria.* The primary mechanism of bacteriocin action is forming pores in the cytoplasmic membrane of sensitive bacteria, but they can also interfere with essential enzyme activities in some species. In addition, several strains of Bifidobacteria have been found to produce bacteriocin-like compounds toxic to both Gram-positive and Gram-negative bacteria.[12] Interestingly, probiotics also stimulate intestinal epithelial cells to produce antimicrobial substances (Section "Probiotics benefit host nutrition" of this chapter).

Acid

Probiotic bacteria, especially strains of *Lactobacilli,* produce acetic, lactic, and propionic acid which lower the local pH leading to growth inhibition of a wide range of Gram-negative pathogenic bacteria. Some *Lactobacillus* strains inhibit the growth of *S. enterica* solely by the production of lactic acid.[13] However, antibacterial effects of other strains of *Lactobacilli* may be the result of a combination of lactic acid and additional unknown *Lactobacillus*-derived bactericidal substances.[13,14] Although these putative substances are not yet identified, their antibacterial function appears to involve pH-dependent mechanism(s). One study suggests that lactic acid or low pH acts as a permeabilizer of Gram-negative bacterial outer membranes, allowing other antimicrobial substances to penetrate and increasing the susceptibility of pathogens.[15]

Hydrogen Peroxide

The production of hydrogen peroxide exerts a nonspecific antimicrobial defense mechanism in the normal vaginal ecosystem. Several *Lactobacillus* strains of vaginal origin have been found to produce hydrogen peroxide to inhibit gonococci growth in the female genital tract.[16] Additionally, inhibition of *Gardnerella vaginalis* by *Lactobacillus* strains is through the combinational effects of hydrogen peroxide, lactic acid, and bacteriocins.[17]

Competitive Inhibition of Pathogen and Toxin Adherence to the Intestinal Epithelium

Probiotics in the gastrointestinal tract decrease adhesion of both pathogens and their toxins to the intestinal epithelium. Several strains of *Lactobacilli* and *Bifidobacteria* are able to compete with pathogenic bacteria, including *S. enterica, Yersinia enterocolitica*[18] enterotoxigenic *E. coli,*[19] and enteropathogenic *E. coli*[20] for intestinal epithelial cell binding. In some cases probiotics can displace pathogenic bacteria even when the pathogens have attached to intestinal epithelial cells prior to probiotic treatment.[18]

Since one of the mechanisms underlying pathogenic bacteria binding to intestinal epithelial cells is interaction between bacterial lectins and carbohydrate moieties of glycoconjugate receptor molecules on the cell surface, studies have been performed to determine whether probiotics block these binding sites of the adhesion receptor.

Investigations using proteinase treatment and carbohydrate competition have confirmed that probiotic binding to intestinal epithelial cells is mediated by lectin-like adhesions and proteinaceous cell surface components.[21, 22, 23] For example, mannose and Galβ1-3GalNAc-specific adhesions are required for binding of *Lactobacilli* and *Bifibobacteria* to intestinal epithelial cells and mucus.[21,22] Thus, probiotic inhibition of pathogen adherence to intestinal cells may well be mediated in part by competition for lectin binding sites on glycoconjugate receptors on the cell surface.

In addition to inhibiting bacterial pathogen adhesion to intestinal epithelial tissue, probiotics can also be clinically useful to prevent pathogens from binding to surgical implants. This activity could be mediated by the production of biosurfactants. For example, *Lactobacilli fermentum* RC-14 inhibits adhesion of *Staphylococcus aureus* to surgical implants, and thus decreases the incidence of implant infections.[24]

Blockade of bacterial enterotoxin binding has also been shown as a mechanism for potential probiotic therapeutic strategies. The virulence factor of Enterotoxigenic *E. coli* strains is a heat-labile enterotoxin, which induces traveler's diarrhea by binding to ganglioside GM1 on the surface of intestinal epithelial cells. By using a toxin-receptor blockade strategy, an engineered probiotic bacterium was generated by expressing glycosyltransferase genes from *Neisseria meningitides* or *Campylobacter jejuni* in a harmless *E. coli* strain (CWG308). The recombinant *E. coli*-produced chimeric lipopolysaccharide (LPS) could neutralize heat-labile enterotoxin and cholera toxin in vitro, prevent enterotoxin-induced fluid secretion in ligated rabbit ileal loops in vivo.[25] and reduce mortality by virulent *Vibrio cholerae* infection in infant mice.[26]

In summary, the production of antibacterial products and blockade of carbohydrate binding sites for pathogens on intestinal epithelial cells represent key mechanisms by which probiotics influence the intestinal microbial environment.

PROBIOTICS INDUCE PROTECTIVE RESPONSES IN INTESTINAL EPITHELIAL CELLS

The intestinal epithelium is critical for maintaining normal intestinal function through formation of a regulated physiological barrier against pathogenic microbes and detrimental substances in the intestinal lumen. Disruption of the integrity of this monolayer occurs in several diseases, such as inflammatory bowel disease (reviewed in [27,28]) and some bacterial and viral infections (reviewed in [29]). The presumed first target of probiotic action is the intestinal epithelial cell, and substantial evidence indicates that probiotic bacteria stimulate intestinal epithelial cell responses, including restitution of damaged epithelial barrier, production of antibacterial substances and cell protective proteins, blockade of cytokine-induced intestinal epithelial cell apoptosis. Many of these responses result from probiotic stimulation of specific intracellular signaling pathways in the epithelial cells.

Barrier Function

The intestinal barrier function, one of the defensive mechanisms of the intestinal epithelium, requires effective tight junctional complexes between intestinal epithelial cells. Disruption of the tight junctional structure or function leads to interruption of the intestinal integrity. Recent studies provide significant evidence suggesting probiotic effects on initiating repair of barrier function after injury. For example, probiotic *E. coli* Nissle 1917 promotes tight junctional barrier function following enteropathogenic *E. coli*-induced disruption in the T84 human intestinal epithelial cell line.[30] This protective response appears to be mediated by overexpression and redistribution of the tight junctional proteins zonula occludens (ZO)-2 and protein kinase C (PKC) ζ to the cell surface to restore the tight junction complex. *Lactobacillus rhamnosus* GG (LGG) and LGG-derived soluble proteins (p40 and p75) also protect intestinal barrier function from hydrogen peroxide-induced insult through enhancing membrane translocation of tight junctional complex proteins, including ZO-1, occludin, PKCβ1 and PKCε in an extracellular signal-regulated kinase (ERK)1/2 mitogen-activated protein kinase (MAPK)-dependent manner.[31] Other probiotic bacteria, such as *L. casei DN-114 001*[32] and VSL#3, a probiotic mixture of eight probiotic bacteria (*L. plantarum, L. acidophilus, L. casei, L. delbrueckii, B. infantis, B. breve, B. longum* and *Streptococcus salivarius* subsp. *Thermofilus*), inhibit enteropathogenic *E. coli*-induced increase in paracellular permeability and prevent *S. dublin*-induced tight junction dissolution and ZO-1 redistribution, respectively, in T84 cells. Furthermore, *L. acidophilus* and *B. thetaiotaomicron* have been reported to prevent cytokine-induced increases of intestinal epithelial paracellular permeability, which may play significant pathological roles in human intestinal epithelial cells. Activation of p38/MAPK and Akt signal transduction pathways in the epithelial cells have been implicated as key mediators of these protective effects.[33]

Production of Cytoprotective and Antibacterial Substances

In addition to the physical barrier function, the intestinal epithelium actively regulates the intestinal microenvironment through production of cytoprotective and antibacterial substances.

Heat shock proteins are constitutively expressed in epithelial cells and induced by stress to maintain intestinal homeostasis and defense against injury. A recent report demonstrated that soluble factors present in LGG culture supernatant induce cytoprotective heat shock protein synthesis in intestinal epithelial cells in a p38 and JNK/MAPK-dependent manner.[34]

β-defensin is an inducible antimicrobial peptide synthesized by the intestinal epithelial cells to prevent bacterial adherence and invasion. Probiotic *E. coli* Nissle 1917 increases β-defensin expression in intestinal epithelial cells through regulation of NFκB and AP-1-dependent transcriptional pathways.[35] By studying deletion mutants, this group further found that flagellin, a factor present in the bacterial culture supernatant, is the major stimulator of *E. coli* Nissle 1917 induced β-defensin expression.[36] In addition to β-defensin, probiotic bacteria promote production of other antimicrobial substances. For example, *B. thetaiotaomicron* stimulates Paneth cells release of Angiogenin 4 (Ang4), which exhibits bactericidal activity against several pathogens.[37] Mucins, synthesized and secreted by intestinal goblet cells, form a protective layer against noxious substances and pathogens in the gastrointestinal tract. The VSL#3 probiotic mixture and soluble factors released from bacteria increase mucin gene expression in

T84 and HT29 intestinal epithelial cells in a MAPK-dependent manner [38]. Furthermore, the VSL#3 probiotic mixture increases mucin section in rat colon in vivo. However, VSL#3 bacterial secreted products, but not bacteria, stimulate mucin secretion in LS 174T colonic epithelial cells. [39] Thus, enhancing antibacterial activity of the intestinal epithelium is an important potential mechanism for probiotic bacteria regulation of host defense responses.

Prevention of Cytokine-Induced Apoptosis

Another potential mechanism conferring clinical efficacy of probiotics is prevention of cytokine-induced epithelial damage by promoting intestinal epithelial cell survival. Apoptosis is a major factor in the colonic inflammatory response and the pathogenesis of IBD.[40] LGG has been used to investigate molecular mechanisms by which probiotics regulate intestinal epithelial cell survival for treating and/or preventing IBD. LGG prevents cytokine-induced apoptosis in both human and mouse intestinal epithelial cells through activating anti-apoptotic Akt signal in a phosphatidylinositol-3′-kinase (PI3K)-dependent manner and inhibiting pro-apoptotic p38/MAPK activation. Furthermore, soluble factors recovered from LGG culture broth supernatant activate Akt and prevent cytokine-mediated apoptosis.[41] This anti-apoptotic activity induced by LGG-derived soluble factors appears to be mediated by two novel proteins (p75 and p40), which were recently purified and cloned from LGG culture supernatant.[42] In both cultured cells and ex vivo colon organ culture models, anti-apoptotic function and signal transduction pathways mediated by soluble LGG factors were inhibited by antibodies to these proteins. These findings suggest that it may be possible to identify specific probiotic bacterial products for prevention and/or treatment of gastrointestinal diseases. Therefore, one important finding from this series of studies has been the recognition of bacterial specificity of biological effects through specific interactions with the host. Thus perhaps making selection of probiotics for future clinical trials linked to a mechanistic understanding of desired outcomes will increase their likelihood of success.

Maintaining Normal Perception of Visceral Pain

One potential area for clinical application of probiotics is on relief of abdominal symptoms related to abnormal colonic transit and motility and irritable bowel syndrome, which may impact 10–12% of the population.[43] A recent study in mice and rats showed that the *L. acidophilus* NCFM exerts analgesic function through up-regulation of μ-opioid and cannabinoid receptor in intestinal epithelial cells. This effect contributes to the modulation and restoration of the normal perception of visceral pain.[44] Thus, this study provides important insight into the mechanisms of probiotic effects on the regulation of the enteric nervous system with potential therapeutic implications and applications.

In summary, the intestinal epithelium serves as a major target for probiotics to benefit the host health by prevention and/or treatment of intestinal diseases. Probiotics regulate intestinal epithelial cell function through molecular and cellular mechanisms that enhance intestinal epithelial barrier function, increase synthesis of protective and antibacterial proteins, enhance cell survival, and modulate enteric neurological functions.

PROBIOTICS REGULATE CROSSTALK BETWEEN INTESTINAL EPITHELIAL CELLS AND THE IMMUNE RESPONSES

Intestinal epithelial cells play important immunomodulatory roles through complex interactions with immune cells to induce appropriate innate or adaptive immunity. Probiotics exert inhibitory effect on inflammatory cytokine and chemokine production to directly affect immune cells. For example, *B. anamalis* MB5 and LGG and factors present in bacterial culture supernatant decrease enterotoxigenic *E. coli*-induced gene expression of interleukin (IL)-8, IL-1β, tumor necrosis factor (TNF), and chemokines essential for neutrophil migration, including growth-related oncogene (Gro)-α and epithelial neutrophil-activating peptide-78.[19]

Nuclear factor (NF) κB signaling is a critical mediator of intestinal epithelial cell crosstalk with immune cells. Low-level NFκB activation by toll-like receptors (TLR), a class of membrane receptors that sense extracellular microbes and trigger antipathogen signaling cascades, in intestinal epithelial cells defends against most pathogens to maintain intestinal homeostasis. Deficiency of NFκB in intestinal epithelial cells causes increased intestinal epithelial apoptosis, impaired expression of antimicrobial peptides and chronic inflammation. Furthermore, inflammatory colitis induced by NFκB inhibition in intestinal epithelial cells depends on TNF receptor 1 and MyD88, a down stream target of TLR, which indicates that TLR activation of NFκB by intestinal bacteria is essential for maintaining intestinal homeostasis.[45] Another group also showed that mice deficient in MyD88 have defects in their ability to repair DSS-induced mucosal damage. Furthermore, the presence of bacterial flora in damaged mucosa induces expression of several cytoprotective factors, including IL-6, KC-1, and heat shock proteins.[46] Thus bacterial activation of TLR signaling pathways plays a critical role in directing colonic tissue repair process.

Results from experimental models of colitis show that TLR 2, 4 and 9 are required for some probiotics to exert their anti-inflammatory effects in vivo.[47,48] Such a mechanism permits the epithelial cell to serve as a sentinel to coordinate the appropriate level of immune response to overlying bacteria.[49] However, it is not clear whether activation of TLRs on intestinal epithelial cells serves as a mechanism of probiotic actions (activation of TLRs by probiotics for regulating immune cells is discussed in Section Differential activation of TLR by probiotics in immune cells). Thus, further studies are needed to determine the role of TLR expression on epithelial cells and their potential for anti-inflammatory cytokine regulation induced by probiotics.

Studies also indicate that excessive activation of NFκB induces increased cytokine and chemokine production by intestinal epithelial cells, leading to inflammation. Probiotics have been reported to inhibit NFκB-induced pro-inflammatory cytokine and chemokine production by intestinal epithelial cells. Probiotic bacteria, *L. reuteri*, LGG, *B. infantis* and *L. salivarius* for example, suppress TNF- or *S. typhimurium*-induced IL-8 gene expression and secretion by intestinal epithelial cells in a NFκB-dependent manner.[50, 51, 52]

Further studies reveal that *L casei* suppresses invasive *Shigella flexneri*-induced transcription of inflammatory cytokines, chemokines and adhesion molecules in intestinal epithelial cells through modulation of the ubiquitin/proteasome pathway to stabilize IκB and thus inhibit NFκB nuclear translocation.[53] Another mechanism of probiotic regulation of NFκB transcriptional activity in the nucleus is through activation of peroxisome proliferators activated receptor (PPAR)-γ.[54]*B. thetaiotaomicron* induces nuclear export of the RelA subunit of NFκB associated with PPAR-γ.

Therefore, NFκB regulation by probiotics may serve as a checkpoint to integrate appropriate protective responses between epithelial cells and immune cells to maintain intestinal homeostasis.

PROBIOTICS REGULATE HOST IMMUNE FUNCTIONS

Commensal bacterial flora plays a key role in defining and maintaining the delicate balance between necessary and excessive defense mechanisms including innate and adaptive immune responses. Similar to other flora interacting with the immune system, probiotic bacteria are internalized by M cells to interact with dendritic cells and follicle associated epithelial cells, initiating responses mediated by macrophages and T and B lymphocytes (reviewed in [55,56]). Both in vitro and in vivo studies show effects of probiotics on host immune functions: up-regulation of immune function may improve the ability to fight infections or inhibit tumor formation; down-regulation may prevent the onset of allergy or intestinal inflammation. One of the mechanisms of probiotics regulating immunomodulatory functions is through activation of TLRs.

Enhancing Host Innate Immunity

Innate immunity includes a suite of cellular and biomedical mechanisms that prevent invasion of both pathogenic and commensal microorganism. Probiotics have the potential to stimulate innate immune responses against microorganisms and dietary antigens, newly encountered by the host through several mechanisms. Intestinal dendritic cells can retain commensal bacteria by selectively activating B lymphocytes to produce IgA to reduce mucosal penetration by bacteria. The dendritic cells carrying commensals are restricted to the intestinal mucosal lymphoid tissues to avoid potential systemic immune responses.[57] Furthermore, use of probiotics may reinforce innate function as a recent report suggests that *B. animalis*-enriched formula increases fecal sIgA levels in infants.[58] Interestingly, in addition to significant elevation of fecal sIgA by nonviable LGG treatment, spleen cells of mice fed with nonviable LGG show enhanced secretion of IL-6, which augments IgA antibody responses at the mucosal surface.[59]

Stimulation of active immune responses without inducing inflammation is another mechanism to protect the host from excess injury. LGG stimulates only moderate expression of costimulatory molecules, low production of TNF and CCL20, and no production of IL-2, IL-12, IL-23 and IL-27 in dendritic cells compared with vigorous Th-1 type responses to pathogenic *S. pyogenes*.[60] Similar differential modulation of dendritic cells has been reported between *Klebsiella pneumoniae* and *L. rhamnosus*,[61] suggesting differential responses of dendritic cells to pathogenic and nonpathogenic probiotic bacteria.

Modulation of Pathogen-Induced Inflammatory Responses

The host innate defenses must modulate response to the appropriate level of threat provided by a given pathogen. If the response is too weak, the infection may not be cleared, leaving the host susceptible to systemic infection. However, if it is too strong, the result may be excess tissue damage. A significant mechanism of probiotic protection from pathogen-induced injury and inflammation is modulating the balance of pro- and anti-inflammatory cytokine production.

Increasing Anti-Inflammatory Cytokine Production

Dendritic cell maturation results in increased secretion of cytokines and the expression of molecules required for T and B cell activation. Most studies show probiotic bacteria induce dendritic cells to produce anti-inflammatory cytokines, including IL-10, which suppress the Th1 response. For example, the probiotic mixture, VSL#3 induces IL-10 production in human and murine dendritic cells.[62,63] Furthermore, dendritic cells activated by microbial products enhance antigen presentation to naïve T cells to T regulatory cells (Tregs) for cytokine production. *L. reuteri* and *L. casei* prime human monocyte-derived dendritic cells to drive the development of Tregs to produce high levels of IL-10.[64]

However, the role of IL-10 production in preventing Th1 responses by probiotics is controversial, and the mechanisms by which probiotics inhibit Th1-type cytokine production may be through both IL-10 dependent and independent mechanisms. *B infantis* and *Lactobacillus* spp fail to block production of Th1-type cytokines, such as IL-12 and interferon (IFN)-γ, in IL-10 knock-out mice.[65,66] However, inhibition of two other Th1-type cytokines, IL-12 and TNF, by probiotics is not affected by the absence of IL-10.

Suppressing Proinflammatory Cytokine Production

Probiotics also inhibit pro-inflammatory cytokine production. LGG inhibits LPS and *H. pylori*-stimulated TNF production by murine macrophages. Furthermore, LGG-conditioned cell culture media decreases TNF production, indicating that soluble molecules derived from LGG exert this immunoregulatory role.[67] Studies further showed that LGG and *L. rhamnosus* GR-1 and their cell culture supernatants induce high levels of granulocyte-colony stimulating factor (G-CSF) production from macrophages compared to those induced by pathogenic *E. coli* GR-12. This increased G-CSF production from macrophages is required for inhibition of *E. coli* or LPS-induced TNF production in macrophages and in mice. The suppression of TNF production by G-CSF is mediated through STAT3 and subsequent inhibition of c-Jun-N-terminal kinases (JNKs).[68]*L. casei* strain Shirota (LcS) down-regulates LPS-induced IL-6 and IFN-γ production by peripheral blood mononuclear cells isolated from normal and chronic colitis mice.[69] Furthermore, *E. coli* Nissle 1917 inhibits peripheral blood T-cell cycle progression and expansion, increases IL-10 and decreases TNF, IFN-γ and IL-2 release by these cells.[70]

Up-Regulation of Host Immune Responses to Defend Against Infection

Probiotics stimulate host immunological functions including Th1 responses through dendritic cell-directed T-cell activation. During colonization of mice with *B. fragilis*, dendritic cells take up and retain a bacterial polysaccharide (PSA). This PSA promotes maturation of dendritic cells, Th1-type cytokine production including IL-4, IL-12, and IFN-γ, and subsequent CD4+ T cell expansion.[71]*L. gasseri, L. reuteri*, and *L. johnsonii* up-regulate IL-12 and IL-18 production from dendritic cells, and *Lactobacilli*-exposed dendritic cells skew CD4+ and CD8+ T cells to Th1 and Tc1 polarization to increase IFN-γ production.[72] Thus probiotics and commensal flora are involved in maintaining intestinal homeostasis by promoting a balance between pro- and anti-inflammatory mucosal responses.

Regulation of Immune Responses by Probiotic DNA

In addition to the direct interactions between probiotic bacteria and immune cells, DNA from probiotic bacteria modulates both human and mouse immune function. DNA isolated from the probiotic VSL#3 mixture decreases LPS-activated IL-8 production and TNF and IFN-γ release in vivo and in vitro. VSL#3 DNA also inhibits p38 MAP kinase and delays NFκB activation.[73] The unmethylated dinucleotides, CpG, commonly found in bacterial and other nonmammalian genomes activate innate immunity through TLR9.[74] Importantly, administration of unmethylated probiotic- or *E. coli*-derived DNA protects against injury in the DSS model of colitis in a TLR-dependent manner.[48] Mammalian or methylated bacterial DNA shows no preventative effect and the therapeutic advantage of CpGs is likewise lost in TLR9-deficient mouse.

Differential Activation of TLRs by Probiotics in Immune Cells

Similar to pathogenic bacteria, probiotic bacteria possess molecular recognition patterns detected by TLRs, yet these organisms do not normally initiate pathogenic inflammatory responses. At least 10 TLRs are currently known, and specific molecular patterns have been identified for many of the receptors. Human T cells cultured with the probiotic organism *E. coli* Nissle 1917 express increased levels of both TLR2 and TLR4. Furthermore, in TLR2 and TLR4 knockout mice, *E coli* Nissle 1917 fails to improve colitis and modulate cytokine production when compared to wild-type mice.[47] In contrast, the probiotic VSL#3 mixture reduces the severity of DSS-induced colitis in wild type, TLR2 and TLR4 deficient mouse models, but not in the TLR9 deficient mouse, indicating that TLR9 signaling mediates this mixture's regulation of the host immune response.[48] Thus different probiotic bacteria stimulate distinct TLRs on host cells.

Given the evidence that both pathogenic and commensal bacterial molecular patterns are recognized by TLRs, understanding how probiotic bacteria escape triggering an inflammatory cascade has biological and clinical relevance. We speculate the following factors which may contribute to different effects of activation of TLRs by probiotics compared to pathogenic bacteria: (1) Accessibility of probiotic bacteria to interact with TLRs in different cellular positions on polarized intestinal epithelial cells. It has been reported that apical but not basolateral stimulation of TLR9 in intestinal epithelial cells inhibits of NFκB activation.[75] (2) Probiotics may contain some components, which pathogenic bacteria do not possess to induce the differential activation of TLRs. For example, although the structural differences between LPS from pathogenic and nonpathogenic bacteria are not clear, they are recognized differentially by TLR4 to induce inflammation.[76] (3) Probiotics-induced cellular responses may be due to synergistic effects of TLRs, which cannot be or are differentially regulated by pathogenic bacteria.

Synergic responses of TLRs have been reported in that using multiple ligands to stimulate TLRs1/2, TLRs2/6, 4, 5, or TLRs7/8 induces high levels of cytokine secretion compared to individual TLR activation.[77]

In summary, probiotics exert both up- and down-regulatory effects on immune responses. TLR-regulated signaling pathways appear to be one of the mechanisms for these immunoregulatory actions. However, further studies are needed to determine the basis for observed differences among the signals induced by probiotics and pathogens, which use similar receptors to induce divergent responses.

SUMMARY

Information reviewed in this chapter suggests several mechanisms by which probiotics promote maintenance of host homeostasis. Probiotics produce enzymes to benefit host nutrition, generate antibacterial substance, and compete for pathogen-binding sites on epithelial cells. Probiotics promote intestinal epithelial cell survival, enhance barrier function, and stimulate protective responses by regulating signaling pathways such as Akt, MAPK, and NFκB. They also enhance the innate immunity and prevent pathogen-induced inflammation through activating distinct TLR-regulated signaling pathways in immune and other cells. However, it is clear that we have just scratched the surface of understanding the delicate interactions between probiotics and the host. The use of advanced cellular and molecular approaches will improve our mechanistic understanding of the relationships of the genetics of probiotic microbes to their functions, and the influences of the host microenvironment on the probitotic actions. These living therapeutic agents require specific biological niches that are regulated by a number of factors including host diet.[78] Furthermore, to improve the efficacy of this approach for diseases, new insights regarding the mechanisms involved in regulating "bioavailability" and "biosafety" of probiotics are needed. The discovery of molecular and cellular mechanisms of action will provide the basis for targeted use of probiotics or manipulation of their gene products for disease prevention or therapeutic effects, which we have thus far not fully realized.

Acknowledgements The authors want to thank Dr. Mark Frey at Vanderbilt University for his suggestions in manuscript preparation.

REFERENCES

1. Lilly DM, Stillwell RH. Probiotics: growth-promoting factors produced by microorganisms. *Science* 1965;147:747–8.
2. Walker WOG, Morelli L, Antoine J. Progress in the science of probiotics: from cellular microbiology and applied immunology to clinical nutrition. *Eur J Nutr* 2006;45:1–18.
3. Yan F, Polk DB. Commensal bacteria in the gut: learning who our friends are. *Curr Op Gastroenterol* 2004;20:565–71.
4. Yan F, Polk DB. Probiotics as functional food in the treatment of diarrhea. *Curr Opin Clin Nutr Metab Care* 2006;9:717–21.
5. Xu J, Bjursell MK, Himrod J, et al. A genomic view of the human-*Bacteroides thetaiotaomicron* symbiosis. *Science* 2003;299:2074–6.
6. Hooper LV, Wong MH, Thelin A, Hansson L, Falk PG, Gordon JI. Molecular analysis of commensal host-microbial relationships in the intestine. *Science* 2001;291:881–4.

7. Servin AL. Antagonistic activities of lactobacilli and bifidobacteria against microbial pathogens. *FEMS Microbiol Rev* 2004;28:405–40.
8. Makarova K, Slesarev A, Wolf Y, et al. Comparative genomics of the lactic acid bacteria. *Proc Natl Acad Sci USA* 2006;103:15611–6.
9. Chaillou S, Champomier-Verges MC, Cornet M, et al. The complete genome sequence of the meat-borne lactic acid bacterium *Lactobacillus sakei* 23K. *Nat Biotechnol* 2005;23:1527–33.
10. Altermann E, Russell WM, Azcarate-Peril MA, et al. Complete genome sequence of the probiotic lactic acid bacterium *Lactobacillus acidophilus* NCFM. *Proc Natl Acad Sci USA* 2005;102:3906–12.
11. Pridmore RD, Berger B, Desiere F, et al. The genome sequence of the probiotic intestinal bacterium *Lactobacillus johnsonii* NCC 533. *Proc Natl Acad Sci USA* 2004;101:2512–7.
12. Collado MC, Hernandez M, Sanz Y. Production of bacteriocin-like inhibitory compounds by human fecal Bifidobacterium strains. *J Food Prot* 2005;68:1034–40.
13. Makras L, Triantafyllou V, Fayol-Messaoudi D, et al. Kinetic analysis of the antibacterial activity of probiotic lactobacilli towards *Salmonella enterica* serovar Typhimurium reveals a role for lactic acid and other inhibitory compounds. *Res Microbiol* 2006;157:241–7.
14. De Keersmaecker SC, Verhoeven TL, Desair J, Marchal K, Vanderleyden J, Nagy I. Strong antimicrobial activity of *Lactobacillus rhamnosus* GG against *Salmonella typhimurium* is due to accumulation of lactic acid. *FEMS Microbiol Lett* 2006;259:89–96.
15. Alakomi HL, Skytta E, Saarela M, Mattila-Sandholm T, Latva-Kala K, Helander IM. Lactic acid permeabilizes gram-negative bacteria by disrupting the outer membrane. *Appl Environ Microbiol* 2000;66:2001–5.
16. St Amant DC, Valentin-Bon IE, Jerse AE. Inhibition of *Neisseria gonorrhoeae* by *Lactobacillus* species that are commonly isolated from the female genital tract. *Infect Immun* 2002;70:7169–71.
17. Mastromarino P, Brigidi P, Macchia S, et al. Characterization and selection of vaginal *Lactobacillus* strains for the preparation of vaginal tablets. *J Appl Microbiol* 2002;93:884–93.
18. Candela M, Seibold G, Vitali B, Lachenmaier S, Eikmanns BJ, Brigidi P. Real-time PCR quantification of bacterial adhesion to Caco-2 cells: competition between bifidobacteria and enteropathogens. *Res Microbiol* 2005;156:887–95.
19. Roselli M, Finamore A, Britti MS, Mengheri E. Probiotic bacteria Bifidobacterium animalis MB5 and *Lactobacillus rhamnosus* GG protect intestinal Caco-2 cells from the inflammation-associated response induced by enterotoxigenic *Escherichia coli* K88. *Br J Nutr* 2006;95:1177–84.
20. Sherman PM, Johnson-Henry KC, Yeung HP, Ngo PS, Goulet J, Tompkins TA. Probiotics reduce enterohemorrhagic *Escherichia coli* O157:H7- and enteropathogenic *E. coli* O127:H6-induced changes in polarized T84 epithelial cell monolayers by reducing bacterial adhesion and cytoskeletal rearrangements. *Infect Immun* 2005;73:5183–8.
21. Mukai T, Kaneko S, Matsumoto M, Ohori H. Binding of *Bifidobacterium bifidum* and *Lactobacillus reuteri* to the carbohydrate moieties of intestinal glycolipids recognized by peanut agglutinin. *Int J Food Microbiol* 2004;90:357–62.
22. Sun J, Le GW, Shi YH, Su GW. Factors involved in binding of *Lactobacillus plantarum* Lp6 to rat small intestinal mucus. *Lett Appl Microbiol* 2007;44:79–85.
23. Tallon R, Arias S, Bressollier P, Urdaci MC. Strain- and matrix-dependent adhesion of *Lactobacillus plantarum* is mediated by proteinaceous bacterial compounds. *J Appl Microbiol* 2007;102:442–51.
24. Gan BS, Kim J, Reid G, Cadieux P, Howard JC. *Lactobacillus fermentum* RC-14 inhibits *Staphylococcus aureus* infection of surgical implants in rats. *J Infect Dis* 2002;185:1369–72.
25. Paton AW, Jennings MP, Morona R, et al. Recombinant probiotics for treatment and prevention of enterotoxigenic *Escherichia coli* diarrhea. *Gastroenterology* 2005;128:1219–28.
26. Focareta A, Paton JC, Morona R, Cook J, Paton AW. A recombinant probiotic for treatment and prevention of cholera. *Gastroenterology* 2006;130:1688–95.
27. Strober W, Fuss I, Mannon P. The fundamental basis of inflammatory bowel disease. *J Clin Invest* 2007;117:514–21.
28. Xavier RJ, Podolsky DK. Unravelling the pathogenesis of inflammatory bowel disease. *Nature* 2007;448:427–34.
29. Clayburgh DR, Shen L, Turner JR. A porous defense: the leaky epithelial barrier in intestinal disease. *Lab Invest* 2004;84:282–91.

30. Zyrek AA, Cichon C, Helms S, Enders C, Sonnenborn U, Schmidt MA. Molecular mechanisms underlying the probiotic effects of *Escherichia coli* Nissle 1917 involve ZO-2 and PKCzeta redistribution resulting in tight junction and epithelial barrier repair. *Cell Microbiol* 2007;9:804–16.

31. Seth A, Yan F, Polk DB, Rao RK. Probiotics ameliorate hydrogen peroxide-induced epithelial barrier disruption by PKC and MAP kinase-dependent mechanism. *Am J Physiol Gastrointest Liver Physiol* 2008; 294:G1060–69.

32. Parassol N, Freitas M, Thoreux K, Dalmasso G, Bourdet-Sicard R, Rampal P. *Lactobacillus casei* DN-114 001 inhibits the increase in paracellular permeability of enteropathogenic *Escherichia coli*-infected T84 cells. *Res Microbiol* 2005;156:256–62.

33. Resta-Lenert S, Barrett KE. Probiotics and commensals reverse TNF-alpha- and IFN-gamma-induced dysfunction in human intestinal epithelial cells. *Gastroenterology* 2006;130:731–46.

34. Tao Y, Drabik KA, Waypa TS, et al. Soluble factors from *Lactobacillus* GG activate MAPKs and induce cytoprotective heat shock proteins in intestinal epithelial cells. *Am J Physiol Cell Physiol* 2006;290:C1018–30.

35. Wehkamp J, Harder J, Wehkamp K, et al. NF-kappaB- and AP-1-mediated induction of human beta defensin-2 in intestinal epithelial cells by *Escherichia coli* Nissle 1917: a novel effect of a probiotic bacterium. *Infect Immun* 2004;72:5750–8.

36. Schlee M, Wehkamp J, Altenhoefer A, Oelschlaeger TA, Stange EF, Fellermann K. Induction of human beta-defensin 2 by the probiotic *Escherichia coli* Nissle 1917 is mediated through flagellin. *Infect Immun* 2007;75:2399–407.

37. Hooper LV, Stappenbeck TS, Hong CV, Gordon JI. Angiogenins: a new class of microbicidal proteins involved in innate immunity. *Nat Immunol* 2003;4:269–73.

38. Otte JM, Podolsky DK. Functional modulation of enterocytes by gram-positive and gram-negative microorganisms. *Am J Physiol Gastrointest Liver Physiol* 2004;286:G613–26.

39. Caballero-Franco C, Keller K, De Simone C, Chadee K. The VSL#3 probiotic formula induces mucin gene expression and secretion in colonic epithelial cells. *Am J Physiol Gastrointest Liver Physiol* 2007;292:G315–22.

40. Sartor RB. Mucosal immunology and mechanisms of gastrointestinal inflammation. In: Feldman M, Friedman LS, Sleisenger MH, eds. Sleisenger and Fordtran's Gastrointestinal and Liver Disease: Pathophysiology, Diagnosis, Management. 7th ed. Philadelphia: Saunders; 2002:21–51.

41. Yan F, Polk DB. Probiotic bacterium prevents cytokine-induced apoptosis in intestinal epithelial cells. *J Biol Chem* 2002;277:50959–65.

42. Yan F, Cao H, Cover TL, Whitehead R, Washington MK, Polk DB. Soluble proteins produced by probiotic bacteria regulate intestinal epithelial cell survival and growth. *Gastroenterology* 2007;132:562–75.

43. Camilleri M. Probiotics and irritable bowel syndrome: rationale, putative mechanisms, and evidence of clinical efficacy. *J Clin Gastroenterol* 2006;40:264–9.

44. Rousseaux C, Thuru X, Gelot A, et al. *Lactobacillus acidophilus* modulates intestinal pain and induces opioid and cannabinoid receptors. *Nat Med* 2007;13:35–7.

45. Nenci A, Becker C, Wullaert A, et al. Epithelial NEMO links innate immunity to chronic intestinal inflammation. *Nature* 2007;446:557–61.

46. Rakoff-Nahoum S, Paglino J, Eslami-Varzaneh F, Edberg S, Medzhitov R. Recognition of commensal microflora by toll-like receptors is required for intestinal homeostasis. *Cell* 2004;118:229–41.

47. Grabig A, Paclik D, Guzy C, et al. *Escherichia coli* strain Nissle 1917 ameliorates experimental colitis via toll-like receptor 2- and toll-like receptor 4-dependent pathways. *Infect Immun* 2006;74:4075–82.

48. Rachmilewitz D, Katakura K, Karmeli F, et al. Toll-like receptor 9 signaling mediates the anti-inflammatory effects of probiotics in murine experimental colitis. *Gastroenterology* 2004;126:520–8.

49. Cario E, Brown D, McKee M, Lynch-Devaney K, Gerken G, Podolsky DK. Commensal-associated molecular patterns induce selective toll-like receptor-trafficking from apical membrane to cytoplasmic compartments in polarized intestinal epithelium. *Am J Pathol* 2002;160:165–73.

50. Ma D, Forsythe P, Bienenstock J. Live *Lactobacillus reuteri* is essential for the inhibitory effect on tumor necrosis factor alpha-induced interleukin-8 expression. *Infect Immun* 2004;72:5308–14.

51. O'Hara AM, O'Regan P, Fanning A, et al. Functional modulation of human intestinal epithelial cell responses by *Bifidobacterium infantis* and *Lactobacillus salivarius*. *Immunology* 2006;118:202–15.

52. Zhang L, Li N, Caicedo R, Neu J. Alive and dead *Lactobacillus rhamnosus* GG decrease tumor necrosis factor-alpha-induced interleukin-8 production in Caco-2 cells. *J Nutr* 2005;135:1752–6.

53. Tien MT, Girardin SE, Regnault B, et al. Anti-inflammatory effect of *Lactobacillus casei* on Shigella-infected human intestinal epithelial cells. *J Immunol* 2006;176:1228–37.

54. Kelly D, Campbell JI, King TP, et al. Commensal anaerobic gut bacteria attenuate inflammation by regulating nuclear-cytoplasmic shuttling of PPAR-g and RelA. *Nat Immunol* 2004;5:104–12.

55. Kraehenbuhl JP, Corbett M. Immunology. Keeping the gut microflora at bay. *Science* 2004;303:1624–5.

56. Winkler P, Ghadimi D, Schrezenmeir J, Kraehenbuhl JP. Molecular and cellular basis of microflora-host interactions. *J Nutr* 2007;137:756S-72S.

57. Macpherson AJ, Uhr T. Induction of protective IgA by intestinal dendritic cells carrying commensal bacteria. *Science* 2004;303:1662–5.

58. Bakker-Zierikzee AM, Tol EA, Kroes H, Alles MS, Kok FJ, Bindels JG. Faecal SIgA secretion in infants fed on pre- or probiotic infant formula. *Pediatr Allergy Immunol* 2006;17:134–40.

59. He F, Morita H, Kubota A, et al. Effect of orally administered non-viable *Lactobacillus* cells on murine humoral immune responses. *Microbiol Immunol* 2005;49:993–7.

60. Veckman V, Miettinen M, Pirhonen J, Siren J, Matikainen S, Julkunen I. *Streptococcus pyogenes* and *Lactobacillus rhamnosus* differentially induce maturation and production of Th1-type cytokines and chemokines in human monocyte-derived dendritic cells. *J Leukoc Biol* 2004;75:764–71.

61. Braat H, de Jong EC, van den Brande JM, et al. Dichotomy between *Lactobacillus rhamnosus* and *Klebsiella pneumoniae* on dendritic cell phenotype and function. *J Mol Med* 2004;82:197–205.

62. Drakes M, Blanchard T, Czinn S. Bacterial probiotic modulation of dendritic cells. *Infect Immun* 2004;72:3299–309.

63. Hart AL, Lammers K, Brigidi P, et al. Modulation of dendritic cell phenotype and function by probiotic bacteria. *Gut* 2004;53:1602–9.

64. Smits HH, Engering A, van der Kleij D, et al. Selective probiotic bacteria induce IL-10-producing regulatory T cells in vitro by modulating dendritic cell function through dendritic cell-specific intercellular adhesion molecule 3-grabbing nonintegrin. *J Allergy Clin Immunol* 2005;115:1260–7.

65. Pena JA, Rogers AB, Ge Z, et al. Probiotic *Lactobacillus* spp. diminish *Helicobacter hepaticus*-induced inflammatory bowel disease in interleukin-10-deficient mice. *Infect Immun* 2005;73: 912–20.

66. Sheil B, MacSharry J, O'Callaghan L, et al. Role of interleukin (IL-10) in probiotic-mediated immune modulation: an assessment in wild-type and IL-10 knock-out mice. *Clin Exp Immunol* 2006;144:273–80.

67. Pena JA, Versalovic J. *Lactobacillus rhamnosus* GG decreases TNF-a production in lipopolysaccharide-activated murine macrophages by a contact-independent mechanism. *Cell Microbiol* 2003;5:277–85.

68. Kim SO, Sheikh HI, Ha SD, Martins A, Reid G. G-CSF-mediated inhibition of JNK is a key mechanism for *Lactobacillus rhamnosus*-induced suppression of TNF production in macrophages. *Cell Microbiol* 2006;8:1958–71.

69. Matsumoto S, Hara T, Hori T, et al. Probiotic Lactobacillus-induced improvement in murine chronic inflammatory bowel disease is associated with the down-regulation of pro-inflammatory cytokines in lamina propria mononuclear cells. *Clin Exp Immunol* 2005;140:417–26.

70. Sturm A, Rilling K, Baumgart DC, et al. *Escherichia coli* Nissle 1917 distinctively modulates T-cell cycling and expansion via toll-like receptor 2 signaling. *Infect Immun* 2005;73:1452–65.

71. Mazmanian SK, Liu CH, Tzianabos AO, Kasper DL. An immunomodulatory molecule of symbiotic bacteria directs maturation of the host immune system. *Cell* 2005;122:107–18.

72. Mohamadzadeh M, Olson S, Kalina WV, et al. *Lactobacilli* activate human dendritic cells that skew T cells toward T helper 1 polarization. *Proc Natl Acad Sci USA* 2005;102:2880–5.

73. Jijon H, Backer J, Diaz H, et al. DNA from probiotic bacteria modulates murine and human epithelial and immune function. *Gastroenterology* 2004;126:1358–73.

74. Krieg AM. *CpG motifs: the active ingredient in bacterial extracts?* Nat Med 2003;9:831–5.

75. Lee J, Mo JH, Katakura K, et al. Maintenance of colonic homeostasis by distinctive apical TLR9 signalling in intestinal epithelial cells. *Nat Cell Biol* 2006;8:1327–36.

76. Hajjar AM, Ernst RK, Tsai JH, Wilson CB, Miller SI. Human Toll-like receptor 4 recognizes host-specific LPS modifications. *Nat Immunol* 2002;3:354–9.

77. van Heel DA, Ghosh S, Butler M, et al. Synergistic enhancement of Toll-like receptor responses by NOD1 activation. *Eur J Immunol* 2005;35:2471–6.

78. Sonnenburg JL, Xu J, Leip DD, et al. Glycan foraging in vivo by an intestine-adapted bacterial symbiont. *Science* 2005;307:1955–9.

6 Safety Issues of Probiotic Ingestion

David R. Mack

Key Points

- Probiotics as fermented foods have been ingested for a long period of time and are generally recognized to be safe for human ingestion.
- Safety of ingesting higher numbers of probiotic microorganisms over a prolonged period of time for medical therapeutics is important.
- A large number of study subjects have ingested probiotic organisms without reported incidents.
- There are reports of individuals who have developed adverse events due to the ingestion of probiotics as medical interventions.
- This chapter provides insight into potential safety issues for probiotics.

Key Words: Probiotics safety, adverse events, resistance infection.

INTRODUCTION

It is understood that the microbiome of the intestinal tract does not tolerate microbes within, but these microbes are essential for the intestinal development and maturation [1] and for the maintenance of epithelial homeostasis [2]. The human intestinal microbial diversity is surprisingly limited to 9 of the potential 55 described divisions, but with great diversity found at the level of species and strains. In fact, only a limited number of the organisms are currently identified [3]. Thus, the organisms currently used as probiotics are those that are relatively simple to identify and grow in sufficient quantities at a cost that make the economic concerns possible for companies in this field of health care. Significant information determined from the interactions of noninfectious microbes in sterile cell culture and in germ-free animal models has allowed the identification of complex alterations in host gene expression mediated through microbial interactions [1], but we are truly at the beginning of gaining knowledge with regards to manipulation of the human intestinal microbiome in vivo. Thus, when considering the development of adverse events following administration of probiotics one must consider

From: *Nutrition and Health: Probiotics in Pediatric Medicine*
Edited by: S. Michail and P.M. Sherman © Humana Press, Totowa, NJ

both the microbial organism and the host organism as two equally important and intertwining protagonists in this relationship.

PROBIOTIC MICROBE ISSUES

The most common adverse events related to probiotics reported in studies are minor in nature and include bloating, diarrhea, constipation, and nausea [4]. Microbes have inherent properties transcribed from genetic material of their chromosomes and plasmids, which are responsible for their functioning within a given environment and thus provide the basis for the potential for adverse events. Furthermore, as the organisms are part of a production and delivery process the manufacturing process must also be considered with regard to safety issues.

ANTIBIOTIC RESISTANCE

Lactobacillus, among other species, is known to contain chromosomal genes that encode for antibiotic resistance. Since vancomycin tends to be used as an antibiotic of "last resort" for bacteria with multiple resistances, resistance to vancomycin is a focus of concern. Some *Lactobacillus* species commonly used in the food industry's fermentation process include *L. casei*, *L. rhamnosus*, *L. curvatus*, *L. plantarum*, *L. coryneformis* and *L. fermentum*. However, studies have shown that the chromosomally encoded vancomycin-resistance gene in *Lactobacillus* is nontransferable [5,6] in contrast to genes encoded on plasmids. However, the importance of manufacturers documenting antimicrobial testing is highlighted by findings of acquired antibiotic resistance genes in isolates intended for probiotic usage [7].

Enterococcus strains are used in the food industry as starter cultures for cheeses and yogurts and as probiotics. However, in contrast to *Lactobacillus* and *Bifidobacterium* strains, some *Enterococcus* strains are known to cause serious infections in humans. This problem is compounded because these strains can acquire virulence determinants, such as vancomycin resistance. Eaton and Gasson [8] found fewer virulence determinants in starter culture strains compared to food strains and, in turn, fewer virulence determinants in food strains compared to medically isolated strains. Acquisition of *E. faecalis* plasmid encoded virulence determinants, including the possibility of antibiotic resistance, occurred between starter strains and medical strains during in vitro experiments. Whether there is risk of virulence determinant acquisition and development of disease over the lifetime of an individual ingesting 10^{11} cfu/day of nonvirulent probiotic strain of *Enterococcus* who may be carrying a nosocomial acquired *Enterococcus* strain with multiple virulence determinants is not known and is a hypothetical concern. Nevertheless, there is opinion that caution should be exercised in the use of *Enterococcus* as a probiotic [9].

INFECTION

The most serious adverse event to probiotic administration currently known is that of infection. The very properties one wants to harness a probiotic, which are nontoxin producing and noninvasive microorganisms, largely explains their good safety profile for infectious events. *Lactobacillus* strains are found in approximately 0.1–0.4% of positive blood cultures with *L. casei* and *L. rhamnosus* the most common among a large number of species accounting for identified cases [10]. Without known virulence factors [11], sepsis or deep tissue infections resulting from ingestion of *Lactobacillus*-containing probiotics is thought to be rare [11–14]. There are supportive retrospective analyses in general population surveys. For instance, in Finland, *L. rhamnosus* strain GG was introduced into dairy products in 1989. By 1999, annual consumption had increased considerably to an average 10^{11} colony forming units/person/year) [15]. Finland required all positive blood isolates be recorded into a national database, allowing for retrospective study of *Lactobacillus* sepsis in their population. When the database was examined for the years 1990–2000, Salminen et al. [15] found only 48 confirmed cases of *Lactobacillus* sepsis, only a portion of which were identical to *L. rhamnosus* strain GG. The authors concluded there was no association with the increase in *L. rhamnosus* strain GG intake and the incidence of *L. rhamnosus* GG sepsis.

A large number of clinical trials have not documented sepsis related to probiotic ingestion. However, case reports exist in the literature of serious systemic infections with ingestion of probiotic bacteria. Representative examples of case reports include that of *L. rhamnosus* endocarditis and sepsis in a 67-year-old man with mitral valve regurgitation and dental caries, who chewed probiotics and then presented with endocarditis after a dental procedure [16]. Molecular analysis of the *Lactobacillus* strain isolated from his blood was indistinguishable from the probiotic taken by mouth. In another report, a 75-year-old woman with a history of atrial fibrillation and stroke developed *L. paracasei* endocarditis. Molecular analysis showed the organism was a *L. paracasei* strain also used in the fermentation process of dairy products [17]. In a 74-year-old woman with type 2 diabetes mellitus, a liver abscess and pleuropulmonary infection caused by a *L. rhamnosus* with a molecular profile similar to *L. rhamnosus* strain GG are also reported [18]. This same strain has also been reported to cause infections in infants, including an infant who developed sepsis in the postoperative period following repair of a double-outlet right ventricle and pulmonary stenosis, and in a 6-year-old female with cerebral palsy and microcephaly [19]. Both patients had central venous catheters in place and the authors discuss gut translocation as potentially responsible for the infection, compared to the contamination of the central venous access devices [19]. Moreover, Salminen and colleagues documented 22 cases of *L. rhamnosus* GG blood infections [20], showing these infections do occur. Of interest, is a study evaluating the efficacy of probiotic administration in reducing nosocomial infection in the pediatric intensive care unit setting. Rising concern about the use of *L rhamnosus* GG and an interim analysis revealing a trend toward increased nosocomial infections in those subjects receiving *L. rhamnosus* GG (but statistically nonsignificant) compared to placebo led to premature closure of the study [21].

Other probiotic organisms have also been associated with the development of sepsis. Four of eight cases of *Bacillus subtilis* bacteremia were associated with the absorption of an oral preparation containing *B. subtilis* spores, which was administered empirically to reduce tube-feeding related diarrhea in cancer patients [22]. Another case of *B. subtilis* sepsis was described in an elderly patient with cancer [23].

Saccharomyces boulardii is not normally found in humans, but is a yeast isolated from the lychee fruit. Its properties of growing at 37°C and being intrinsically antibiotic-resistant have led to its use as a probiotic in humans. This probiotic has been studied in different patient groups, including those with antibiotic-associated diarrhea without reports of fungemia [24]. However, a case series of six critically ill adult patients with central venous lines who developed fungemia following administration of *S. boulardii* as a probiotic has been published [25]. In this series, there was an additional seventh patient in the same critical care unit as the others who developed *Saccharomyces* central line sepsis despite no oral administration of the probiotic [25]. A review of a number of other cases of *Saccharomyces* sepsis in both children and adults related to use of this probiotic are reported [26]. Patients were very ill and cared for in an intensive care unit setting, similar to *B. subtilis* probiotic-related sepsis cases. There were reasons for infections based on factors such as host compromise and central line usage leading to the suggestion that a central venous catheter is a contraindication to the use of yeast probiotics in this type of patient [24].

Bifidobacterium sepsis and other serious infections, such as meningitis, are rare events and are related to immunocompromised and medically fragile patients, including neonates [27,28]. One study examining the side effects and safety of two strains of *B. longum* in 39 healthy adults using an in vitro safety assay determined the phagocytic activity of peripheral blood mononucleocytes as higher in the placebo group [29]. Whether this has any clinical relevance was not studied, but no higher rate of adverse effects was found in the treatment group compared with the placebo. To date, no reports of sepsis being associated with *Bifidobacterium* administration as probiotics are known, but as their usage increases it may not be surprising if isolated cases are reported.

There are now a few studies with specific safety issues such as growth and weight gain in infants as primary outcomes. For infant studies, growth is a primary determinant of safety. The study of Saavedra et al. [30] was one of the first of such studies. The authors employed a formula containing *B. lactis* (strain Bb 12) and *Streptococcus thermophilus* in 131 healthy infants aged 6 months and older. In this study, there was no difference in growth between infants taking a formula with the two different probiotic bacteria and those infants on an identical formula that did not contain the probiotics. Another study involved 201 healthy 4–10 month-old infants recruited from multiple day-care centers. The infants were fed formulas with either *B. lactis* BB-12 or *L. reuteri* SD 2112 and the investigators did not detect any differences when examining growth, behaviors, or stools compared to an identical formula without added probiotics [31]. Evaluation of *B. longum* BL999 in infants from 2 weeks of age until 6 months of age has shown similar findings [32].

PRODUCT VIABILITY

One dilemma faced by the probiotic manufacturing industry is the delivery of live, viable microorganisms. Probiotic products contained in dairy products have a limited shelf-life, compared to freeze-dried probiotic products in the form of powders and pills. Viability of probiotic products is extended with cold conditions utilized during storage, distribution, and retailing, but this adds to the cost and in some cases it may not be possible. The rancid smell and altered taste of outdated dairy products alerts the consumer quickly, but loss of viability is not obvious for pills and powders of freeze-dried probiotics. At one time, heat-killed intact probiotics were considered to be a solution to overcome this problem, but studies demonstrating live, viable probiotics with superior efficacy to heat-inactivated probiotics in both in vitro and clinical studies have largely dispelled this notion [33–35]. Studies initiated during this era also alerted to the adverse effects of ingestion of heat-killed probiotics. In a study comparing one study group that ingested live, viable *L. rhamnosus* strain GG with another group that ingested heat-killed *L. rhamnosus* GG for the prevention of allergies in infants, Kirjavainen and colleagues [36] reported increased gastrointestinal symptoms and diarrhea in those ingesting the formula with the heat-killed product, which led the Review Ethics Board to prematurely discontinue the study. In another study comparing micronutrients, micronutrients were combined with either a heat-inactivated *L. acidophilus* probiotic strain or placebo, and the impact on the prevalence of diarrhea in an at-risk group of children was assessed. The benefits of the micronutrients were negated by the addition of heat-inactivated probiotics. The prevalence of diarrhea in children receiving the combination of micronutrients and heat-killed probiotic was the same as placebo with both being worse than micronutrients given alone [37]. Thus, the importance of ingestion of viable probiotics is important not only from an efficacy point of view but also from the adverse effects associated with the ingestion of dead probiotics.

CONTAMINANTS

Some probiotic products evaluated at the retailer level have grown different microorganisms and different numbers of stated organisms than were supposed to be present [38–40]. These findings clearly demonstrate that production of high concentration of viable probiotic products demands considerable expertise and stringent quality control procedures that need to be in place to avoid contamination of consumer products.

Excipients used in the manufacturing process present in probiotic preparations may also cause problems. For instance, some children receiving probiotics have developed anaphylactic reactions from cow's milk protein allergens present in the probiotic product [41]. There are culture methods to grow lactic acid bacteria that will effectively eliminate residual cow milk protein allergens, but unless the probiotic product specifically states allergen-free or the specific culture conditions, it behooves parents of patients with cow's milk protein allergy who want to use probiotic products to actively seek assurance from manufacturers that a given product does contain an offending allergen. Thus, advocacy for these products will need to be much the same as for parents who have children with other serious food allergies (e.g., peanuts).

METABOLIC PRODUCTS

d-Lactic Acid

Human metabolism produces the l(+)-isomer of lactic acid. If d(−)-lactate is present in humans, it is then as a consequence of bacterial metabolism of carbohydrates producing d(−)-lactate directly or indirectly from l(+)-lactate through a dl-lactate racemase [42]. Not all microbes possess this ability (e.g., *B. lactis* strain BB12), but some *Lactobacillus* species do possess the racemase enzyme and, thus, can convert l(+)-lactate to d(−)-lactate [43]. Human cells metabolize and excrete d(−)-lactate poorly, with the very young newborn and neonate being at particular risk due to the lack of full renal excretory capability and decreased barrier function of the intestinal tract. When excessive build-up of d(−)-lactate occurs there is a metabolic acidosis, the clinical effects of which can be difficult to detect.

One study evaluated otherwise healthy infants and the safety of ingesting a probiotic capable of d(−)-lactate production. About 24 6-month-old infants were randomly selected from a larger group of subjects receiving 10^8 colony-forming units of *L. reuteri* strain ATCC 55730 since birth as part of a double blind, multicenter trial for the prevention of allergy. Comparison of blood levels of d(−)-lactate between those receiving placebo and the probiotic were similar at the 6-month time age of the infants [44].

Most patients reporting with d-lactic acidosis have been those with short gut syndrome, which occurs following mesenteric thrombosis, midgut volvulus, or Crohn's disease [45,46]. Other patients who have developed this problem include those who have undergone intestinal bypass surgery and patients with small-bowel bacterial overgrowth [45,46]. One common feature among these patients is excessive carbohydrate exposure to d(−)-lactate-producing bacteria. For patients developing d-lactic acidosis, recolonization with bacteria that are not d(−)-lactate producers has proven beneficial [47]. On the whole, administration of d(−)-lactate producing probiotics should be carefully considered in patients at risk of developing d-lactic acidosis, such as those with previous bowel surgery and subsequent short gut syndrome and in the very young newborn or neonate until appropriate safety data becomes available for specific probiotic strains.

Biogenic Amines

Biogenic amines (e.g., histamine, tyramine) are low-molecular weight organic molecules present in many foods and also produced in large quantities by microorganisms through the activity of amino acid decarboxylases. Ingestion of large quantities can be mistaken for allergic reactions as the signs and symptoms include facial flushing, sweating, rash, burning taste in the mouth, diarrhea and cramps with severe reactions including respiratory distress, swelling of the tongue and throat, and blurred vision [48]. One of the better-recognized presentations is that of ingestion of fish from the family *Scombridae* (e.g., tuna), although the accumulation of histamine and adverse events can be prevented through constant cool temperature control [48]. Although some species of *Lactobacilli* are capable of forming biogenic amines, there is great variability in this ability and the addition of probiotics organisms to foods must consider this ability [49,50]. In addition, hygienic procedures adopted during production of probiotic containing foods, availability of precursors, and physicochemical properties will be involved in the accumulation of the biogenic amines [51]. To date, there are no reported cases of such potentially harmful compounds found in fermented milk prepared with lactobacilli [11].

SPECIAL CONSIDERATIONS

Infants

Colonization patterns are determined by the mode of parturition, the environment (i.e., neonatal units, home deliveries), and whether the child is breast-fed or bottle-fed [52]. Among premature infants, the gut of the very low birth weight (VLBW) infant is colonized by less than three bacterial species at the tenth day of life, and common enteric species *Bifidobacterium* and *Lactobacillus* are found in only 5% infants at one month of age [53]. Generally speaking, probiotics have not been found to establish intestinal colonization for long periods of time [54]. However, exposure of younger infants may lead to long-term colonization. For instance, in a study evaluating the colonization of infants whose mothers' ingested *L. rhamnosus* strain GG during late pregnancy, but stopped at the time of delivery, all four vaginally delivered infants had the probiotic detectable in the stool for six months, three for one year, and in one infant until two years of age [55]. This finding suggests that the manipulation of the intestinal microbiome in the very young could have greater potential for alteration of health and potential for ameliorating disease as compared to the administration of the probiotics to older people with a more established microbiota. On the other hand, the finding also raises the possibility of long-term adverse unintended consequences.

The question of administration of probiotic products to neonates and young infants is driven by both short-term benefits, such as reducing the risk of necrotizing enterocolitis that might occur with the administration of probiotics to preterm infants [56], and other long-term benefits, such as the prevention of atopic eczema, which some investigators have reported [57]. Importantly, administration of probiotics to this age group has not caused increased rates of sepsis [56], but long-term consequences are still unknown. Rather than administering probiotics to neonates and young infants with alacrity and focusing only on the potential for benefit, there are calls by Pediatric Gastroenterology Organizations [58,59] for both short-term and long-term studies before probiotics are recommended as the standard of care. Concerns about potential for overstimulation of the inflammatory response and detrimental long-term effects related to autoimmunity, allergies, and atopy have been raised [60]. Although these remain speculative at this time, clearly additional and appropriate safety trials are needed.

Intestinal Disease

The intestinal mucosal barrier is effective in the compartmentalization of the various noxious substances, potentially deleterious and helpful commensal microbes from overwhelming access to the host. Breaks in the mucosal barrier may pose a threat to this function. Despite speculation of this potential threat, by and large, this does not appear to be a major risk factor on its own. For instance, active Crohn's disease [61] and ulcerative colitis [62–66] patients have been administered probiotics as the sole therapy without reports of sepsis. However, there are reports of patients with active inflammatory bowel disease who have developed sepsis with *Lactobacillus* species [67,68]. In these reports of patients with *Lactobacillus* sepsis, active disease was being treated with immunomodulators (i.e., prednisone, prednisone + cyclosporine), with even prednisone determined to be a mortality risk factor in inflammatory bowel disease [69]. Translocation of probiotics across inflamed intestinal mucosa has also been suspected in two cases of *L. rhamnosus* GG sepsis reported in infants with short gut syndrome [70].

Immunocompromised Patients

There is precedent for probiotic use in certain patient groups in this category of diseases. For instance, bacterial probiotics have been administered to patients with

Table 6.1
Proposed risk factors for probiotic sepsis (From [83])

Major risk factors
Immune compromise, including a debilitated state or malignancy
Premature infants
Minor risk factors
Central venous catheter
Impaired intestinal epithelial barrier, e.g., diarrheal illness, intestinal inflammation
Concomitant administration of broad spectrum antibiotics to which probiotic is resistant
Probiotics with properties of high mucosal adhesion or known pathogenicity
Cardiac valvular disease (*Lactobacillus* probiotics only)

The presence of a single major or more than one minor risk factor merits caution in using probiotics.

AIDS [71,72], cancer [73,74], and in the peri-operative period of patients undergoing organ transplantation [75] with rare reports of infections due to the probiotic agent being administered [22,23,76]. The use of yeast probiotics appears to be of greater risk with adverse event case reports in posttransplantation, HIV, during corticosteroid therapy, and in a child with leukemia [77–82]. It must be stressed that no minimum blood counts or immune parameters defining the safe administration of bacterial probiotics to immunocompromised patients are known.

CONCLUSION

Over the past decade, consumption of high numbers of concentrated probiotics for the prevention of treatment of medical conditions and for health maintenance has increased rapidly. It appears that for most organisms used as probiotics, ingestion in the human intestinal tract is safe. Patients that are very sick, those with chronic underlying diseases, and those who have artificial, implanted devices should be cautious in their use of certain *Lactobacillus* species and yeast probiotics.

There are no consensus guidelines defining safe parameters for the use of probiotics in special patient populations. However, Boyle and colleagues [83] have proposed a set of risk factors for probiotic sepsis (see Table 6.1). For those promoting probiotics and having a mandate for public safety, advocacy for regulations to ensure quality control of products, studies on efficacy, declaration of excipients in the production of the probiotics, and appropriate safety studies should all be encouraged. For those prescribing and supporting the use of probiotics for medical conditions, it would seem wise to counsel patients on the risks, much in the same manner as patients are currently counseled regarding side effects of pharmaceutical agents that require a prescription.

REFERENCES

1. Hooper LV, Wong MH, Thelin A, et al. Molecular analysis of commensal host–microbial relationships in the intestine. *Science* 2001:291:881–884.
2. Rakoff-Nahoum S, Paglino J, Eslami-Varzaneh F et al. Recognition of commensal microflora by toll-like receptors is required for intestinal homeostasis. *Cell* 2004:118:229–241.

3. Ley RE, Peterson DA, Gordon JI. Ecological and evolutionary forces shaping microbial diversity in the human intestine. *Cell* 2006;124:837–848.

4. Shen B, Brzezinski A, and Fazio VW, et al. Maintenance therapy with a probiotic in antibiotic-dependent pouchitis: experience in clinical practice. *Aliment Pharmacol Ther* 2005;22:721–728.

5. Tynkkynen S, Singh KV, Varmanen P. Vancomycin resistance factor of *Lactobacillus rhamnosus* GG in relation to enterococcal vancomycin resistance (van) genes. *Int J Food Microbiol* 1998;41:195–204.

6. Swenson JM, Facklam RR, Thornsberry C. Antimicrobial susceptibility of vancomycin-resistant *Leuconostoc, Pediococcus*, and *Lactobacillus* species. *Antimicrob Agents Chemother* 1990;34:543–549.

7. Klare I, Konstabel C, Werner G, et al. Antimicrobial susceptibilities of *Lactobacillus, Pediococcus* and *Lactococcus* human isolates and cultures intended for probiotic or nutritional use. *J Antimicrob Chemother* 2007;59:900–912.

8. Eaton TJ, Gasson MJ. Molecular screening of *Enterococcus* virulence determinants and potential for genetic exchange between food and medical isolates. *Appl Environ Microbiol* 2001;67:1628–1635.

9. Holzman D. Virulence factor transfers among the Enterococci suggest risk for probiotics. *ASM News* 2001;67:293–294.

10. Cannon JP, Lee TA, Bolanas JT, et al. Pathogenic relevance of *Lactobacillus*: a retrospective review of over 200 cases. *Eur J Clin Microbiol Infect Dis* 2005;24:31–40.

11. Bernardeau M, Guguen M, Vernoux JP. Beneficial lactobacilli in food and feed: long-term use, biodiversity and proposals for specific and realistic safety assessments. *FEMS Microbiol Rev* 2006;30:487–513.

12. Saxelin M, Chuang N-H, Chassy B, et al. Lactobacilli and bacteremia in southern Finland, 1989–1992. *Clin Infect Dis* 1996;22:564–566.

13. Gasser F. Safety of lactic acid bacteria and their occurrence in human clinical infections. *Bull Inst Pasteur* 1994;92:45–67.

14. Hammerman C, Bin-Nun A, Kaplan M. Safety of probiotics: comparison of two popular strains. *BMJ* 2006;333:1006–1008.

15. Salminen MK, Tynkkynen S, Rautelin H, et al. *Lactobacillus bacteremia* during a rapid increase in probiotic use of *Lactobacillus rhamnosus* GG in Finland. *Clin Infect Dis* 2002;35:1155–1160.

16. MacKay A, Taylor M, Kibbler C, et al. *Lactobacillus endocarditis* caused by a probiotic microorganism. *Clin Microbiol Infect* 1999;5:290–292.

17. Soleman N, Laferl H, Kneifel W, et al. How safe is safe? – A case of *Lactobacillus paracasei* sp. paracasei endocarditis and discussion of the safety of lactic acid bacteria. *Scand J Infect Dis* 2003;35:759–762.

18. Rautio M, Jousimies-Somer H, Kauma H, et al. Liver abscess due to a *Lactobacillus rhamnosus* strain indistinguishable from *L. rhamnosus* strain GG. *Clin Infect Dis* 1999;28:1159–1160.

19. Land MH, Rouster-Stevens K, Woods CR, et al. *Lactobacillus sepsis* associated with probiotic therapy. *Pediatrics* 2005;115:178–181.

20. Salminen MK, Rautelin H, Tynkkynen S, et al. *Lactobacillus bacteremia*, species identification, and antimicrobial susceptibility of 85 blood isolates. *Clin Infect Dis* 2006;42:e35–44.

21. Honeycutt TC, El Khashab M, Wardrop RM III, et al. Probiotic administration and the incidence of nosocomial infection in pediatric intensive care: a randomized placebo-controlled trial. *Pediatr Crit Care Med* 2007;8:452–458.

22. Richard V, Van der Auwera P, Snoeck R, et al. Nosocomial bacteremia caused by *Bacillus* species. *Eur J Clin Microbiol Infec Dis* 1988;7:783–785.

23. Oggioni MR, Pozzi G, Galieni P, et al. Recurrent septicemia in an immunocompromised patient due to probiotic strains of *Bacillus subtilis*. *J Clin Microbiol* 1998;36:325–326.

24. Czerucka D, Piche T, Rampal P. Review article: yeast as probiotics – *Saccharomyces boulardii*. *Aliment Pharmacol Ther* 2007;26:767–778.

25. Lherm T, Monet C, Nougiere B, et al. Seven cases of fungemia with *Saccharomyces boulardii* in critically ill patients. *Intensive Care Med* 2002;28:797–801.

26. Munoz P, Bouza E, Cuenca-Estrella M, et al. *Saccharomyces cerevisiae* fungemia: an emerging infectious disease. *Clin Infect Dis* 2005;40:1625–1634.

27. Book I. Isolation of non-sporing anaerobic rods from infections in children. *J Med Microbiol* 1996;45:21–26.

28. Hata D, Yoshida A, Ohkubo H, et al. Meningitis caused by Bifidobacterium in an infant. *Pediatr Infect Dis J* 1988;7:669–671.
29. Makelainen H, Tahvonen R, Salminen S, et al. In vivo safety assessment of two *Bifidobacterium longum* strains. *Microbiol Immunol* 2003;47:911–914.
30. Saavedra JM, Abi-Hanna A, Moore N, et al. Long-term consumption of infant formulas containing live probiotic bacteria: tolerance and safety. *Am J Clin Nutr* 2004;79:261–267.
31. Weizman Z, Asli G, Alsheikh A. Effect of a probiotic infant formula on infections in child case centers: comparison of two probiotic agents. *Pediatrics* 2005;115:5–9.
32. Puccio G, Cajozzo C, Meli F, et al. Clinical evaluation of a new starter formula for infants containing live *Bifidobacterium longum* BL999 and probiotics. *Nutrition* 2007;23:1–8.
33. Yan F, Polk DB. Probiotic bacterium prevents cytokine-induced apoptosis in intestinal epithelial cells. *J Biol Chem* 2002;277:50959–50965.
34. Olah A, Belagyi T, Issekutz A, et al. Randomize clinical trial of specific Lactobacillus and fibre supplement to early enteral nutrition in patients with acute pancreatitis. *Br J Surg* 2002;89:1103–1107.
35. Rayes N, Seehofer D, Hansen S, et al. Early enteral supply of lactobacillus and fiber versus selective bowel decontamination: a controlled trial in liver transplant recipients. *Transplantation* 2002;74:123–127.
36. Kirjavainen PV, Salminen SJ, Isolauri E. Probiotic bacteria in the management of atopic disease: underscoring the importance of viability. *J Pediatr Gastroenterol Nutr* 2003;36:223–227.
37. Sharieff W, Bhutta Z, Schauer C, et al. Micronutrients (including zinc) reduce diarrhoea in children: The Pakistan Sprinkles Diarrhoea Study. *Arch Dis Child* 2006;91:573–579.
38. Hoa NT, Baccigalupi L, Huxham A, et al. Characterization of Bacillus species used for oral bacteriotherapy and bacterioprophylaxis of gastrointestinal disorders. *Appl Environ Microbiol* 2001;67:3819–3823.
39. Coeuret V, Gueguen M, Vernoux JP. Numbers and strains of Lactobacilli in some probiotic products. *Int J Food Microbiol* 2004;97:147–156.
40. Milazzo I, Speciale A, Masmeci R, et al. Identification and antibiotic susceptibility of bacterial isolates from probiotic products available in Italy. *New Microbiol* 2006;29:281–291.
41. Lee TT, Morisset M, Astier C, et al. Contamination of probiotic preparations with milk allergens can cause anaphylaxis in children with cow milk allergy. *J Allergy Clin Immunol* 2007;119:746–747.
42. Mack DR. d(−)-lactic acid producing probiotics, d (−)-lactic acidosis and infants. *Can J Gastroenterol* 2004;18:671–675.
43. Hove H, Mortensen PB. Colonic lactate metabolism and d-lactic acidosis. *Dig Dis Sci* 1995;40:320–30.
44. Connolly E, Abrahamsson T, Bjorksten B. Safety of d(−)-lactic acid producing bacteria in the human infant. *J Pediatr Gastroenterol Nutr* 2005;41:489–492.
45. Uribarri J, Oh MS, Carroll HJ. d-lactic acidosis. A review of clinical presentation, biochemical features, and pathophysiologic mechanisms. *Medicine (Baltimore)* 1998;77:73–82.
46. Hove H. Lactate and short chain fatty acid production in the human colon: implications for d-lactic acidosis, short-bowel syndrome, antibiotic-associated diarrhoea, colonic cancer, and inflammatory bowel disease. *Danish Med Bull* 1998;45:15–33.
47. Uchida H, Yamamoto H, Kisaki Y et al. d-lactic acidosis in short bowel syndrome managed with antibiotics and probiotics. *J Pediatr Surg* 2004;39:634–636.
48. Scomboid fish poisoning associated with tuna steaks – Louisiana and Tennessee, 2006. MMWR 2007;56:817-819.
49. Straub BW, Kicherer M, Schilcher SM, et al. The formation of biogenic amines by fermentation organisms. *Z Lebensm Unters Forssch* 1995;201:79–82.
50. Pessione E, Mazzoli R, Guiffrida MG, et al. A proteomic approach to studying biogenic amine producing lactic acid bacteria. *Proteomics* 2005;5:687–698.
51. Suzzi G, Gardini F. Biogenic amines in dry fermented sausages: a review. *Int J Food Microbiol* 2003;15:41–54.
52. Fanaro S, Chierici R, Guerrini P, et al. Intestinal microflora in early infancy: composition and development. *Acta Pediatr Suppl* 2003;91:48–55.
53. Gewolb IH, Schwalbe RS, Taciak VL, et al. Stool microflora in extremely low birthweight infants. *Arch Dis Child Fetal Neonatal Ed* 1999;80:F167–F173.

54. Favier CF, Vaughan EE, De Vos WM, et al. Molecular succession of bacterial communities in human neonates. *Appl Environ Microbiol* 2002;68:219–226.
55. Schultz M, Gottl C, Young RJ, et al. Administration of oral probiotic bacteria to pregnant women causes temporary infantile colonization. *J Pediatr Gastroenterol Nutr* 2004;38:293–297.
56. Deshpande G, Rao S, Patole S. Probiotics for prevention of necrotizing enterocolitis in preterm neonates with very low birthweight: a systematic review of randomized controlled trials. *Lancet* 2007;369: 1614–1620.
57. Kalliomaki M, Salminen S, Poussa T, et al. Probiotics and prevention of atopic disease: 4-year follow-up of a randomized placebo-controlled trial. *Lancet* 2003;361:1869–1871.
58. Agostoni A, Axelson I, Goulet O, et al. Probiotic bacteria in dietetic products for infants: a commentary by the ESPGHAN Committee on Nutrition. *J Pediatr Gastroenterol Nutr* 2004;39:365–374.
59. NASPGHAN Nutrition Report Committee. Michail S, Sylvester F, Fuchs G, Issenman R. Clinical efficacy of probiotics: review of evidence with focus on children. J Pediatr Gastroenterol Nutr 2006;43:550–557.
60. Neu J. Perinatal and neonatal manipulation of the intestinal microbiome: a note of caution. *Nutr Rev* 2007;65:282–285.
61. Fujimori S, Tatuguchi A, Gudis T, et al. High dose probiotic and prebiotic cotherapy for remission induction of active Crohn's disease. *J Gastroenterol Hepatol* 2007;22:1199–1204.
62. Kato K, Mizuno S, Umesaki Y, et al. Randomized placebo-controlled trial assessing the effect of bifidobacteria-fermented milk on active ulcerative colitis. *Aliment Pharmacol Ther* 2004;20:1133–1141.
63. Bibiloni R, Fedorak RN, Tannock GW, et al. VSL#3 probiotic-mixture induces remission in patients with active ulcerative colitis. *Am J Gastroenterol* 2005;100:1539–1546.
64. Guslandi M, Giollo P, Testoni PA. A pilot trial of *Saccharomyces boulardii* in ulcerative colitis. *Eur J Gastroenterol Hepatol* 2003;15:697–698.
65. Furrie E, Macfarlane S, Kennedy A, et al. Synbiotic therapy (*Bifidobacterium longum*/Synergy 1) initiates resolution of inflammation in patients with active ulcerative colitis: a randomized controlled pilot trial. *Gut* 2005;54:242–249.
66. Tursi A, Brandimarte G, Giorgetti GM, et al. Low-dose balsalazide plus a high-potency probiotic preparation is more effective than balsalazide alone or mesalazine in the treatment of acute-mild-to-moderate ulcerative colitis. *Med Sci Monit* 2004;10:Pl126–Pl131.
67. Cukovic-Cavka S, Likic R, Francetic I, et al. *Lactobacillus acidophilus* as a cause of liver abscess in a NOD2/CARD15-positive patient with Crohn's disease. *Digestion* 2006;73:107–110.
68. Farina C, Arosio M, Mangia M. *Lactobacillus casei* subsp rhamnosus sepsis in a patient with ulcerative colitis. *Clin Gastroenterol* 2001;33:251–252.
69. Lichtenstein GR, Feagan BG, Cohen RD, et al. Serious infections and mortality in association with therapies for Crohn's disease: TREAT registry. *Clin Gastroenterol Hepatol* 2006;4:621–630.
70. Kunz AN, Noel JM, Fairchok MP. Two cases of *Lactobacillus bacteremia* during probiotic treatment of short gut syndrome. *J Pediatr Gastroenterol Nutr* 2004;38:457–458.
71. Cunningham-Rundles S, Ahrne S, Bengmark S. Probiotics and immune response. *Am J Gastroenterol* 2000;95:S22–S25.
72. Salminen MK, Tynkkynen S, Rautelin H, et al. The efficacy and safety of probiotic *Lactobacillus rhamnosus* GG on prolonged, noninfectious diarrhea in HIV patients on antiretroviral therapy: a randomized, placebo-controlled, crossover study. *HIV Clin Trials* 2004;5:183–191.
73. Benchimol EI, Mack DR. Probiotics in relapsing and chronic diarrhea. *J Pediatr Hematol Oncol* 2004;26:515–517.
74. Urbancsek H, Kazar T, Mezes I, et al. Results of a double-blind, randomized study to evaluate the efficacy and safety of *Acidophilus* in patients with radiation-induced diarrhea. *Eur J Gastroenterol Hepatol* 2001;13:391–396.
75. Rayes N, Seehofer D, Theruvath T, et al. Supply of pre- and probiotics reduces bacterial infection rates after liver transplantation-a double-blind trial. *Am J Transplant* 2005;5:125–130.
76. LeDoux D, LaBombardi VJ, Karter D. *Lactobacillus acidophilus* bacteremia after use of a probiotic in a patient with AIDS and Hodgkin's disease. *Int J STD AIDS* 2006;17:280–282.
77. Riquelme AJ, Calvo MA, Guzman AM, et al. *Saccharomyces cerevisiae* fungemia after *Saccharomyces boulardii* treatment in immunocompromised patients. *J Clin Gastroenterol* 2003;36:41–43.

78. Lestin F, Pertschy A, Rimek D. Fungemia after oral treatment with *Saccharomyces boulardii* in a patient with multiple co-morbidities. *Dtsch Med Wochenschr* 2003;128:2531–2533.

79. Bassetti S, Frei R, Zimmerli W. Fungemia with *Saccharomyces cerevisiae* after treatment with *Saccharomyces boulardii*. *Am J Med* 1998;105:71–72.

80. Fredenucci I, Chomarat M, Boucaud C, et al. *Saccharomyces boulardii* fungemia in a patient receiving ultra levure therapy. *Clin Infect Dis* 1998;27:222–223.

81. Zunic P, Lacotte J, Pegoix M, et al. *Saccharomyces boulardii* fungemia. A propos of a case. *Therapie* 1991;46:498–499.

82. Cesaro S, Chinello P, Rossi L, et al. *Saccharomyces cerevisiae* fungemia in a neutropenic patient treated with *Saccharomyces boulardii*. *Support Care Cancer* 2000;8:504–505.

83. Boyle RJ, Robins-Browne RM, Tang MLK. Probiotic use in clinical practice: what are the risks. *Am J Clin Nutr* 2006;83:1256–1264.

Section B
Probiotics and Infants

7 Neonatal and Infant Microflora

Josef Neu

Key Points

- The intestine of the newborn is sterile at birth, but it is rapidly colonized with microorganisms from maternal and environmental sources.
- Intestinal microbiota has a profound effect on the individual's nutrition and development of the gastrointestinal tract, and in the maintenance of the integrity of the mucosal surface.
- Establishment of normal microflora is important for physiologic, nutritional, and immune development.
- Perturbations of the intestinal ecosystem, especially during early development, may have consequences that extend well beyond the neonatal period.

Key Words: Necrotizing enterocolitis, probiotics, premature infants, preterm, neonates.

INTRODUCTION

Symbiosis between bacteria and multicellular organisms through the millennia has been a prominent feature of life on earth, with perturbations in one affecting the physiology and even the genetics and evolution of the other. In humans, the microbiota of the adult is found primarily in the colon and distal small intestine and exceeds the total number of somatic and germ cells by at least an order of magnitude. The number of different microbial species residing in the intestine is estimated to be between 500 and 1000, with most being unculturable. The number of microbial genes (the microbiome) may exceed the total number of human genes by a factor of 100.[1] For the most part this is a mutually beneficial relationship, as evidenced by the important role commensal bacteria play in nutrition,[2] angiogenesis,[3] and mucosal immunity.[4,5] This chapter is intended to present various aspects of neonatal intestinal microbial colonization, the effects of microbes on the development of the gastrointestinal (GI) tract, the role of early microflora and its manipulation on short-term and later disease development, and the role and mechanisms of probiotics and their related agents on short- and long-term health.

From: *Nutrition and Health: Probiotics in Pediatric Medicine*
Edited by: S. Michail and P.M. Sherman © Humana Press, Totowa, NJ

COLONIZATION OF THE NEONATAL INTESTINE

Normal Colonization

In contrast to the adult, the intestine of the newborn is sterile at birth, but it is rapidly colonized (in less than 24 h)[6] with microorganisms from maternal and environmental sources. Bacteria from the mother, then obligate anaerobes, and later, the Bifidobacterium and Bacteroides become established in the GI tract.[7] Newborns fed with formula will have a predominance of Bacteroides with some Bifidobacterium. In full-term infants a diet of breast milk induces the development of a flora rich in *Bifidobacterium* spp.[8] Facultative anaerobes (such as Streptococci and Coliforms) decline during the weaning period as obligate anaerobes such as Bacteroides establish a foothold, eventually becoming the predominant community residing in the intestine. Recent studies utilizing molecular techniques for phylogenetic analysis show that microbial diversity changes very rapidly in the few days after birth, the acquisition of unculturable bacteria expanding rapidly after the third day, underlining the importance of nonculture-based techniques for analysis.[9]

Bacterial colonization of preterm infants differs from that of healthy full-term infants because of the methods of neonatal care. Recent studies suggest that Bifidobacterial colonization is different in preterm versus term infants.[10] It appears that sufficient gut maturity is critical for Bifidobacterial implantation and prematurity delays this implantation. Bifidobacterial implantation occurs after a corrected gestational age of approximately 34 weeks. Bifidobacteria appear to have beneficial effects and inhibit certain pathogens. Whether this delay plays a role in diseases such as necrotizing enterocolitis (NEC) remains speculative and whether any individual-specific pattern of colonization in preterm infants relates to pathology remains to be determined.

Pathogenic Colonization

The potentially hostile microbial environment of the neonatal intensive care unit (NICU) can be reflected in the pathogenic colonization[9] of the infant's mucosal surfaces, the largest and the most susceptible of which is the GI tract. Widespread prophylaxis with antibiotics (Ampicillin being the most commonly used), exposure to waterborne microbes in NICU hardware, parenteral nutrition, and feeding in incubators or under radiant warmers, may delay or impair colonization with normal nonpathogenic microbes. Antibiotics are commonly used shortly after birth in premature infants because the etiology of respiratory distress cannot be immediately determined (it could be bacterial pneumonia) and the cause of premature labor might be due to infection. The effect of this widespread practice on the microbial ecology and the developing GI tract is unknown, but recent studies in neonatal rodents demonstrate that the use of the ampicillin-like antibiotic, clomoxyl, noticeably alters the GI tract developmental gene expression and intestinal barrier transcriptome.[11] Studies in rodents demonstrate increased susceptibility of the GI tract to chemical-induced damage after decolonization with antibiotics.[12] The short- and long-term effects of these alterations in the GI microbiota with antibiotics should be the subject of intense research because their implications may be pertinent throughout the lifetime of the individual and will be addressed in greater detail at the end of this chapter.

PHYSIOLOGIC, NUTRITIONAL, AND IMMUNE RELEVANCE OF ESTABLISHMENT OF NORMAL MICROFLORA

Physiologic Relevance

Profound physiological changes occur in the intestinal ecosystem during early development. An example of such a change that normally occurs is in the angiogenins—potent antimicrobial peptides released from the Paneth cells of the crypt.[3] Commensal bacterial, through "cross talk," are critical for Paneth cell production of angiogenins. In mice raised in a conventional environment, angiogenin mRNA expression is markedly increased at the time of weaning from mother's milk to an adult diet. This change occurs to a much lesser degree in germ-free mice.[3] It is also thought that commensal bacteria influence normal villus development. One dramatic example is seen in the growth of the villus capillaries in the rodent small intestine grown in a germ-free environment versus normal growth in an environment containing normal mixed biota or even in only one species of commensal bacterium (*Bacteroides thetaiotaomicron*).[5]

Nutritional Relevance

We are in the early stages of understanding the importance of bacteria in providing nutrients to the host. One example of this beneficial relationship is the fermentative salvage of unabsorbed lactose[13] in the distal intestine in premature babies (which have low lactase activity). The end-products of this pathway are short-chain fatty acids such as acetate, propionate, and butyrate.[14] These can alter intestinal interepithelial tight junctions [8], stimulate intestinal blood flow, affect intestinal proliferation and differentiation, and can be utilized for energy or synthetic processes [6]. Other beneficial nutritional effects of commensal bacteria include lipid hydrolysis, protein breakdown into small peptides and amino acids, and vitamin production[6]

Immunologic Relevance

The lumen of the GI tract is normally filled with an array of organisms that are separated from the highly immunoreactive subepithelium and internal milieu by only a single layer of epithelial cells and a layer of protective mucus. The constantly produced mucus is made up of glycoproteins and offer many attachment sites for the commensal bacteria.[15] Therefore, in normal circumstances, the bacteria stay on the surface of the mucus at the entrance of the villi (not in the crypts) and do not adhere to the intestinal cells. A genetically coded repertoire (or "innate repertoire") of potential mucin adhesion sites for the bacteria generates a highly individualized colonization process. Furthermore, inside the gastrointestinal ecosystem, bacteria are able to communicate with their environment and with other bacteria by the process known as "quorum sensing."[16] This interaction leads to the defense against colonization by new external strains of bacteria. Interplay between the attachability of microbes that the intestine is exposed to in early life as well as the nutrient intake (especially mothers milk) is likely to play an important role that provides attachment sites and stimulates their development.

MICROBES IN HUMAN MILK: WHAT IS THEIR SIGNIFICANCE?

Human breast milk is known to contain lactic acid bacteria that may have beneficial effects on the neonatal GI tract.[17,18] The fact that breast milk is not sterile, even when collected aseptically, suggests that breast milk may influence neonatal colonization as well as intestinal function. A recent study[19] demonstrated that aseptically collected breast milk samples contain a total concentration of microbes of $<10^3$ colony forming units per milliliter. While the origin of these bacteria may be debated, these bacteria may originate from the mother's skin or the infant's mouth; the presence of microbes in all the samples studied support that a discrete micriobiota is found in breast milk. In addition, this study demonstrated microbial DNA in breast milk, which along with bacteria are thought to be transported to the mother's breast from her GI tract after bacterial translocation through her intestinal mucosa and subsequent uptake by mononuclear cells. Whether the microbial DNA actually plays a role that is similar to live microbes with attachment of and stimulus of toll-like receptors in intestinal cells is debatable. The physiologic relevance of this potentially exciting finding requires additional elucidation.

NEONATAL INTESTINE DERIVED SYSTEMIC INFLAMMATORY RESPONSE SYNDROME (SIRS)

The intestinal microbiota has a profound effect on the individual's nutrition and development of the gastrointestinal tract, and in the maintenance of the integrity of the mucosal surface.[20] Breakdown of this barrier is a well-known cause of SIRS, which can ultimately lead to multiple organ dysfunction syndrome[11,12]. We are also beginning to appreciate why some microorganisms secrete products that cause damage under certain conditions, while others actually offer protection [14,15,16,17]. On the basis of the profound immunoreactivity of the gastrointestinal submucosa and liver, along with the exquisite vulnerability of the neonatal intestinal surface to translocation of inflammatory agents, it is likely that the intestinal microbiota play a critical role in the prevention and pathogenesis of not only neonatal intestinal diseases such as NEC but also liver failure, chronic lung disease, and central nervous problems such as periventricular leukomalacia, which have all been associated with systemic inflammation. [21,22,23] Figure 7.1 provides a conceptual framework of how disruption of the intestinal microbial environment might lead to mucosal disruption. Increased permeability at the interepithelial junctions is caused by microbial toxins, and this leads to subsequent overproduction of proinflammatory mediators with a systemic inflammatory response. The end-result can be injury not only to the intestine but also to distal organs such as the liver, lung, and brain.

ROLE OF PROBIOTICS

There is considerable information emerging about the potential benefit of probiotics. Probiotics appear to affect the development of NEC in high-risk premature infants (reviewed in more detail in Chapter 9). Furthermore, their use in the perinatal and early neonatal period also appears to affect later development of autoimmune and allergic diseases. Here, we will review some of these actions of probiotics.

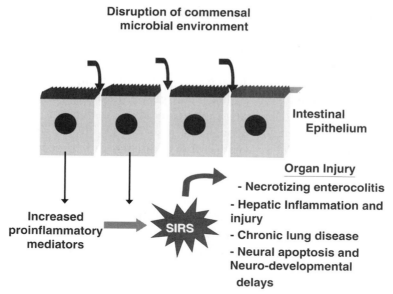

Fig. 7.1. A conceptual framework of how disruption of the intestinal microbial environment might lead to mucosal disruption.

NECROTIZING ENTEROCOLITIS (NEC)

NEC is the most common severe clinical gastrointestinal emergency that affects primarily newborns. In the newborn, heterogeneity of NEC exists. Compared to preterms, NEC in term and late preterm infants has a greater association with other predisposing factors such as low APGAR scores, chorioamnionitis, exchange transfusions, prolonged rupture of membranes, congenital heart disease, and neural tube defects.[24] Another entity (sometimes confused with NEC), spontaneous intestinal perforations, frequently is not accompanied by significant intestinal necrosis, occurs earlier than NEC, and is associated with the use of glucocorticoids and indomethacin, but probably not enteral feeding.[25,26]

The more classic form of NEC occurs most commonly in infants less than 32 weeks gestation, presents after the first week after birth, has been associated with aggressive enteral feeding, and does not appear to be associated with primary hypoxia-ischemia (such as might be seen in babies with low apgar scores).The incidence of NEC is inversely proportional to the gestational age, with 90% cases occurring in premature babies. The incidence is clearly related with prematurity with a sharp decrease in incidence around 35–36 weeks of GA or weight >1500 g.

The pathogenesis of NEC remains enigmatic, but immaturity of the gastrointestinal tract and colonization with microbes associated with an inflammatory response appear to be involved in the pathophysiologic cascade of this disease.[27] The development of innate and adaptive immune systems of human premature infants as related to the pathogenesis of NEC remains largely unexplored. However, recent evidence supports several aspects of innate immunity to be involved. One of the first lines of defense against ingested pathogens and toxins is luminal digestion in the stomach and duodenum. Immature physiochemical luminal factors include a lower hydrogen ion output in the stomach[28] and low pancreatic proteolytic enzyme activity.[29] A relatively low enterokinase activity and subsequent low tryptic activity is likely to suppress the hydrolysis of toxins that have the ability to damage the intestine. Thus, immature luminal digestion can predispose to entry of pathogens from the environment and allow colonization by pathogens in the distal gastrointestinal tract. In fact, recent studies suggest that further decreasing the already low acid output of the stomach by use of H2 blockers in premature neonates is associated with a higher incidence of NEC.[30] It remains speculative whether this is directly due to decreased pathogen entry via the upper GI tract or other chemical changes in the intestinal lumen secondary to altered acidity.

The motility of the small intestine in premature infants is considerably less organized than that in term infants.[31] This is caused by an intrinsic immaturity of the enteric nervous system that delays transit, causing subsequent bacterial overgrowth and distension from gases that are the byproducts of fermentation. It is likely that this immature motility contributes to the milieu in which the interaction of nutrients, immature host defenses, increased intraluminal pressure, and other factors initiate the cascade of events including transgression of microbes or their toxic products through an immature intestinal mucosal barrier, which eventually culminates in an inflammatory cascade leading to NEC.[32,33,34] Immature neonates have higher intestinal permeability than older children and adults.[35] Preterm infants born at less than 33 weeks of gestation have higher serum concentrations of β-lactoglobulin than term infants given equivalent milk feedings.[36] The permeability of the preterm human intestine to intact carbohydrate markers such as lactulose also exhibits a developmental pattern of increased permeability with maturation.[35] Little is currently known about the maturation in human infants of tight junction proteins such as occludin and claudins, which constitute the major paracellular barrier of the epithelium.[37]

Similar to sepsis and adult respiratory stress syndrome, NEC seems to involve a final common pathway that includes the endogenous production of inflammatory mediators involved in the development of intestinal injury.[38] Endotoxin lipopolysaccharide (LPS), platelet-activating factor (PAF), tumor necrosis factor (TNF), and other cytokines together with prostaglandins and leukotrienes and nitric oxide are thought to be involved in the final common pathway of NEC pathogenesis.[32,38]

Preterm human infants randomly assigned to receive a daily feeding supplement of a probiotic mixture (*Bifidobacteria infantis*, *Streptococcus thermophilus*, and *Bifidobacteria bifidus* in one study, and *Lactobacillus acidophilus* and *Bifidobacterium infantis* in another) had a relative risk reduction in mortality, incidence of NEC, and late onset of sepsis.[39,40] In a large multicenter trial conducted in 12 Italian NICUs on 565 patients, a statistically significant beneficial effect of probiotic (*Lactobacillus* GG) on NEC was not elicited.[41] Whether the differences in outcomes in these studies are associated with the use of different probiotic preparations, a different baseline incidence of NEC in the different NICUs, or other factors such as breast milk feeding remain speculative. These studies are summarized in Table 7.1.

Table 7.1.
Randomized Studies of Probiotics and NEC

Author and journal reference	Patient population	Major outcome
Dani, C. *Biology of the Neonate* 2002;82:103–108	Probiotic group = 295 patients; placebo group = 290 patients; gestational age <33 weeks or <1500 g birth weight	Four cases of NEC in probiotic group and eight in placebo (1.4 vs. 2.8%). Only results after 7 days of probiotics were included in the analysis
Lin, H. *Pediatrics* Jan 2005;115(1):1–4	Probiotic group = 180 patients and control 187 patients: <1,500 gm surviving beyond the seventh day after birth	NEC in probiotic group = 2/180 (1.1%) and = 10/187 in control group (5.3%) ($p = 0.04$)
Bin-Nun, A. *Journal of Pediatrics* 2005 (Aug);147(2):192–196	Probiotic group = 72, control group = 73	NEC = 3/72 (4%) in probiotic group and 12/73 (16.4%) in control group ($p = 0.03$)

ILLNESSES MANIFESTED IN LATER CHILDHOOD

The attention given to microbes as causative agents of disease has overshadowed their potentially beneficial roles, especially those of the commensal intestinal microbiota. Figure 7.2 depicts pediatric diseases whose pathogenesis has been related to abnormal intestinal colonization. The escalating use of antibiotics during infancy as well as the mounting antibiotic load in our food supply has likely altered the intestinal microenvironment over the past half century, especially in developed countries where marked increases in autoimmune, allergic, and atopic diseases have emerged over the same time period.[42] Antibiotic usage during infancy has been linked with the pathogenesis of asthma,[43] allergies,[44] atopy,[45] and Type 1 diabetes,[46,47] but clear cause-and-effect relationships are yet to be established.

TYPE 1 DIABETES

The dramatic increase in Type 1 diabetes over the past 50 years especially in countries with relatively high per capita incomes and clean hygienic conditions and where antibiotics are readily available suggests an environmental role.[48] The GI tract, in addition to being the digestive–absorptive organ, is also the largest immune organ of the body. Its massive surface provides the greatest potential for interaction between the external and internal milieus. Approximately 30 years ago, an attempt to raise infant rats under germ-free conditions resulted in the serendipitous generation of rats that had the propensity to develop diabetes associated with insulitis caused by autoimmunity (Presentation by Clifford Chappel and Errol Marliss at the BB rat meeting Ottawa, Canada December 2004). Such was the genesis of the biobreeding (BB) rat. Studies have verified that the BB rat, prior to the onset of diabetes, exhibits a highly permeable intestine associated

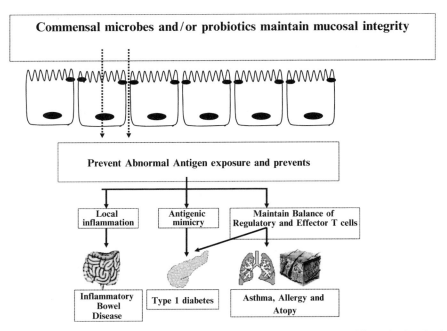

Fig. 7.2. Pediatric diseases whose pathogenesis has been related to abnormal intestinal colonization.

with low levels of intestinal claudin, a major intercellular tight junction protein.[49] Intestinal myeloperoxidase activities and goblet cell density are also higher in the diabetes-prone rats than in the controls, supporting an early intestinal inflammatory response. Likewise in humans, data supports that humans with a propensity to develop Type 1 diabetes as well as other autoimmune diseases have an abnormal intestinal barrier: they have the so-called leaky gut.[49, 50, 51]Similar to studies in the BB rat, a recent report evaluating jejunal biopsy samples from children with Type 1 diabetes demonstrated several signs of enhanced intestinal immune activation associated with interepithelial junction abnormalities seen on electron microscopy, which is entirely consistent with a "leaky intestine" allowing greater exposure of the intestinal immune system to antigens. The role of early antibiotics (in prevention or causation)[46,47] and probiotics (in prevention)[52] are becoming exciting areas of research interest.

ATOPIC ECZEMA

Studies showing probiotic administration to mothers and infants around the time of birth resulting in lower atopic eczema when they are older[53] support the concept that maintenance of a "friendly" intestinal microenvironment improves later tolerance. The administration of probiotics in these infants is also associated in infancy with a higher plasma antiinflammatory IL-10 concentration.[53] Of note is that in studies following these patients for several years, a borderline nearly statistically significant increase in allergic rhinitis and asthma was detected in the group receiving the probiotics. In the 7-year follow-up, the cumulative risk for developing eczema during the first 7 years of life was significantly lower in the Lactobacillus GG group than in the placebo group (42.6% vs. 66.1%; RR, 0.64; 95% CI, 0.45–0.92). There were 17 of 116 (15%) cases of allergic rhinitis (6 cases in the placebo and 12 cases in the Lactobacillus GG group; RR, 2.30; 95% CI, 0.93–5.70) and 12 of 116 (10%) cases of asthma (3 cases in the placebo and 9 cases in the Lactobacillus GG group; RR, 3.44; 95% CI, 0.98–12.1) at 7 years of age.[54] Thus, the long-term beneficial effect of probiotics remains unclear and additional studies are needed to determine their long-term safety and efficacy.

MECHANISMS OF PROBIOTIC ACTION: TOLL RECEPTORS

The mechanisms of how probiotics (live, inactivated, or their products, e.g., TLR ligands) might prevent intestinal as well as nonintestinal pathology remain an area of intense recent investigation. Microbial components that are TLR receptor ligands have been demonstrated to be protective if given prior to administration of agents that are injurious to the intestine.[12,55,56] Inactivated probiotic bacteria or their products may provide similar beneficial effects to live bacteria.[49,57] Because premature infants have poor intestinal motility, they are susceptible to intestinal bacterial overgrowth resulting in higher than desired stimuli or perhaps even translocation, sepsis, and long-term complications in the host. Inactivated probiotic bacteria and their components (cell walls, DNA, culture medium extracts, or TLR ligands) may provide an exciting and potentially safer alternative because the dose of these agents can be readily controlled in these highly susceptible babies.

Studies of the interaction between resident microbiota and toll-like receptors (TLRs) are beginning to shed light on how the healthy intestinal surface defuses the threat of commensal bacteria in the lumen, and how this interaction is actually required to maintain the architectural integrity of the epithelium. One study reported nonvirulent Salmonella strains whose direct interaction with model human epithelia attenuate IL-8 production elicited by various proinflammatory stimuli.[58] The mechanisms were found to be through abrogation of polyubiquitination of IκBα degradation.[58]

Commensal bacteria secrete molecules such as LPS and lipoteichoic acid, which in turn interact in the normal intestine with a population of surface TLRs. The resultant ongoing signaling, when provided at apparently low doses, paradoxically enhances the ability of the epithelial surface to withstand chemical or inflammatory mediator induced injury while also priming the surface for enhanced repair responses.[12,59] Therefore, either the disruption of TLR signaling or the removal of TLR ligands (derived from intestinal microorganisms) compromises the ability of the intestinal surface to protect and repair itself in the face of inflammatory or infectious insult.[12,59,60] These studies and especially the recent finding that LPS can induce tolerance to cytokine (IL-1β and TNFα) mediated IL-8 production in human adult and fetal intestinal epithelium[59] raises the question whether LPS exposure (or other TLR ligand) provided at low doses might actually offer a paradoxical protection for the highly vulnerable neonatal intestine.

MECHANISMS OF PROBIOTIC ACTION: THE "OLD FRIENDS" HYPOTHESIS

The intestinal epithelium must discriminate between pathogenic and nonpathogenic organisms as well as food antigens. It must "tolerate" the commensal flora present in the lumen and maintain mucosal homeostasis by controlled inflammatory responses, as well as sensing danger signals of potentially harmful pathogens so that appropriate immune responses of the underlying lamina propria are activated. The "old friends" hypothesis states that the presence of normal microbes ("old friends") stimulates a low-grade upregulation of T-regulatory cells that produce IL-10 and TGFß, which in turn diminishes the effects of proinflammatory processes.[61] In addition to decreasing a response that would eliminate the "old friends," this regulatory response also maintains tolerance to "self." This is likely to be one of the critical mechanisms underlying the benefits of maintaining GI commensal microorganisms as well as the supplementation with probiotics. Maintaining a strong relationship between the "old friends" and the human host GI tract may thus be the basis of prevention of several of the aforementioned diseases.

MECHANISMS OF PROBIOTIC ACTION: TOLERANCE AND CD4+ CD25+ REGULATORY T CELLS

Central to tolerance is a class of the so-called regulatory T cells (Treg), a class of lymphocytes that diminish immune responses. These are defined by their coexpression of CD4 and CD25 molecules (CD4+ CD25+). Those exhibiting the Forkhead P3 (FoxP3) transcription factor and associated cytokines (e.g., TGFß)[62,63,64] are especially active. Recently, reports have demonstrated that FoxP3 is expressed specifically by CD4 + CD25 + Treg cells.[65] It has been proposed that a progressive decline in the percentage of FoxP3 positive and hence most actively TGF-β producing CD4+ CD25+ Treg cells contributes to the development of insulitis in NOD female mice. During the prediabetic stage, a balance between pathogenic T cells and CD4+ CD25+ Treg cells that reside in the pancreatic lymph nodes and islets is maintained. However, as FoxP3 and TGFß positive expressing T cells decline within the pool of CD4+ CD25+ Treg cells, a minimum threshold is surpassed and pathogenic β-cell specific T effectors are permitted to expand and drive the response to an overt diabetic state.[66]

Several studies have demonstrated a relationship between a lack of CD4+ CD25+ cells in the intestine and the development of inflammatory bowel disease,[67,68,69] possibly related to changes in the normal microbiota, as described above. However, most of the currently available studies only provide circumstantial evidence of a conjunction between the GI microbiota to the Treg/Teff balance and Type 1 diabetes.

Thus, the intestinal microbiome interacts closely with the innate and adaptive immune system representing a largely unexplored area, especially during early life, which is likely to yield important new information for the prevention and treatment of diseases that manifest in not only the neonatal period and infancy but also well into childhood and adult life.

CAVEATS TO THE MANIPULATION OF THE INTESTINAL MICROBIOME IN EARLY INFANCY

Antibiotics

Antibiotics are increasingly prescribed in both the antenatal and neonatal periods. Used antenatally, their effective use reduces the incidence of life-threatening infections, such as group B streptococcal septicemia in the newborn.[70] In the NICU, widespread use of antibiotics, parenteral nutrition, and feeding in incubators and radiant warmers, may also delay or impair their colonization process. The all too common use of preemptive antibiotics in premature infants is empiric and based on traditional dogma rather than on scientific evidence.

Although the emergence of resistant strains and short-term pathology related to infection by these resistant strains is a concern, there is a paucity of studies of long-term outcome. The organisms initially colonizing the gut at birth may establish chronic persistence in many children, in contrast to effective and prompt clearance if encountered in later infancy, childhood, or adulthood. This is supported by studies showing that probiotic bacteria administered after 6 months to human infants have very limited persistence,[71] whereas those given perinatally have been shown to persist in some infants for months or years.[72,73]

Individual members of the gut flora specifically induce gene activation within the host, modulate mucosal and systemic immune function, and likely have an additional impact on metabolic programming during this highly vulnerable period.[4,74] Recent studies in neonatal rodents demonstrate that the use of the ampicillin-like antibiotic, clomoxyl, noticeably alters the GI tract developmental gene expression and intestinal barrier transcriptome.[11] The long-term implications of these alterations in the GI microbiota and intestinal genes are unknown and deserve further investigation.

Concern about changes in the microbial ecology of the GI tract in early life should not be limited to the NICU. On a global scale, dramatic changes have occurred in the pattern of initial colonization of the intestine in the first days of life in infants from developed world countries, and as previously described, evidence is accumulating that these changes may be linked to the later development of autoimmune and allergic diseases.[48,75,76]

Probiotics

There is emerging information about the potential benefit of pre and probiotics. Their use has been shown to decrease the duration and severity of several diseases of the GI tract.[77] On the basis of these studies and the apparent relative safety of such agents, considerable enthusiasm for the routine use of probiotics in neonates has emerged despite lack of knowledge about long-term effects. The very fact that both beneficial and detrimental effects are seen years after administration of probiotics during pregnancy and the neonatal period[53,54,72] should raise concern that other long-term effects such as immunosuppression in later life may also occur. Of concern for public health is that patterns of colonization in germ-free mice also have profound effects on fat deposition, circulating leptin levels, and insulin resistance.[78] Thus, careful attention needs to be paid to long-term effects, which include development of infections, cancer, obesity, and autoimmunity.

SUMMARY

New information about the importance of normal establishment and maintenance of the intestinal ecosystem during the immediate neonatal period and early life is emerging. Perturbations of this ecosystem, especially during its early development, may have consequences that extend well beyond the neonatal period and manifest as diseases in later life. Although it is tempting to rush toward reengineering of the intestinal microflora with use of agents such as pro and prebiotics during infancy, a cautious approach on the basis of sound scientific data is warranted.

REFERENCES

1. Xu J, Gordon JI. Honor thy symbionts. *Proc Natl Acad Sci USA* 2003;100(18):10452–9.
2. Hooper LV, Midtvedt T, Gordon JI. How host–microbial interactions shape the nutrient environment of the mammalian intestine. *Annu Rev Nutr* 2002;22:283–307.
3. Hooper LV, Stappenbeck TS, Hong CV, Gordon J. Angiogenins: a new class of microbicidal proteins involved in innate immunity. *Nat Immunol* 2003;4(3):269–73.
4. Hooper LV. Bacterial contributions to mammalian gut development. *Trends Microbiol* 2004;12(3):129–34.
5. Stappenbeck TS, Hooper LV, Gordon JI. Developmental regulation of intestinal angiogenesis by indigenous microbes via Paneth cells. *Proc Natl Acad Sci USA* 2002;99(24):15451–5.
6. Bourlioux P, Koletzko B, Guarner F, Braesco V. The intestine and its microflora are partners for the protection of the host: report on the Danone Symposium "The Intelligent Intestine," held in Paris, June 14, 2002. *Am J Clin Nutr* 2003;78(4):675–83.
7. Benno Y, Suzuki K, Suzuki K, Narisawa K, BruceWR, Mitsuoka T. Comparison of the fecal microflora in rural Japanese and urban Canadians. M*icrobiol Immunol* 1986;30(6):521–32.
8. Fanaro S, Chierici R, Guerrini P, Vigi V. Intestinal microflora in early infancy: composition and development. *Acta Paediatr Suppl 2003 Sep;91(441):48–55;* 2003;91(441):48–55.
9. Park HK, Shim SS, Kim SY, et al. Molecular analysis of colonized bacteria in a human newborn infant gut. *J Microbiol* 2005;43(4):345–53.
10. Butel MJ, Suau A, Campeotto F, et al. Conditions of bifidobacterial colonization in preterm infants: a prospective analysis. *J Pediatr Gastroenterol Nutr* 2007;44(5):577–82.
11. Schumann A, Nutten S, Donnicola D, et al. Neonatal antibiotic treatment alters gastrointestinal tract developmental gene expression and intestinal barrier transcriptome. *Physiol Genomics* 2005;23(2):235–45.
12. Rakoff-Nahoum S, Paglino J, Eslami-Varzaneh F, Edberg S, Medzhitov R. Recognition of commensal microflora by toll-like receptors is required for intestinal homeostasis. *Cell* 2004;118(2):229–41.
13. Kien CL. Digestion, absorption, and fermentation of carbohydrates in the newborn. *Clin Perinatol* 1996;23(2):211–28.
14. Sanderson IR. Short chain fatty acid regulation of signaling genes expressed by the intestinal epithelium. *J Nutr* 2004;134(9):2450S–4S.
15. Snyder JD, Walker WA. Structure and function of intestinal mucin: developmental aspects. *Int Arch Allergy Appl Immunol* 1987;82(3–4):351–6.
16. Swift S, Vaughan EE, de Vos WM. Quorum Sensing within the gut ecosystem. *Microbial Ecol Health Dis* 2000;12(4):81–92.
17. Martin R, Langa S, Reviriego C, et al. Human milk is a source of lactic acid bacteria for the infant gut. *J Pediatr* 2003;143(6):754–8.
18. Martin R, Olivares M, Marin ML, Fernandez L, Xaus J, Rodriguez JM. Probiotic potential of 3 Lactobacilli strains isolated from breast milk. *J Hum Lact* 2005;21(1):8–17.
19. Perez PF, Dore J, Leclerc M, et al. *Bacterial imprinting of the neonatal immune system: lessons from maternal cells? Pediatrics* 2007;119(3):E724–32.

20. Caicedo RA, Schanler RJ, Li N, Neu J. The developing intestinal ecosystem: implications for the neonate. *Pediatr Res* 2005;58(4):625–8.
21. Volpe JJ. Neurobiology of periventricular leukomalacia in the premature infant. *Pediatr Res* 2001;50(5):553–62.
22. Speer CP. Inflammatory mechanisms in neonatal chronic lung disease. *Eur J Pediatr* 1999;158(Suppl. 1): S18–22.
23. Speer CP. Pre- and postnatal inflammatory mechanisms in chronic lung disease of preterm infants. *Paediatr Respir Rev* 2004;5(Suppl. A):S241–4.
24. Martinez-Tallo E, Claure N, Bancalari E. Necrotizing enterocolitis in full-term or near-term infants: risk factors. *Biol Neonate* 1997;71(5):292–8.
25. Stark AR, Carlo WA, Tyson JE, et al. Adverse effects of early dexamethasone treatment in extremely-low-birth-weight infants. *N Engl J Med* 2001;344(2):95–101.
26. Attridge JT, Clark R, Walker MW, Gordon PV. New insights into spontaneous intestinal perforation using a national data set: (2) two populations of patients with perforations. *J Perinatol* 2006;26(3):185–8.
27. Neu J. Neonatal necrotizing enterocolitis: an update. *Acta Paediatr Suppl* 2005;94(449):100–5.
28. Hyman PE, Clarke DD, Everett SL, et al. Gastric acid secretory function in preterm infants. *J Pediatr* 1985;106(3):467–71.
29. Antonowicz I, Lebenthal E. Developmental pattern of small intestinal enterokinase and disaccharidase activities in the human fetus. *Gastroenterology* 1977;72(6):1299–303.
30. Guillet R, Stoll BJ, Cotten CM, et al. Association of H2-blocker therapy and higher incidence of necrotizing enterocolitis in very low birth weight infants. *Pediatrics* 2006;117(2):e137–42.
31. Berseth CL. Gastrointestinal motility in the neonate. *Clin Perinatol* 1996;23(2):179–90.
32. Hsueh W, Caplan MS, Qu XW, Tan XD, De Plaen IG, Gonzalez-Crussi F. Neonatal necrotizing enterocolitis: clinical considerations and pathogenetic concepts. *Pediatr Dev Pathol* 2003;6(1):6–23.
33. Neu J. Necrotizing enterocolitis: the search for a unifying pathogenic theory leading to prevention. *Pediatr Clin North Am* 1996;43(2):409–32.
34. Martin CR, Walker WA. Intestinal immune defences and the inflammatory response in necrotising enterocolitis. *Sem Fetal Neonatal Med Inflam Perinatal Dis* 2006;11(5):369–77.
35. Beach RC, Menzies IS, Clayden GS, Scopes JW. Gastrointestinal permeability changes in the preterm neonate. *Arch Dis Child* 1982;57(2):141–5.
36. Roberton DM, Paganelli R, Dinwiddie R, Levinsky RJ. Milk antigen absorption in the preterm and term neonate. *Arch Dis Child* 1082;57(5):369–72.
37. Nusrat A, Turner JR, Madara JL. Molecular physiology and pathophysiology of tight junctions. IV. Regulation of tight junctions by extracellular stimuli: nutrients, cytokines, and immune cells. *Am J Physiol Gastrointest Liver Physiol* 2000;279(5):G85107.
38. Markel TA, Crisostomo PR, Wairiuko GM, Pitcher J, Tsai BM, Meldrum DR, Cytokines in necrotizing enterocolitis. *Shock* 2006;25(4):293–337 l.
39. Bin-Nun A, Bromiker R, Wilschanski M, et al. Oral probiotics prevent necrotizing enterocolitis in very low birth weight neonates. *J Pediatr* 2005;147(2):192–6.
40. Lin HC, Su BH, Chen AC, et al. Oral probiotics reduce the incidence and severity of necrotizing enterocolitis in very low birth weight infants. *Pediatrics* 2005;115(1):1–4.
41. Dani C, Biadaioli R, Bertini G, Martelli E, Rubaltelli FF. Probiotics feeding in prevention of urinary tract infection, bacterial sepsis and necrotizing enterocolitis in preterm infants. *A prospective double-blind study. Biol Neonate* 2002;82(2):103–8.
42. Bach JF. A toll-like trigger for autoimmune disease. *Nat Med* 2005;11(2):120–1.
43. Wickens K, Pearce N, Crane J, Beasley R. Antibiotic use in early childhood and the development of asthma. *Clin Exp Allergy 1999 Jun;29(6):766–71 Related Articles, Links* 1999;29(6):766–71.
44. Yan F, Polk DB. Commensal bacteria in the gut: learning who our friends are. *Curr Opin Gastroenterol* 2004;20(6):565–71.
45. Johnson CC, Ownby DR, Alford SH, et-al. Antibiotic exposure in early infancy and risk for childhood atopy. *J Allergy Clin Immunol* 2005;115(6):1218–24.
46. Brugman S, Klatter FA, Visser JT, et al. Antibiotic treatment partially protects against type 1 diabetes in the Bio-Breeding diabetes-prone rat. Is the gut flora involved in the development of type 1 diabetes? *Diabetologia* 2006;49(9):2105–8.

47. Schwartz RF, Neu J, Schatz D, Atkinson MA, Wasserfall C. Comment on: Brugman S et al. (2006) Antibiotic treatment partially protects against type 1 diabetes in the bio-breeding diabetes-prone rat. Is the gut flora involved in the development of type 1 diabetes? *Diabetologia* 2007;50(1):220–1.

48. Bach JF. The effect of infections on susceptibility to autoimmune and allergic diseases. *N Engl J Med* 2002;347(12):911–20.

49. Zhang L, Li N, Caicedo R, Neu J. Alive and dead *Lactobacillus rhamnosus* GG decrease tumor necrosis factor-alpha}-induced interleukin-8 production in caco-2 cells. *J Nutr* 2005;135(7):1752–6.

50. Mazmanian SK, Liu CH, Tzianabos AO, Kasper DL. An immunomodulatory molecule of symbiotic bacteria directs maturation of the host immune system. *Cell* 2005;122(1):107–18.

51. Meddings JB, Jarand J, Urbanski SJ, Hardin J, Gall DG. Increased gastrointestinal permeability is an early lesion in the spontaneously diabetic BB rat. *Am J Physiol* 1999;276(4 Pt 1):G951–7.

52. Ljungberg M, Korpela R, Ilonen J, Ludvigsson J, Vaarala O. Probiotics for the prevention of beta cell autoimmunity in children at genetic risk of type 1 diabetes – the PRODIA study. *Ann NY Acad Sci* 2006;1079:360–4.

53. Kalliomaki M, Salminen S, Arvilommi H, Kero P, Koskinen P, Isolauri E. Probiotics in primary prevention of atopic disease: a randomised placebo-controlled trial. *Lancet* 2001;357(9262):1076–9.

54. Kalliomaki M, Salminen S, Poussa T, Isolauri E. Probiotics during the first 7 years of life: a cumulative risk reduction of eczema in a randomized, placebo-controlled trial. *J Allergy Clin Immunol* 2007;119(4):1019–21.

55. Rachmilewicz D, Katakura K, Karmeli F, et al. Toll-like receptor 9 signaling mediates the anti-inflammatory effects of probiotics in murine experimental colitis. *Gastroenterology* 2004;126(2):520–8.

56. Katakura K, Lee J, Rachmilewitz D, Li G, Eckmann L, Raz E. Toll-like receptor 9-induced type I IFN protects mice from experimental colitis. *J Clin Invest* 2005;115(3):695–702.

57. Pessi T, Sutas Y, Saxelin M, Kallioinen H, Isolauri E. Antiproliferative effects of homogenates derived from five strains of candidate probiotic bacteria. *Appl Environ Microbiol* 1999;65(11):4725–8.

58. Neish AS, Gewirtz AT, Zeng H, et al. Prokaryotic regulation of epithelial responses by inhibition of IkappaB-alpha ubiquitination. *Science* 2000;289(5484):1560–3.

59. Savidge TC, Newman PG, Pan WH, et al. Lipopolysaccharide-induced human enterocyte tolerance to cytokine-mediated interleukin-8 production may occur independently of TLR-4/MD-2 signaling. *Pediatr Res* 2006;59(1):89–95.

60. Madara J. Building an intestine – architectural contributions of commensal bacteria. *N Engl J Med* 2004;351(16):1685–6.

61. Rook GA, Brunet LR. Microbes, immunoregulation, and the gut. *Gut* 2005;54(3):317–20.

62. Sakaguchi SSN, Asano M, Itoh M, Toda M. Immunologic self-tolerance maintained by activated T cells expressing IL-2 receptor alpha-chains (CD25). Breakdown of a single mechanism of self-tolerance causes various autoimmune diseases. *J Immunol* 1995;155(3):1151–64.

63. Wing K, Suri-Payer E, Rudin A. CD4+ CD25+-regulatory T cells from mouse to man. *Scand J Immunol* 2005;62(1):1–15.

64. Sakaguchi S. Naturally arising Foxp3-expressing CD25+ CD4+ regulatory T cells in immunological tolerance to self and non-self. *Nat Immunol* 2005;6(4):345–52.

65. Fontenot JD, Rudensky AY. A well adapted regulatory contrivance: regulatory T cell development and the forkhead family transcription factor Foxp3. *Nat Immunol* 2005;6(4):331–7.

66. Wildhaber BE, Yang H, Spencer AU, Drongowski RA, Teitelbaum DH. Lack of enteral nutrition – effects on the intestinal immune system. *J Surg Res* 2005;123(1):8–16.

67. Maul J, Loddenkemper C, Mundt P, et al. Peripheral and intestinal regulatory CD4+ CD25(high) T cells in inflammatory bowel disease. *Gastroenterology* 2005;128(7):1868–78.

68. Gad M. Regulatory T cells in experimental colitis. *Curr Top Microbiol Immunol* 2005;293:179–208.

69. Maloy KJ, Antonell LR, Lefevre M, Powrie F. Cure of innate intestinal immune pathology by CD4 + CD25 + regulatory T cells. *Immunol Lett* 2005;97(2):189–92.

70. Benitz WE. Perinatal treatment to prevent early onset group B streptococcal sepsis. *Sem Neonatol* 2002;7(4):301–14.

71. Favier CF, Vaughan EE, De Vos WM, Akkermans ADL. Molecular monitoring of succession of bacterial communities in human neonates. *Appl Environ Microbiol* 2002;68(1):219–26.

72. Kalliomaki M, Salminen S, Poussa T, Arvilommi H, Isolauri E. Probiotics and prevention of atopic disease: 4-year follow-up of a randomised placebo-controlled trial. *Lancet* 03;361(9372):1869–71.

73. Lodinová-Zádníková R, Cukrowska B, Tlaskalova-Hogenova H. Oral administration of probiotic *Escherichia coli* after birth reduces frequency of allergies and repeated infections later in life (after 10 and 20 years). *Int Arch Allergy Immunol* 2003;131:209–11.

74. Sudo N, Chida Y, Aiba Y, et al. Postnatal microbial colonization programs the hypothalamic-pituitary-adrenal system for stress response in mice*J Physiol (Lond)* 2004;558(1):263–75.

75. Shi HN, Walker A. Bacterial colonization and the development of intestinal defences. *Can J Gastroenterol* 2004;18(8):493–500.

76. Matricardi PM. *Prevalence of atopy and asthma in eastern versus western Europe: why the difference? Ann Allergy Asthma Immunol* 2001;87(6 Suppl. 3):24–7.

77. Vanderhoof JA, Young RJ. The role of probiotics in the treatment of intestinal infections and inflammation. *Curr Opin Gastroenterol* 2001;17(1):58–62.

78. Backhed F, Ding H, Wang T, et al. The gut microbiota as an environmental factor that regulates fat storage. *PNAS* 2004;101(44):15718–23.

8   Probiotics in Infant Dietetics

Carlo Agostoni and Filippo Salvini

Key Points

- Although probiotics used as supplements in infant's formula and foods have been recently studied for several clinical effects, real fields of application still remain limited.
- There are no definitive data on possible long-term effects on intestinal colonization and its consequences on immune and gastrointestinal functions.
- Only strains for which identity, safety, and genetic stability have been demonstrated by culture and molecular analysis should be used in dietetic products for infants.
- The administration of probiotics appears to be safer in infants older than 5 months of age because there is a more mature immune response, an established intestinal colonization, and a history of exposure to environmental microorganisms.

Key Words: Infant formula, probiotics, safety.

INTRODUCTION

During the past several years there has been an increasing interest in probiotic products and their beneficial effects on human health. Therefore, it is important to examine the existing evidence on presumptive beneficial effects and safety properties of different probiotic preparations on infants and their health.

Many claims regarding the health-promoting effects of probiotic preparations have been suggested; some of these therapeutic effects are well demonstrated, while many are only potential with yet unclear and unestablished benefits.

At the beginning, it was necessary to standardize the use of probiotics in humans and establish which species of bacteria could be used as probiotics in commercial products for infants and toddlers. To this end "The joint FAO/WHO Expert Consultation on Evaluation of Health and Nutritional Properties of Probiotics in Food Including Powder Milk with Live Lactic Acid Bacteria" (LAB) was created.[1] This expert committee concluded that probiotic strains belong to two genera, *Lactobacillus* and *Bifidobacterium*, which must survive the passage through the digestive tract and proliferate in the large bowel. *Lactobacillus* species from which probiotic strains have been isolated include

From: *Nutrition and Health: Probiotics in Pediatric Medicine*
Edited by: S. Michail and P.M. Sherman © Humana Press, Totowa, NJ

Lactobacillus acidophilus, *L. johnsonii*, *L. casei*, *L. rhamnosus*, *L. gasseri*, and *L. reuteri*. *Bifidobacterium* strains include *B. bifidum*, *B. longum*, and *B. infantis*, *Saccharomyces boulardii*, *Escherichia coli*, and *Enterococcus* strains are used as probiotics in nonfood formats. It was also recommended that strain identification should be performed by phenotypic tests followed by genetic identification, and cultures should be maintained, stocked under appropriate conditions, and checked periodically. Since none of the in vitro tests can predict the activities of a strain, clinical trials following standards of scientific quality are necessary. In addition, safety must be considered, including the risk of infection and antibiotic-resistant transmission.

The Scientific Committee on Food of the European Commission recommended that infant formulae with probiotics should only be marketed if their benefits and safety have been evaluated according to the principles outlined by the same Committee.[2]

In fact, probiotics must have basic requirements for the development of marketable products. First of all, probiotic bacteria must survive in sufficient numbers (established from 10^6 to 10^9 colony forming units [cfu/g]) in the product. Their physical and genetic stability during storage must be guaranteed and all their properties must be maintained during the manufacturing and storage of the products. In addition, probiotics should not have any negative effects on the taste and aroma of the dairy products.[2]

In summary, the main criteria to classify a microorganism as a probiotic are given as follows: human origin, nonpathogenic, resistant to processing, stable in acid and bile, should adhere to target epithelial tissue, should survive in the gastrointestinal tract, produce antimicrobial substances, and should modulate the immune system and influence metabolic activities. Beneficial effects of probiotics seem to be strain-specific and dose-dependent.

This chapter will discuss the efficacy of infant foods and formula containing probiotics in the treatment and prevention of some illnesses, analyzing randomized controlled trials (RCTs) and meta-analysis published from 1991 to 2007 (the MEDLINE database).

EFFECTS OF METABOLITES PRODUCED BY PROBIOTIC BACTERIA IN FERMENTED MILK

Milk contains not only nutrients like carbohydrates, fat, proteins, minerals, and vitamins that allow growth, development, and tissue differentiation but also growth factors epidermal growth factor (EGF), hormones (gastrin, insulin, insulin growth factor (IGF)-I, and IGF-II), and protective molecules such as immunoglobulin. Furthermore, during gastrointestinal digestion, enzymatic milk protein hydrolysis occurs—a process that generates peptides with specific biological activities. The enzymatic degradation can contribute to the formation of endopeptidase and exopeptidases that belong to the proteolytic system of LAB. The two main species that are included in LAB are *Lactobacillus* and *Bifidobacterium*.

Therefore, fermented milk, obtained by incubation at high temperature with LAB, could be considered a rich source of bioactive peptides that modulate several human beings' functions.

The effects of probiotic bacteria are therefore attributable to all those bioactive peptides generated in fermented milk[3].

These molecules exert local effects interacting with target sites at the luminal side of the intestine, but a systemic effect can be hypothesized due to their absorption and immune-modulation, favoring antiallergic processes, such as Th1-type immunity (↑ IL-2; INF-g), generation of TNF-b, which has an essential role in the suppression of Th2- induced allergic inflammation, and production of secretory IgA.[4].

Examples of these activated peptides contained in fermented milk products are ACE-inhibitory peptides that have an antihypertensive effect and a hemodynamic function, or casein peptides that stimulate the activities of immune system cells (immunomodulating function). Other effects of different bioactive peptides are the following: modulation of absorption processes in the intestine by opioid peptides, inhibition of platelets aggregation by antithrombotic peptides, carriage of minerals, especially calcium, by casein phosphopeptides, and antimicrobial and antiinflammatory effect (anti- TNFa effect).[5]

In different studies, in order to characterize the effects of metabolites produced by LAB, supernatants of different fermented milk products (prepared through ultracentrifugation) have been analyzed and compared to unfermented milk supernatants. For example, in a work by Thoreux et al.5 trophic action and nutrient efficiency of fermented milk were investigated in vitro on IEC-6 intestinal cell in culture. The conclusion of this study was that fermented milk supernatants were more effective than those of unfermented milk in stimulating mitochondrial function, DNA synthesis, and cAMP production (a second messengers of trophic activation), suggesting the existence of specific trophic effects dependent on LAB species. Milk fermentation then produces potent trophic factors that promote cell growth, proliferation, and differentiation. In vivo studies are necessary to confirm these effects.

PROBIOTICS IN INFANT FOOD: RCTS ON CLINICAL EFFECTS

Acute Diarrhea

Among the potential health benefits attributed to probiotic bacteria, only a few have been confirmed for pediatric age in RCTs. The best documented beneficial effects of fermented milk were found in the treatment of infectious gastroenteritis caused by rotavirus and of antibiotic-associated diarrhea (AAD). The rationale for this effect is based on the fact that probiotics are able to modify the microflora composition and act against enteric pathogens.

Moreover, probiotics were found to enhance the colonization resistance of the gut microflora by intestinal pathogens like *Salmonella* sp., *Clostridium difficile*, and *Helicobacter pylori*. Mechanisms of this action could include alteration of intestinal conditions (pH, bacteriocins production, short-chain fatty acids) to be less favorable for pathogens, alteration of toxin binding sites, upregulation of mucin production, interference with pathogen attachment to intestinal epithelial cells, among others. Other studies have shown that probiotics stimulate nonspecific and specific immune responses to pathogens like lymphocyte proliferation, phagocytosis, antibodies, and cytokine[5,7,8] production. For example, *L. rhamnosus GG* and *L. plantarum 299v* can inhibit the binding of *E. coli* to intestinal epithelial cells by stimulation of synthesis and secretion of mucins. Furthermore, probiotics protect against structural and functional damage caused by enteric pathogens on enterocytes by interfering with the crosstalk between the pathogen and the host cell.

In industrialized and developing countries, acute gastroenteritis is one of the most important public health problems in term of morbidity, mortality, and economic costs, especially in the first two years of life. Incidence of acute diarrhea in developing countries range from 6 to 12 episodes per year in children below 5 years of age compared to 1.3–2.3 episodes in developed countries. In nonindustrialized countries, acute diarrhea with dehydration remains one of the most common causes of death. Generally, gastroenteritis is a self-limited disease and the main intervention consists of oral rehydration solution in order to prevent dehydration. In complicated cases it is necessary to prevent or treat the metabolic acidosis and electrolyte disturbances with intravenous replacement of fluids. Nutritional support and continuation of breastfeeding is recommended during acute diarrhea.[9,10]

Rehydration solution does not reduce the frequency and consistency of stools and does not modify the duration of diarrhea. Probiotics could be a beneficial product in adjunct to the standard treatment of acute diarrhea. Many RCTs have been published to address this issue (Table 8.1).

L. rhamnosus GG is the most extensively studied strain for the treatment of infectious diarrhea in children. In a study by Isolauri et al.[11] the effect of *L. rhamnosus GG* on recovery from acute diarrhea in 71 well-nourished Finnish children between 4 and 45 months of age was determined. Children randomly received *L.GG*-fermented milk or *L.GG* freeze-dried powder or placebo twice daily. In the first two groups the mean duration of diarrhea was significantly shorter. A second study was conducted on 49 children aged 6–35 months with rotavirus gastroenteritis[12] who randomly received *L. casei* strain GG, *L. casei rhamnosus*, or a combination of *Streptococcus Thermophilus* and *L. bulgaricus* (Yalacta) twice daily for 5 days. In this study, the mean duration of diarrhea was shorter in the *L.GG* group (1.8 days) while it was 2.8 days in the *L. rhamnosus* group, and 2.6 days in the Yalacta group. Furthermore, *L.GG* supplementation was associated with an enhancement of IgA secretion, and demonstrated importance in promoting immunity against rotavirus infections.

The use of *Lactobacillus GG* for the treatment of acute diarrhea was also studied in a clinical trial conducted in 1997 in the Republic of Karelia on 123 children aged 1–36 months, which confirmed the efficacy of *L.GG* in the reduction of duration of watery diarrhea compared to placebo. This effect was significant for rotavirus diarrhea and not confirmed for bacterial infections.[13] Furthermore, to investigate the efficacy of *L.GG* administered in the oral rehydration solution during acute gastroenteritis, a multicenter double-blind placebo-controlled study was conducted on children aged 1 month to 3 years from 11 centers in 10 countries. Children were divided into two groups: group A ($n = 140$) received an oral solution and placebo and group B ($n = 147$) received the same oral solution and a live preparation of *L.GG*. The conclusions of this study were that administering oral rehydration solution containing live *L.GG* to children with acute diarrhea was safe and resulted in a shorter duration of diarrhea, lesser chance of a protracted course, and faster discharge from the hospital.[14]

Other strains of *L. rhamnosus* than *L. rhamnosus GG* have been demonstrated to be effective in the treatment of acute infectious diarrhea. In fact, an RCT involving 87 children between 2 months and 6 years of age, who were randomly assigned to receive a mixture of three L rhamnosus strains (573L/1 573L/2 573L/3) or placebo, showed a reduction in the duration of rotavirus diarrhea in supplemented children, but not of diarrhea of other etiology.[15]

Table 8.1
Probiotics in infant food and diarrhea: RCTs

Study	N	Age (months)	Probiotics	Outcome	Effect
Isolauri et al., Pediatrics 1991	71	4–45	L. casei GG fermented milk vs. L. casei GG freeze-dried powder vs. pasteurized yogurt	Duration of diarrhea (mean; SD)	1.4; 0.8 days 1.4; 0.8 days 2.4; 1.1 days ($p < 0.001$)
Majamaa et al., JPG 1995	49	6–35	L. casei GG vs. L. casei rhamnosus (Lactophilus) vs. Sreptococcus thermophilus + L. delbrukii bulgaricus (Yalacta)	Duration of diarrhea (mean; SD)	1.8; 0.8 days 2.8; 1.2 days 2.6; 1.4 days ($p = 0.04$)
Shonikova et al., Acta Pediatrica 1997	123	1–36	L. casei GG vs. placebo	Duration of diarrhea (mean; SD)	2.7; 2.2 days 3.7; 2.8 days ($p = 0.03$)
Guandalini et al., JPGN 2000	287	1–36	Placebo vs. L. casei GG	Duration of diarrhea (mean; SD)	71.9;35.8 h 58.3; 27.6 h ($p = 0.03$)[a]
Szymanski et al., Aliment Pharmacol Ther 2005	87	2–72	L. Rhamnosus GG vs. placebo	Duration of diarrhea (mean; SD)	84; 56 h 96;72 h ($p = 0.36$)[b]
Pedone et al., Clin Practice 1999	287	6–36	L. casei DN 114 001 (108 cfu/mL) vs. placebo	Duration of diarrhea (mean)	4.3 vs. 8 days ($p = 0.009$)
Pedone et al., Clin Practice 2000	928	6–24	L. casei DN 114 001 vs. placebo	Incidence of diarrhea (%)	15.9 vs. 22 days ($p = .03$)
Rosenfeldt et al., Pediatr Infect Dis J 2002	43	9–44	L. rhamnosus 19070–2 L. reuteri DSM 12246 vs. placebo	Duration of diarrhea (mean)	82 vs. 101 h ($p = 0.07$)

(continued)

Table 8.1
(continued)

Study	N	Probiotics	Age (months)	Outcome	Effect
Weizman et al., *Pediatrics* 2005	201	Placebo vs. *B. lactis* (Bb-12) vs. *L. reuteri*	4–10	Incidence (*n* episodes) and duration of diarrhea (mean)	0.31 vs. 0.13 vs. 0.02 / 0.59 vs. 0.37 vs. 0.15
Salazar-Lindo et al., *BMC Pediatrics* 2004	179	*LGG* (1 billion (109) cfu/mL) vs. placebo	3–36	Duration of diarrhea (mean; SD)	No significant differences
Sarker et al., *Pediatrics* 2005	230	*L. paracasei* ST11 vs. placebo	4–24	Duration of diarrhea (mean; SD)	No significant differences
Costa et al., JPGN 2003	124	*LGG* vs. placebo	1–24	Duration of diarrhea (mean; SD)	No significant differences
Kurugol et al., *Acta Paediatrica* 2005	200	*S. boulardii* vs. placebo	3–84	Duration of diarrhea (mean)	4.7 vs. 5.5 days ($p = 0.03$)
Villarruel et al., *Acta Paediatrica* 2007	100	*S. boulardii* vs. placebo	3–24	Duration of diarrhea (mean)	4.7 vs. 6.16 days ($p < 0.05$)
Billoo et al., *World J Gastroenterol* 2006	100	*S. boulardii* vs. placebo	2–144	Duration of diarrhea (mean)	3.6 vs. 4.8 days ($p = 0.001$)

d = days; h = hours; Effect (mean ± SD)

[a] In Rotavirus infections 76.6; 41.6 vs. 56.2; 16.9 h ($p < 0.008$).

[b] In Rotavirus infections 76; 35 vs. 115; 67 h ($p = 0.03$).

Another strain of Lactobacillus showing some effect on acute diarrhea in children is the *L. casei DN-114 001*,[15] as demonstrated in a study conducted in France on 287 healthy children aged between 6 and 36 months (mean age 19 months) attending day care centres and supplemented daily with fermented milk containing 10^8 cfu/ml of this probiotic, standard yoghurt, or a jellied milk. Although the incidence of diarrhea was not different between the groups, the severity of diarrhea over the 6-month study was significantly decreased with *L. casei DN 114 001* supplementation. In particular, this probiotic caused a reduction in the total duration of cumulative episodes of diarrhea[16].

A similar multicenter randomized double-blind trial compared the same probiotic with traditional yoghurt. This study included 928 children of ages 6–24 months supplemented daily for over 4 months; the study demonstrated a statistically significant difference between the two groups in the incidence of diarrhea with a reduction in the *L. casei* group. This difference was observed during the supplementation period and was no longer significant 6 weeks after the end of supplementation. No significant differences were found in the duration of diarrhea. These results suggested an additional positive effect of this strain of probiotics, when consumed daily, in preventing acute diarrhea, compared to standard yoghurt alone; this effect could be related to its ability to reduce rotavirus shedding[17].

Two other studies conducted by Rosenfeldt in Denmark examined two probiotic strains (*L. rhamnosus* and *L. reuteri*) and their efficacy in the treatment of acute watery gastroenteritis. The first study involved 69 children in the age group of 6–36 months, hospitalized for acute diarrhea[18]. In patients who received a mixture of these two probiotics, the diarrheal phase of illness was reduced by 20% (although not statistically significant). The positive effect was more evident in patients treated within the first 60 h of illness. After the early intervention the duration of diarrhea was significantly shorter with a reduction in the length of hospitalization. The second study was conducted on 43 children with mild gastroenteritis attending day care centers and supplemented with the same mixture of these strains of probiotics. Similarly, there was a reduction in the duration of diarrhea, more evident when the probiotic was administered early in the course of disease[19].

Efficacy of *L. reuteri* was tested in another study[20] that compared two probiotic agents in preventing infections in children attending day care centers. This study was conducted on 201 children who were randomly fed formula supplemented with *Bifidobacterium lactis* (Bb-12), formula with *L. reuteri*, or formula with no probiotics (control group). The control group experienced more episodes of diarrhea with longer duration.

Studies described until now have been conducted in developed countries and in children with mostly mild viral gastroenteritis. It is also important to evaluate the effect of probiotics on infant's diarrhea in an environment with more severe acute diarrhea caused by etiologic agents other than rotavirus. Hence, a Brazilian randomized, double-blinded, placebo-controlled clinical trial was conducted on 179 infants aged between 3 and 36 months who received formula containing one billion (10^9) cfu/ml of *L.GG* or a milk formula without this strain.[21] No significant difference was found in the duration or severity of diarrhea, duration of hospitalization, or total oral solution intake. These infants presented with mild to moderate dehydration, in a slight compromise of nutritional status, and in more than 55% of patients an enteropathogen could be identified with an important proportion of mixed infections. In conclusion, no positive effect of probiotic treatment was demonstrated in this study as opposed to Isolauri's experience in Finland, suggesting that *L.GG* has a beneficial effect on mild viral acute diarrhea that is more common in developed countries. As a matter of fact, there was a lack of efficacy in diarrhea caused by severe bacterial or mixed infections in developing countries. It is possible that *L.GG* is unable to colonize the gut of patients in the presence of bacterial pathogens. Another RCT using *L.GG* was conducted in a tropical developing country, and it demonstrated no significant reduction in the duration of diarrhea in infants in the age group of 3–36 months, with severe watery diarrhea. It has been noted that in this study the dose of probiotic was lower relative to the other studies, suggesting the importance of a dose-effect [22].

More recently, *L. paracasei* ST11 has been found to be beneficial in the management of children with nonrotavirus-induced diarrhea but is ineffective in rotavirus infection. This study was conducted in Bangladesh on 230 infants from 4 to 24 months of age who were randomly fed lyopholized ST11, or placebo. The treatment with this strain of probiotic was associated with significant reduction of cumulative stool output, stool frequency, and oral rehydration solution intake in children with nonrotavirus diarrhea [23].

Yeast has been considered useful as a probiotic for the treatment of acute diarrhea in children. Kurugol et al.[24] examined the effect of *S. boulardii* in 200 children from 3 months to 7 years of age who were randomized to receive the probiotic in a granulated form in a daily dose of 250 mg or placebo for 5 days. The duration of diarrhea was significantly reduced in the supplemented group and the effect of *S. boulardii* on watery diarrhea became apparent after the second day of treatment. The probiotic also reduced the duration of hospital stay. The effectiveness of *S. boulardii* in children less than 2 years old has been evaluated in a randomized placebo-controlled trial[25]; the study involved 100 children between 3 and 24 months of age with acute mild to moderate diarrhea. The probiotic was orally administrated as an adjuvant to oral rehydration solution for 6 days. *S. boulardii* decreased the duration of diarrhea, accelerated recovery, and reduced the risk of prolonged diarrhea. The results also showed an increased efficacy when *S. boulardii* was administered within the first 48 h of the onset of diarrhea. The role of *S. boulardii* in the management and prevention of diarrhea was confirmed in a trial[26] that enrolled 100 children from 2 months to 12 years of age, with acute watery diarrhea. The duration of diarrhea was 3.6 days in children supplemented with *S. boulardii*, whereas it was 4.8 days in the control group. *S. boulardii* reduced the number of episodes of diarrhea by 50% in the subsequent 2-month period. According to these trials, *S. boulardii* is a useful and safe probiotic for the treatment of acute diarrhea in infants and children, but further multicenter double-blind placebo-controlled trials need to be conducted to confirm these observations.

FERMENTED FORMULA FOR INFANTS AND ACUTE DIARRHEA

Formulae containing fermented metabolites rather than live microbiota have also been studied in the treatment and prevention of acute diarrhea. Fermentation metabolites interact with the intestinal epithelium and with gastrointestinal-associated lymphoid tissue (GALT) and can stimulate the endogenous bifidobacterial flora and their immunomodulating properties.

An infant formula fermented with *B. breve* c50 and *Streptococcus thermophilus* 065 was found to be effective in reducing the severity of acute diarrhea among healthy 4–6 month-old infants[27]. In this study, incidence, duration of episodes, and number of admissions to hospital did not differ between the group fed with fermented formula and the one fed with nonfermented formula, but there were fewer cases of dehydration, fewer medical consultations, fewer oral solution prescriptions, and fewer switches to other formulae in the group fed with the fermented formula. This outcome may be linked to the bifidobacterial effects of fermentation products and their interactions with the intestinal immune system.

Use of fermented formula without live bacteria represents a valid option in newborn infants because these formulae might reduce the potential risk of infections associated with the ingestion of live bacteria, especially in immune-compromised states[27].

META-ANALYSIS AND CONCLUSIONS

The number of RCTs published until now on acute diarrhea and probiotics allowed some authors to perform meta-analysis on this topic. In 2001, Szajewska et al.[28] identified 8 RCTs involving 731 children from 1 to 48 months of age, in which probiotics and in particular *L.GG* strain reduced the risk of diarrhea lasting more than 3 days compared to placebo. A second meta-analysis[29] was conducted on studies from 1966 to 2001, and identified 18 papers involving children less than 5 years of age for a total of 1917 patients. Nearly all the trials showed a significant effect of probiotics in reduction of duration of acute nonbacterial diarrhea. The third meta-analysis[30] included 9 studies and examined the efficacy of lactobacillus therapy for acute infectious diarrhea in children of ages 1–37 months. It was concluded that the lactobacilli were safe and effective as a treatment for infectious diarrhea, reducing the duration by approximately two-thirds of a day and reducing the frequency of diarrhea by 1–2 stools on the second day of treatment. According to this meta-analysis the effect of lactobacillus is dose-dependent and not limited to rotavirus infections. Furthermore, it does not seem to be modified by country of study or live versus killed lactobacillus preparation.

In conclusion, some strains of probiotics are effective mainly in reducing the duration of moderate diarrhea. This effect is strain-dependent, with *L.GG* being the most effective, dose-dependent, and more beneficial in watery viral gastroenteritis. Efficacy is still questionable for invasive bacterial diarrhea. Probiotics are more effective when administered early in the course of the disease and more evident in developed countries (there is a substantial difference between developed and developing countries as far as evidence of probiotic effects on diarrhea is concerned).

ANTIBIOTIC-ASSOCIATED DIARRHEA

Antibiotic therapy that can potentially impact gastrointestinal microflora can cause diarrhea. WHO defines AAD as three or more abnormally loose bowel movements in a 24-h period, but definitions used in pediatric and adult trials have varied from 1 to 3 abnormally loose stools per 24–48 h. The severity of this kind of diarrhea can be mild and self-limited or severe. The most serious adverse events related to AAD is *C. difficile* infection that occurs in immunocompromised patients who can develop life-threatening complications with pseudomembranous colitis. The incidence of AAD ranges from 5 to 62% in the general population. Among children, reported incidences of AAD vary from 11 to 62%[31, 32, 33].

The rationale for probiotic use in AAD is the potential for normalizing the unbalanced indigenous microflora, disturbed from antibiotic administration, with specific beneficial probiotic strains. Four mechanisms explain the protective probiotic effects: antagonism by the production of substances that inhibit or kill the pathogen, immunomodulation of the host, competition with the pathogen for adhesion sites or nutritional resource, and inhibition of the production or action of bacterial toxin[31].

RCTs in preventing AAD in children and infants are limited and provide evidence of a moderate beneficial effect of some probiotic strains such as *L.GG, B. Lactis, S. thermophilus*, and *S. boulardii*[32].

Studies addressing the prevention of AAD using probiotic formula or infant probiotic food are limited. A recent[33] double-blinded controlled study was conducted in infants from 6 to 36 months of age randomly assigned to receive a commercial formula containing 10^7 viable cells of *B. lactis* and 10^6 viable cells of *S. termophilus* at the initiation of antibiotic use that continued for 15 days. Controls received nonsupplemented formula for the entire duration. There was a significant difference in the incidence of AAD in infants fed with probiotic supplemented formula (16%) than with nonsupplemented (31%) formula. The probiotic formula was found to decrease the frequency of AAD by 47.7%.

NOSOCOMIAL DIARRHEA

Nosocomial diarrhea is one of the most common problems among hospitalized children worldwide. It is caused by enteric pathogens, especially rotavirus, and reported incidence rates range from 4.5 to 22.6 episodes per 100 hospital admissions. The development of preventive measures is therefore important[34,35]. In 1994, one of the first trials[36] that examined the role of probiotics in the prevention of diarrhea in infants and young children admitted to hospitals for a reason other than diarrhea was conducted on 55 children of ages 5–24 months, with chronic illnesses, who were randomized to receive a standard formula or the same formula supplemented with *B. bifidum* and *S. thermophilus*. Eight (31%) of the 26 children, who received the control formula, while only 2 of 29 (7%), who received the supplemented formula, developed diarrhea during the course of the study. Furthermore, ten (39%) of the control group patients versus three (10%) of the supplemented group children shed rotavirus during the study. These data suggest the effectiveness of these probiotics in reducing the incidence of nosocomial diarrhea and rotavirus shedding in infants admitted to the hospital. A decrease in rotaviral shedding may lead to less environmental exposure and thus lower rates of transmission of the infection in hospitalized children. Further studies are necessary to allow any recommendation of formula with probiotics for the treatment or prevention of nosocomial diarrhea.

INFANTILE COLIC

Infant colic occurs in 3–28% of newborn children and represents one of the most common problems within the first 3 months of life.[37] The pathogenesis is multifactorial and still unclear. The role of intestinal flora composition in the development of colic has been considered. A lower count of intestinal lactobacilli in colicky infants in comparison to healthy infants has been observed.

There is an increasing scientific interest in the beneficial effects of probiotic supplementation in neonates and infants. In fact, probiotics influence the gut microflora composition and can modulate the balance between beneficial and pathogenic bacteria, maintain gut barrier functions, and contribute to the control of inflammatory and immune responses.

In particular, a recent study[38] investigated whether probiotics administered for 6 months postnatally may affect gastrointestinal symptoms, crying, and the compositional development of the gut microflora throughout infancy. The study involved 132 newborn and their mothers, who were also randomized to receive placebo or *L. rhamnosus GG* (as capsules) for 2–4 weeks before delivery; then the supplementation of both mother and infants continued postnatally for 6 months.

Gastrointestinal symptoms such as the number of vomiting episodes, total duration of crying and fussing, or number of solid watery or loose stools, were comparable between the placebo and the supplemented group during the 7th and 12th weeks of life. The effect of probiotic intervention was significant in microflora composition; viable fecal *L.GG* were present at 6 months in 29.2% of infants in the placebo group versus 56.3% in the probiotic group. No significant difference in Bifidobacteria, Bacteriodes, Lactobacillus/Enterococcus, and total bacterial counts were found but there were less clostridia in the placebo group at 6 months of age. At 24 months of age, there were more lactobacilli/enterococci in the placebo group compared to the probiotic group and more clostridia in the placebo group than in the probiotic group. These results suggest that long-term probiotic effects on microbiota during the first months of life require more specific characterization with respect to qualitative and quantitative composition. In this context, *L.GG* may prove to be safe in the long term and may act as a biomarker for the development of healthy intestinal microflora.

On the basis of this concept, one of the endogenous Lactobacillus species, *L. reuteri*, which has been used as a probiotic dietary supplement for other intestinal disorders such as constipation and diarrhea, was studied for the treatment of colic. In particular Savino et al.[39] tested the hypothesis that modulating the gut microflora of colicky infants through the oral administration of probiotics would decrease crying time related to infant colic. Eighty-three breastfed colicky infants were assigned randomly to receive either the probiotic *L. reuteri* (10^8 live bacteria per day) or simethicone (60 mg/day) each day for 28 days. The mothers avoided cow's milk in their diet.

For the probiotic and simethicone groups, daily median crying times were 159 min/day and 177 min/day on the 7th day and 51 min/day and 145 min/day on the 28th day, respectively. This study also analyzed data with respect to family history of atopy; among patients with high risk of atopy, infants receiving *L. reuteri* showed significantly reduced daily crying time, compared with infants receiving simethicone. Similarly, colicky infants without a family history of atopy demonstrated significant improvement in colic symptoms when treated with *L. reuteri* compared to simethicone. Literature data support the hypothesis that infantile colic may be related to food allergy and can represent the first clinical manifestation of atopy[40]; however, this study shows the independent effect of *L. reuteri* relative to the risk of atopy as both infants with or without family history of atopy benefited from the probiotic.

The beneficial effect of probiotics may be related to the action on the altered balance of intestinal lactobacilli in infants with colic. In fact, this probiotic contributes to positively modulate the gut microflora and stimulate the infants' immature immune system.

It is possible that *L. reuteri* can have an antiinflammatory effect and may contribute to modulating the immune responses and motility of the infant's gut.

Another study by Saavedra et al. shows a lower frequency of reported colic and irritability using an infant formula supplemented with *B. lactis* (Bb12) and *S. thermophilus* for children of ages 3–24 months.[41] Additional and larger studies are necessary to confirm these data.

UPPER RESPIRATORY INFECTIONS

Recently, it has been suggested that the immune-modulation induced by lactobacilli could exert a positive effect at distant mucosal sites, other than the intestine, such as the respiratory tract.

Moreover, the potential use of probiotics in upper respiratory tract infections may be derived from their ability to modulate the immune system. In fact, LAB could stimulate B-lymphocytes of the GALT and improve their migration in the upper respiratory tract and lead to more effective IgA secretory production.

Hatakka et al.[42] showed that *Lactobacillus GG* may reduce incidence and severity of respiratory infection in children attending day care centres. In this study, 571 healthy children of ages 1–6 years, attending 18 day care centers in Finland, received daily milk with or without $1.3–2.6 \times 10^8$ cfu of *L.GG*; children fed with *L.GG* had fewer days of absence from day care centers because of illness. There was also a 17% reduction in the number of children suffering from respiratory infections with complications such as lower respiratory tract infections. Antibiotic treatment was reduced by 19%. This effect, even though modest, could have important clinical and socioeconomic consequences.

In a prospective 12-week double-blind RCT, Weizman et al. showed that children (ages, 4–10 months) receiving formula supplemented with *L. reuteri* and attending day care centers experienced fewer febrile episodes, had fewer clinic visits, fewer absences from child care, and had fewer prescriptions for antibiotics.[20]

Further studies are needed to evaluate the effectiveness of different strains of probiotics in this field, especially for children younger than 5 years of age. Some trials have been conducted on adolescents with rhinitis and their results are controversial.

ATOPIC DISEASE

Probiotics may play a role in modulating allergic response. They could improve mucosal barrier function and prevent antigen translocation into the blood stream. According to the hygiene hypothesis, the reduced microbial exposure during infancy and early childhood results in a slower postnatal maturation of the immune system and delay in the progression to an optimal balance of Th1 and Th2 immunity. This balance is crucial for the manifestation of atopy. An abnormal gut flora may lead to a Th2 skewed inflammatory response and a weakened intestinal barrier function with increased exposure to enteric allergens and a subsequently increased risk of atopic disease. This abnormal flora includes reduced number of Bifidobacteriae and a prevalence of Clostridia.[43]

The use of probiotics in the primary prevention of atopic disease is based on their ability to favor antiallergic processes, such as Th1-type immunity (IL-2; INF-g); generation of TNF-b, which has an essential role in the suppression of Th2-induced allergic inflammation; production of IgA, an essential component of the mucosal immune defences (which is deficient in children with allergy4); and the induction of oral tolerance.

Considering the increasing prevalence of atopic disease in the western world, double-blind placebo-controlled trials have been conducted since 1997 on infants with atopic dermatitis (AD) and cow milk allergy, showing that atopic eczema improved in terms of SCORAD index in children consuming infant formula supplemented with probiotics (Table 8.2).

In an RCT, Majamaa et al.[44] randomized 27 infants (ages 2.5–15.7 months) with AD and cow milk allergy to receive an extensively hydrolyzed formula, with or without *L.GG*, for 1 month. A significant clinical improvement of eczema in terms of SCORAD index was observed in the supplemented group (median 26 before start vs. 15 at the end of supplementation). A second similar RCT conducted by Isolauri's group[45] divided 27 infants with AD into 3 groups receiving extensively hydrolyzed formula alone, the same formula supplemented with *L.GG*, or the same formula supplemented with *B. lactis* Bb-12. The SCORAD was 16 during breastfeeding. After 2 months, a significant improvement in skin condition occurred in patients fed with probiotics formulas and SCORAD decreased to 0 in the Bb12 group and to 1in *L.GG* group, while the unsupplemented group had a SCORAD index of 13.4. These results provided the first clinical demonstration of specific probiotic strain capacity to modulate allergic signs. At 6 months, SCORAD index was 0 in all three groups, which means that probiotics lead to an earlier control of allergic inflammation as supported by the reduction of soluble CD4 in serum and eosinophilic protein X (EPX) in the urine of patients receiving the strains of probiotics.

In another double-blind placebo-controlled study,[46] two strains of lactobacilli (*L rhamnosus* 19070–2 and *L reuteri* DSM 122460 as powder dissolved in water) were given together for 6 weeks to 1–13-year-old children with AD. Fifty-four percent (54%) of the children reported improvement of the eczema after probiotic treatment, whereas only 14% improved after placebo. The SCORAD index did not change significantly but the extension of eczema decreased by 25% during probiotic supplementation. The conclusion of the study was that the combination of these two strains was beneficial for the management of AD and the effect was more evident in patients with positive skin prick test response and increased IgE levels. In support of this concept, the effect of probiotics on AD in sensitized children in an RCT[47] involving 60 children of ages 1–10 years, who were randomized to receive probiotics (*L. rhamnosus* + *B. lactis*) or placebo, was studied. SCORAD improvement was noted among the food-sensitized children in the probiotic group compared to the placebo group.

There are two other positive studies related to the use of probiotics in atopic disease. Viljanen et al. conducted the first study[48] on 230 infants with AD and with symptoms

Table 8.2
Probiotics in infant food and AD: RCTs

Study	N	Probiotics	Age	Outcome	Effect
Maajama et al., *J Allergy Clin Immunol*, 1997	27	HE formula vs. HE formula + L.GG (2.5–5 cfu)	2,5–15,7 m	SCORAD index reduction (medians)	21 vs. 19; p = 0.89 26 vs. 15; p = 0.008[a]
Isolauri et al., *Clinical and Exp Allergy*, 2000	27	HE formula vs. HE formula + L.GG vs. HE formula +B. lactis Bb-12	4.6 m (median age)	SCORAD index reduction (medians)	16 (7–25) vs. 13.4 (4.5–18.1) 16(7–25) vs. 1(0.1–8.7) 16(7–25) vs. 0(0–3.8)[b]
Rosenfeldt et al., *J Allergy Clin Immunol*, 2003	43	L. rhamnosus 19070-2 + L. reuteri DSM 122460 (powder dissolved in water) vs. placebo (skimmed milk powder)	1–13 year	Eczema extension (mean)	18.2% vs. 13.7% (p = 0.02)[c]
Viljanen et al., *Allergy*, 2005	230	L. rhamnosus GG vs. Probiotics mix vs. placebo (contained in capsules and mixed in food)	1.4–11.9 m	SCORAD index reduction	Negative value? Yes–26.1 vs.–19.8 (p = 0.036)[d]
Weston et al., *Arch Dis Child*, 2005	53	L. fermentum VRI-033 PCC (freeze-dried powder sachets, mixed in water) vs. placebo	6–18 m	SCORAD index r eduction(% children)	92% vs. 63% (p = 0.01)
Brouwer et al. *Clinical and Exp Allergy*, 2006	50	L.GG vs. L. rhamnosus vs. Placebo	<5 m	SCORAD index	No statistical differences in SCORAD reduction
Taylor et al., *J Allergy Clin Immunol*, 2007	178	L. acidophilus LAVRI-A1 vs. placebo	0–6 m	Incidence of AD (%)	25.8 vs. 22.7 (p = 0.039)

[a] SCORAD index medians before and after treatment in the placebo and supplemented groups, respectively
[b] SCORAD index medians (interquartile range) during breastfeeding and after 2 months of formula feeding in the three groups, respectively
[c] supplemented group
[d] SCORAD index median reduction only in IgE-sensitized infants in the L. GG group vs. placebo

suggestive of cow's milk allergy. In this study, subjects treated with *L. rhamnosus GG* (contained in capsules and mixed in food) alleviated AD symptoms only in IgE-sensitized infants. The second study (Weston et al.)[49] involved 56 children of ages 6–18 months with AD and demonstrated that the probiotic *L. fermentum* VRI-033PCC (freeze-dried powder sachets mixed in water) is beneficial in improving the extent and severity of AD.

An important consideration has been made in a recent study[50] suggesting that supplementation with viable bacterial cells of *L.GG*, rather than heat-inactivated *L.GG*, can be considered beneficial for the management of atopic eczema and cow's milk allergy.

Probiotics have been studied not only for the treatment of AD but also for prevention. Kalliomaki's group conducted the most famous study[51], where dietary supplementation with *Lactobacillus GG* was given to 159 pregnant and lactating mothers, with at least one first-degree relative with atopic eczema, allergic rhinitis, or asthma, and to their offsprings for 6 months. The incidence of atopic eczema in their infants was reduced at 2 years of age. In particular, the frequency of atopic eczema in the probiotic group was half that of the placebo group. In a follow-up study, 4 years later[52], 14 of 53 children receiving lactobacillus developed atopic eczema compared to 25 of 54 receiving placebo. Recently, data on the cumulative effect of the probiotic intervention during the first 7 years of life of the same cohort of children has been published[53]. The cumulative risk for developing eczema during the first 7 years of life was significantly lower in the *L.GG* group than in the placebo group, but there were 17 of 116 cases of allergic rhinitis (6 cases in the placebo vs. 12 in the *L.GG* group) and 12 of 116 cases of asthma (three cases in the placebo and nine in *L.GG* group). While the risk of eczema was significantly reduced in probiotic group, allergic rhinitis and asthma tended to be more common in the probiotic group, calling for further studies.

Recently, another double-blind randomized placebo-controlled trial[54] investigated the role of probiotics in the prevention of IgE-associated eczema. In particular, 188 families with allergic disease were involved. The mothers received probiotic *L. reuteri* ATCC55730 (freeze-dried suspended in refined coconut and peanut oil) daily from gestational week 36 until delivery and their babies consumed the same probiotic from birth to 12 months of age. The results showed that the cumulative incidence of eczema was similar in treated and placebo groups (36% vs. 34%) but the *L. reuteri* group had less IgE-associated eczema during the second year (8% vs. 20%). Skin prick test positivity was also less common in the supplemented group, especially in infants born to allergic mothers (14% vs. 31%). Although no preventive effect on infant eczema occurred, there was less IgE-associated eczema at 2 years of age in the probiotic group and the effect was more pronounced in infants with allergic mothers. As sensitized infants with eczema have increased risk for later development of allergic asthma and rhino conjunctivitis, this study suggests that probiotics could stop or modify the clinical course of allergy. Studies on the outcome in older children are necessary.

In contrast to previous studies, two more recent trials have found no clinical improvement of AD with the use of probiotic supplementation. An RCT[55] found no clinical or immunological effect of probiotics *L.GG and L. rhamnosus* administered orally in a hydrolyzed formula for 3 months in infants less than 5 months old with AD. In particular, no statistically significant effects on SCORAD index, sensitization, inflammatory parameters, or cytokine production between probiotic and placebo group were found.

The same strain of probiotic was found ineffective in another RCT involving 54 infants from 1 to 55 months of age with moderate to severe AD, who were randomly assigned to receive the probiotic or the placebo for a period of 8 weeks. No significant difference between groups was found with respect to clinical symptoms, use of corticosteroids and antihistamines, immunological parameters, or quality of life.

Finally, in another RCT,[56] probiotic (*L. acidophilus* LAVRI-A1 in freeze-dried powder dissolved in water) supplementation for the first 6 months of life failed to reduce the risk of AD and increased the risk of allergen sensitization in high-risk children. In fact, at 6 and 12 months atopic disease rates were similar in the probiotic and placebo groups, and at 12 months the proportion of children with positive skin prick test AD and the rate of sensitization were significantly higher in the probiotic group. The long-term significance of this increase needs to be investigated.

In conclusion, there are promising results on antiatopic effects of some probiotic strains (*L.GG and L. reuteri*) but further studies are necessary to recommend their use in atopic disease and allergy prevention.

RISKS AND SAFETY OF PROBIOTICS IN INFANT FOODS

Probiotics, as living microorganisms, may theoretically pose a risk to human subjects. Given the increasingly widespread use of probiotics, the question of their safety and the risk to benefit ratio have to be assessed. Moreover, because of the paucity of information regarding the mechanisms through which probiotics act, further investigation is needed regarding appropriate regimens of administration and probiotic interactions. Another concern is that the probiotic effects are strain-specific and a strain effect should not be extended to other strains.

However, the tolerance of the available products is excellent but potential side effects are possible especially in susceptible individuals like premature newborns and patients with immunodeficiency[57,58].

There are four types of potential side effects: systemic infections, risk of deleterious metabolic activities, risk of adjuvant side effects and of immune-dysregulation, and risk of gene transfer.

Infections

Probiotics are theoretically nonpathogens and so the risk of infection should be very low. However, the adherence to the intestinal mucosa, which is one of the mechanisms of the probiotic action, may increase the risk of bacterial translocation and virulence. Translocation is defined as the passage of microorganisms from the gastrointestinal tract to extra intestinal sites, such as the mesenteric lymph nodes, liver, spleen, and bloodstream; this mechanism can be the source of infection specially in subjects with underlying conditions that predispose them to infections, such as prematurity, immunosuppression, trauma, and postsurgical conditions.

Recently, case reports have been published on sepsis due to probiotic strains in humans. Sepsis related to probiotics have been described in children and in particular in two premature infants with short gut syndrome fed via ostomy during supplementation with *L.GG*[59].

Land et al.[60] reported two cases of Lactobacillus sepsis associated with probiotic therapy. The first case occurred in a 6-week-old patient with antibiotic-related diarrhea after cardiac surgery, who developed LGG endocarditis on day 99 of hospitalization. The other case occurred in a 6-year-old with cerebral palsy, microcephaly, mental retardation, and seizures, who was feeding through a gastrojejunostomy tube and was admitted to the hospital for *E. coli* urinary tract infection, complicated by an enterococcal central catheter sepsis treated with Vancomycin. From the 25th day of hospitalization, *L.GG* was administered for the treatment of AAD. On the 69th day, the child developed fever and peripheral blood cultures were positive for *Lactobacillus GG*.

It is important to note that all cases of probiotics bacteraemia occurred in patients with underlying immune compromise, chronic disease, or debilitation, and no cases have been described in healthy people.

Deleterious Metabolic Activities

During bacterial colonization of the small bowel, probiotics induce metabolic effects such as deconjugation and dehydroxylation of bile salts and this can result in diarrhea and intestinal lesions.[61] A study by Marteau et al.[62] on healthy humans showed how *L. acidophilus and Bifidobacterium* spp. contained in fermented dairy products could transform conjugated primary bile salts into secondary bile salts: a potential risk for health may occur if deconjugation and dehydroxylation induced by these probiotics are excessive. Further studies on this issue are necessary. Also, excessive degradation of intestinal mucus layer by probiotics may theoretically be a potential risk for development of intestinal lesions.[63] Some researchers have reported that lactobacilli isolated in case reports of infective endocarditis produced enzymes that may enable the breakdown of human glycoproteins and the synthesis and lysis of fibrin clots[64].

Immunological Effects

The important role of microflora in normal immunological development and in immunomodulation can suggest that its manipulations through the probiotic supplementation may have negative immunological effects. Parenteral administration of bacterial cell wall components such as peptide-glycane-polysaccharides from Gram-positive bacteria including lactobacilli can induce side effects mediated by cytokines such as fever, arthritis, or autoimmune disease. It is now well known that probiotics stimulate cytokine secretion. However, oral administration of high doses of LAB did not induce immunological adverse effects in mice and until now no side effects have been reported in humans.

Gene Transfer of Antibiotic Resistance

Many lactobacillus strains are naturally resistant to antibiotics such as vancomycin, macrolides, chloramphenicol, and tetracycline[65], and it is possible that antimicrobial resistance genes may be transferred from probiotic strains to more pathogenic bacteria in the intestinal microbiota like enterococci and Staphylococcus aureus. The gene transfer can be caused by the passage of a plasmid from a probiotic strain to a sensitive strain that becomes antibiotic resistant too. The probability of gene transfer depends on the nature of the donor and the recipient microorganism, on their concentration, and on the selection pressure due to antibiotic treatments. Strains harboring resistant plasmids should not be used in human or animal probiotics, and the ability of a proposed probiotic to act as a donor of conjugate antibiotic resistance genes should be checked as a prudent precaution.[66,67].

SUMMARY AND CONCLUSION

Although probiotics have been recently studied as supplements in infant's formula and foods for several clinical effects, real fields of application still remain limited. There are no definitive data on possible long-term effects on intestinal colonization and its consequences on immune and gastrointestinal functions.

For these reasons the ESPGHAN committee on nutrition2 recommends that only strains for which identity, safety, and genetic stability have been demonstrated by culture and molecular analysis should be used in dietetic products for infants. Furthermore, each strain has to be used as viable bacteria at the optimal dose.

The committee concluded that available data are still not sufficient to support the safety of probiotics in healthy newborns and very young infants with immature immune systems, in immunocompromized subjects, and in premature infants. The administration of probiotics appears to be safer in infants older than 5 months of age because there is a more mature immune response, an established intestinal colonization, and a history of exposure to environmental microorganisms.

In conclusion, the recognized benefits of probiotics on human health, based on evidence and approved by The Committee of ESPGHAN, include the following: a reduced severity of diarrhea, promising results in vitro and in animal models on digestive and immune functions, and indications from human studies on possible short-term preventative and therapeutic intervention for AD.

REFERENCES

1. FAO/WHO (Food and Agriculture Organization/World Health Organization). Joint FAO/WHO expert consultation on evaluation of health and nutritional properties of probiotics in food including powder milk with live lactic acid bacteria. Cordoba, Argentina, 2001.
2. ESPGHAN Committee on Nutrition Medical Position Paper Probiotic Bacteria in Dietetic Products for Infants: a commentary by the ESPGHAN Committee on nutrition. J Paediatr Gastroenterol Nutr, 2004;38:365–374.
3. Menard S, Candalh C, Bambou JC, et al. Lactic acid bacteria secrete metabolites retaining anti-inflammatory proprieties after intestinal transport. *Gut*, 2004;53:821–828.
4. Kalliomaki A, Isolauri E, Probiotics and down-regulation of the allergic response. *Immunol Allergy Clin N Am*, 2004;24:739–752.
5. Thoreux K, Senegas-Balas F, Bernard-Perrone F, Giannarelli S, Denariaz G, Bouley C, Balas D. Modulation of proliferation, second messenger levels, and morphotype expression of the rat intestinal epithelial cell line IEC-6 by fermented milk. *J Dairy Sci*, 1996;79(1):33–43.
6. Aattour N, Bouras M, Tome D, et al. Oral ingestion of lactic-acid bacteria by rats increases lymphocyte proliferation and interferon-gamma production. *Br J Nutr*, 2002;87:367–373.
7. Kaila M, Isolauri E, Soppi E, et-al.. Enhancement of the circulating antibody secreting cell response in human diarrhoea by a human *Lactobacillus* strain. *Pediatr Res*, 1992;32:141–144.

8. Miettinen M, Vuopio-Varkila J, Varkila K. Production of human tumor necrosis factor alpha, inter-leukin-6 and interleukin-10 is induced by lactic acid bacteria. *Infect Immun*, 1996;64: 5403–5405.

9. Guandalini S. Acute diarrhea. In: Walzer WA, Durie PR, Hamilton JR, Walker-Smith JA, Watkins JB, Ed., Pediatric gastrointestinal disease-pathophysiology, diagnosis, management, 3rd ed. Ontario, BC Decker, 2000:28–38.

10. Guarino A, Albano F, Guandalini S, for the ESPGHAN Working group on Acute Diarrhoea. Oral rehy-dration solution: toward a real solution. *J Paediatr Gastroenterol Nutr*, 2001;33:S2–12.

11. Isolauri E, Juntunen M, Rautanen T, et-al.. A human Lactobacillus strain (*Lactobacillus casei* strain GG) promotes recovery from acute diarrhoea in children. *Pediatrics*, 1991;88:90–97.

12. Majamaa H, Isolauri E, Saxelin M and Vesikari T. Lactic acid bacteria in the treatment of acute Rotavirus Gastroenteritis. *J Paediatr Gastroenterol Nutr*, 1995;20:333–338.

13. Shornikova AV, Isolauri E, Burkanova L, Lukovnikova S, Vesikari T. A trial in the Karelian Republic of oral rehydration and Lactobacillus GG for treatment of acute diarrhoea. *Acta Paediatr*, 1997;86(5):460–465.

14. Guandalini S, Pensabene L, Zikri M, et-al.. Lactobacillus GG administered in oral rehydration solution to children with acute diarrhoea: a multicenter European trial. *J Paediatr Gastroenterol Nutr*, 2000;30:54–60.

15. Szymanski H, Pejcz J, Jawien M, Chmielarczyks A, Strus M, Heczko. Treatment of acute infectious diarrhoea in infants and children with a mixture of three *Lactobacillus rhamnosus* strains – a rand-omized, double blind, placebo controlled trial. *Aliment Pharmacol Ther*, 2006;23:247–253.

16. Pedone CA, Bernabeu AO, Postaire, et-al.. The effect of supplementation with milk fermented by *Lactobacillus casei* (strain DN114 001) on acute diarrhoea in children attending day care centres. *Int J Clin Practice*, 1999;53:179–184.

17. Pedone CA, Arnaud CC, Postaire ER, et-al.. Multicenter study of the effects of milk fermented by *Lactobacillis casei* on the incidence of diarrhoea. *Int J Clin Practice*, 2000;54:567–571.

18. Rosenfeldt V, Michaelsen K, Jakobsen M, et-al.. Effect of probiotic Lactobacillus strains in young children hospitalized with acute diarrhoea. *Pediatr Infect Dis J*, 2002;21:411–416.

19. Rosenfeldt V, Michaelsen K, Jakobsen M, et-al.. Effect of probiotic *Lactobacillus* strains on acute diar-rhoea in a cohort of non-hospitalized children attending day-care centers. *Pediatr Infect Dis J*, 2002;21:417–419.

20. Weizman Z, Ghaleb A, Alsheikh A. Effect of probiotic infant formula on infections in child care cent-ers: comparison of two probiotic agents. *Pediatrics*, 2005;115:5–9.

21. Costa-Ribeiro H, Ribeiro T, Mattos A, et-al. Limitation of probiotic therapy in acute, severe dehydrat-ing diarrhoea. *J Paediatr Gastroenterol Nutr*, 2003;36:112–115.

22. Salazar-Lindo E, Langschwager P, Campos-Sanchez M, Chea-Woo E and Sack B. *Lactobacillus casei* strain GG in the treatment of infants with acute watery diarrhoea: a randomized, double blind, placebo controlled clinical trial. *BMC Paediatr*, 2004;4:18.

23. Sarker S, Sultana S, Fuchs G, et-al. *Lactobacillus paracasei* strain ST11 has no effect on Rotavirus but ameliorate the outcome of nonrotavirus diarrhoea in children from Bangladesh. *Pediatrics*, 2005;116:e221–228.

24. Kugurol Z, Koturoglu G. Effects of *Saccharomyces boulardii* in children with acute diarrhoea. *Acta Paediatr*, 2005;94:44–47.

25. Villarruel G, Martinez Rubio D, Lopez F, Cintioni J, Gurevech R, Romero G *Saccharomyces boulardii* in acute childhood diarrhoea: a randomized, placebo-controlled study. *Acta Paediatr*, 2007;96:538–541.

26. Billoo AG, Memon MA, Khaskheli SA, et-al.. Role of a probiotic (*Saccharomyces boulardii*) in man-agement and prevention of diarrhoea. *World J Gastroenterol*, 2006;28:4557–4560.

27. Thibault H, Aubert-Jacquin C and Goulet O. Effect of long-term consumption of a fermented infant formula (with *Bifidobacterium breve c50* and *Streptococus thermophilus 065*) on acute diarrhoea in healthy infants. *J Paediatr Gastroenterol Nutr*, 2004;39:147–152.

28. Szajewska H, Mrukowicz J. Probiotics in the treatment and prevention of acute infectious diarrhoea in infants and children: a systematic review of published randomized, double blind, placebo-controlled trials. *J Paediatr Gastroenterol Nutr*, 2001;33:S17–S25.

29. Huang J, Bousvaros A, Lee J, Diaz A, Davidson E. Efficacy of probiotic use in acute diarrhoea in children a meta-analysis. *Dig Dis Sci*, 2002;47:2625–2634.

30. Van Niel C, Feudtner C, Garrison M, Christakis D. Lactobacillus therapy for acute infectious diarrhoea in children: a meta-analysis. *Pediatrics*, 2002;109:678–684.

31. D'Souza AL, Rajkumar C, Cooke J, et-al.. Probiotics in prevention of antibiotic associated diarrhea: meta-analysis. *BMJ*, 2002;324:1–6.

32. Vanderhoof J, Whitney D, Antonson D, et-al.. *Lactobacillus GG* in the prevention of antibiotic associated diarrhea in children. *J Paediatr*, 1999;135(5):564–535.

33. Correa N, Filho LP, Penna F, Lima F, and Vicoli J. A randomized formula controlled trial of *Bifidobacterium lactis* and *Streptococcus thermophilus* for prevention of antibiotic associated diarrhea in infants. *J Clin Gastroenterol*, 2005;39(5):385–389.

34. Szajewska H, Kotowska M, Mrukowicz JZ, Armanska M, Mikolajczyk W. Efficacy of *Lactobacillus* GG in prevention of nosocomial diarrhea in infants. *J Pediatr*, 2001;138(3):361–365.

35. Mastretta E, Longo P, Laccisaglia A, et-al.. Effect of *Lactobacillus* GG and breast feeding in the prevention of rotavirus nosocomial infection. *J Paediatr Gastroenterol Nutr*, 2002;35:527–531.

36. Saavedra J, Bauman N, Oung I, Perman J, Yolken R. Feeding of *Bifidobacterium bifidum* and *Streptococcus thermophilus* to infants in hospital for prevention of diarrhea and shedding rotavirus. *Lancet*, 1994;344:1046–1049.

37. Lucassen PL, Assendelft WJ, van Eijk JT, et-al. Systematic review of the occurrence of infantile colic in the community. *Arch. Dis Child*, 2001;84:398–403.

38. Rinne M, Kalliomaki M, Salminem S, Isolauri E. Probiotic intervention in the first months of life: short-term effects on gastrointestinal symptoms and long-term effects on gut microbiota. *J Pediatr Gastroenterol Nutr*, 2006 Aug;43(2):200–205.

39. Savino F, Pelle E, Palumeri E, Oggero R, Miniero R. *Lactobacillus reuteri* (American type culture collection strain 55730) versus simethicone in the treatment of infantile colic: a prospective randomized study. *Pediatrics*, 2007;119:e124–130.

40. Bjorksten B, Sepp A, Julge K, et-al.. Allergy development and the microflora during the first year of life. *J Allergy Clin Immunol*, 2001;108:516–520.

41. Saavedra J, Abi-Hanna A, Moore N, Yolken R. Long term consumption of infant formulas containing live probiotic bacteria: tolerance and safety. *Am J Clin Nutr*, 2004;79:261–267.

42. Hattaka K, Savilhati E, Ponka A, et-al.. Effect of long term consumption of probiotic milk on infections in children attending day care centres: double blind, randomised trial. *BMJ*, 2001 June 2;322(7298):1327.

44. Bjorksten B, Naaber P, Sepp E, et-al.. The intestinal microflora in allergic Estonian and Swedish 2-years old children. *Clin Exp Allergy*, 1999;29:342–346.

45. Majamaa H, Isolauri E. Probiotics: a novel approach in the management of food allergy. *J Allergy Clin Immunol*, 1997;99(2):179–185.

46. Isolauri E, Arvola T, Sutas Y, Moilanen E, Salminem S. Probiotics in the management of atopic eczema. *Clin Exp Allergy*, 2000;30:1604–1610.

47. Rosenfeldt V, Benfeldt E, Dam Nielsen S, et-al.. Effect of probiotic Lactobacillus strains in children with atopic dermatitis. *J Allergy Clin Immunol*, 2003;111:389–395.

48. Sistek D, Kelly R, Wickens K, Stanley T, Fitzharris P, and Crane J. Is the effect of probiotics on atopic dermatitis confined to food sensitized children. *Clin Exp Allergy*, 2006;36:629–633.

49. Viljanen M, Savilahti E, Haahtela, et-al. Probiotics in the treatment of atopic eczema/dermatitis syndrome in infants: a double-blind placebo-controlled trial. *Allergy*, 2005;60:494–500.

50. Weston S, Halbert A, Richmond P, Prescott L. Effects of probiotics on atopic dermatitis: a randomised controlled trial. *Arch Dis Child*, 2005;90:892–897.

51. Kirjavainen P, Salminem S, and Isolauri E. Probiotic bacteria in the management of atopic disease: underscoring the importance of viability. *J Paediatr Gastroenterol Nutr*, 2003;36:223–227.

52. Kalliomaki M, Salminem S, Arvilommi H, Kero P, Koskinen P, Isolauri E. Probiotics in primary prevention of atopic disease: a randomised placebo-controlled trial. *Lancet* 2001;357:1076–1079.

53. Kalliomaki M, Salminem S, Poussa T, Arvilommi H, Isolauri E. Probiotics and prevention of atopic disease: 4 year follow-up of a randomised controlled trial. *Lancet*, 2003;361:1869–1871.

54. Kalliomaki M, Salminem S, Poussa T, Isolauri E. Probiotics during the first 7 years of life: a cumulative risk reduction of eczema in a randomised, placebo controlled trial. *J Allergy Clin Immunol*, 2007;119(4):1019–1021.

55. Abrahamsson T, Jakobsson T, Bottcher M, et-al.. Probiotics in prevention of IgE-associated eczema: a double blind randomized placebo controlled trial. *J Allergy Clin Immunol*, 2007;119(5):1174–1180.

56. Brouwer M, Wolt-Plompen A, Dubois A, et-al.. No effects of probiotics on atopic dermatitis in infancy: a randomized placebo-controlled trial. *Clin Exp Allergy*, 2006;36:899–906

57. Taylor A, Dunstan J, Prescott S. Probiotic supplementation for the first 6 months of life fails to reduce the risk of atopic dermatitis and increase the risk of allergen sensitization in high-risk children: a randomized controlled trial. *J Allergy Clin Immunol*, 2007;119(1):184–191.

58. Saavedra J, Abi-Hanna A, Moore N, Yolken R. Long term consumption of infant formulas containing live probiotic bacteria: tolerance and safety. *Am J Clin Nutr*, 2004;79:261–267.

59. Boyle R, Robins-Browne R, and Tang M. *Probiotic use in clinical practise: what are the risks? Am J Clin Nutr*, 2006;83:1256–1264.

60. Kunz AN, Noel JM, Fairchok MP. Two cases of *Lactobacillus bacteraemia* during probiotic treatment of short gut syndrome. *J Pediatr Gastroenterol Nutr*, 2004;38:457–458.

61. Land MH, Rouster-Stevens K, Woods CR, Cannon ML, Cnota J, Shetty AK. Lactobacillus sepsis associated with probiotic therapy. *Pediatrics*, 2005;115(1):178–181.

62. Donohue D, Salminem S, Martial P. Safety of probiotic bacteria. In: Salminen S, von Wright A, Ed., Lactic acid bacteria. Marcel Dekker, New York, 1998:369–384.

63. Marteau P, Gerhardt MF, Myara A, et-al. Bifidobacteria and Lactobacilii ingested in fermented dairy products can metabolized bile salts in the human small intestine. *Microbiol Ecol Health Dis.* 8;151–157.

64. Ruseler V, Lieshout LM, Gosselink MJ, Inability of *Lactobacillus casei* strain GG, *L. acidophilus* and *Bifidobacterium bifidum* to degrade intestinal mucus glycoproteins: clearing the way for mucosa-protective therapy. *Scand J Gastroenterol*, 1995;30:675–680.

65. Olukoya DK, Ebigwei SI, Adebawo OO, Osiyemi FO. Plasmid profile and antibiotic susceptibility patterns of Lactobacillus isolated from fermented food in Nigeria. *Food Microbiol*, 1993;10:279–285.

66. Tynkkynen S, Singh KV, Varmenen P, Vancomycin resistance factor of *Lactobacillus rhamnosus* GG in relation to enterococcal vancomycin resistance van genes. *Int J Food Microbiol*, 1998;41:195–204.

67. Salminem S, Wright A, Morelli L, et-al.. Demonstration of safety of probiotics – a review. *Int J Food Microbiol*, 1998;44:93–106.

68. Vescovo M, Morelli L, and Bottazzi V. Drug resistance Plasmids in *Lactobacillus acidophilus* and *Lactobacillus reuteri. Appl Envir Microbiol*, 1982;43(1):50–56.

Necrotizing Enterocolitis: The Role of Probiotics in Prevention

Zvi Weizman

Key Points

- Necrotizing enterocolitis (NEC) may result from an aberrant intestinal microbial colonization.
- Trials suggest that probiotic supplementation reduces NEC incidence as well as overall mortality.
- Probiotics present a remarkable clinical potential in preventing NEC in premature infants.
- Probiotics do not have a similar effect on death due to definite NEC.
- Future research is necessary to address unanswered issues.

Key Words: Necrotizing enterocolitis, NEC, probiotics, premature infants, preterm, neonates

INTRODUCTION

Necrotizing enterocolitis (NEC) is the most common and most severe gastrointestinal disorder among premature infants, and is associated with significant morbidity and mortality. The incidence of NEC is highly variable worldwide, affecting 2.6–28% of very low birth weight infants [1], and up to 5% of admissions to neonatal intensive care units, with a mortality of 15–30% [2]. Over the past few decades, the frequency of this illness has shown no signs of reduction [3]. Over 90% of affected infants are born preterm, and the risk of developing NEC is inversely related to birth weight and gestational age. Advances in obstetric and neonatal care have improved survival rates for smaller, more premature infants. And as more very low birth weight preterm infants survive the early neonatal period, the population at risk for NEC is constantly increasing [4]. Although most cases of NEC are managed medically, an estimated 20–40% of infants undergo surgery. The case fatality rate with surgical intervention is as high as 50%, and is the highest for the smallest, least mature infants [5]. Despite extensive research, the precise pathophysiology of NEC remains poorly understood. A current multifactorial

From: *Nutrition and Health: Probiotics in Pediatric Medicine*
Edited by: S. Michail and P.M. Sherman © Humana Press, Totowa, NJ

theory postulates that the risk factors of prematurity, formula feeding, bacterial colonization, and ischemia-hypoxia result in the final common pathway of intestinal necrosis and NEC [6]. Prematurity presents immaturity of a variety of intestinal functions, including immune defense, barrier function, circulatory regulation, motility, and digestion.

There is insufficient data on new approaches for the medical management of NEC that might prevent the progression of the disease [2]. Therefore, recent research has focused on the prevention of this challenging clinical entity.

PREVENTION OF NEC

Although mortality rates among infants with NEC may have decreased as a result of improved supportive and medical care, effective well-documented official recommendations for particular preventive measures do not exist.

Several potential preventive strategies have been used in common practice. Feeding of human milk and conservative feeding practices have been shown to reduce the incidence of the disease, especially in high-risk infants [7]. Diet plays a crucial role in intestinal development and defense. Nonnutritive dietary components such as polyamines and epidermal growth factor stimulate intestinal epithelial cell growth and differentiation [8]. Other nutrients such as glutamine and arginine are able to counteract proinflammatory activity [9]. Bowel rest, on the other hand, can lead to intestinal atrophy and encourage inflammatory activity. Hence, it is common to advocate trophic enteral feedings, which promote the activity of digestive hormones and enzymes and enhance intestinal blood flow. Furthermore, infants given early trophic feeds demonstrate improved growth, better feeding tolerance, and fewer infections. At the same time, these infants do not have an increased susceptibility of developing NEC [10]. However, research studies have not yet clearly defined the optimal feeding strategies for high-risk premature infants.

Other potential preventive measures mentioned in the literature include antenatal administration of corticosteroids, IgA supplementation, arginine, erythropoietin, enhancement of platelet-activating factor acetyl hydrolase activity, and the use of platelet-activating factor receptor antagonists [2,11–13]. Although some studies support the role of these substances in reducing the incidence or the severity of NEC, authoritative recommendations for the use of any of these preventive steps are not yet available.

Another potential preventive strategy is to administer probiotic microorganisms. This option is discussed below in detail.

RATIONALE

At delivery, the neonatal digestive tract is nearly sterile. When the newborn infant is exposed to the maternal bacterial flora and the contaminated environment, the gut is assumed to be quickly colonized with a variety of bacterial species. The pattern of the neonatal gut colonization is dramatically influenced by route of delivery, hygiene of the environment, maternal flora, and diet [14,15].

The gut interacts with the intestinal flora to develop protective mechanisms, such as improved barrier function and immune stimulation [16,17]. The maturation and integrity of the neonatal immune system is dependent on exposure to microbial antigens.

In addition, the newborn gut microflora has several key metabolic and nutritional roles, such as the production of vitamins.

In preterm infants, the high rate of caesarean sections, antibiotic administration, interruption of regular feeding habits, and nosocomial flora can all contribute to an abnormal and delayed colonization of the intestine [18]. Immaturity of both immune function and mucosal defense in the gut may result in an exaggerated inflammatory response to factors such as stress, hypoxia-ischemia, virulent microorganisms, and enteral feedings. All these elements might provoke progressive damage to the mucosal epithelial barrier and thereby allow increased bacterial translocation. Colonization of infants with NEC is described as abnormal, compared to healthy preterm infants [19].

Because NEC might result from an aberrant intestinal colonization, research has focused on the preventive benefits of probiotics. Administration of probiotics to preterm infants promotes maturation of intestinal barrier functions and inhibits the adherence and proliferation of pathogenic bacteria.

Administration of some common probiotic agents reduces the incidence of NEC in experimental animals. Using an animal model of NEC, Caplan et al. demonstrated that probiotics may play a role in preventing NEC-like illness in rats. Treated animals had a significant reduction in the incidence of NEC, as well as lower levels of proinflammatory mediators, plasma endotoxin, and phospholipase A2 [20].

CLINICAL TRIALS

The use of probiotics in the clinical setting has been a source of great interest, and the body of evidence for using these agents in the prevention of NEC is growing rapidly. Recently, a systematic review with meta-analysis of randomized controlled clinical trials has been published [21]. The authors aimed to review all randomized controlled trials, evaluating efficacy as well as safety of any probiotic supplementation, in preventing stage 2 [22] or greater NEC in preterm neonates (gestation <33 weeks) with very low birth weight (<1500 g), started within the first ten days, with a duration of at least seven days. They have followed the standard search strategy of the Cochrane Neonatal Review Group. No language restriction was applied. Of 59 potentially relevant citations obtained by the search, only 12 were randomized well-controlled clinical trials in preterm infants involving the use of probiotics. Seven trials, which included 1393 neonates, were eligible for inclusion in the meta-analysis, after extracting data from the publications and obtaining additional data from investigators. [23–29]. All trials included in this meta-analysis had a Jadad quality score of 3 or more. On the basis of the study criteria, five other studies were excluded from the meta-analysis [30–34]. The reasons for this exclusion include insufficient demographic details as well as lack of clinical data regarding the NEC itself, sepsis mortality, and feeding practices.

The characteristics of the seven trials included in the meta-analysis are presented in Table 9.1. The researchers used various types of probiotic agents, either single or combined in a mixture. In addition, there was a wide range of administration patterns in terms of dosing and duration.

The results of the analysis are quite promising. A higher proportion of neonates in the control group developed definite NEC (38 of 690, 6%), compared to the probiotic group (15 of 730, 2%). Meta-analysis of data using a fixed effects model estimated a

Table 9.1

Characteristics of the seven randomized, controlled trials included in a meta-analysis of the effects of probiotics in preventing NEC in premature infants (Reproduced from (19))

	Birthweight/ gestation	Probiotic agents	Dose and duration	Type of milk	Primary outcome
Kitajima (1997)[29]	<1500 gm	BB	0.5×10^9 organisms once daily from first feed for 28 days	MM or FM	Gut colonization by BB
Dani (2002)[23]	3 weeks or <1500 gm	LBGG (discloflor)	6×10^9 CFU once daily from first feed till discharge	MM or DM or FM	UTI, sepsis, necrotising enterocolitis
Costalos (2003)[26]	28–32 weeks	SB	10^9/kg twice daily from first feed for 30 days	FM	Gut function, stool colonization
Bin-Nun (2005)[25]	<1500 gm	BI, ST, BBB	BI0 35×10^9 CFU, ST0.35$\times 10^9$ CFU, BBB 0.35 $\times 10^9$ CFU once daily from first feed to 36 weeks corrected age	MM or FM	Necrotising enterocolitis
Lin (2005)[24]	<1500 gm	LBA, BI	LBA 1004356 and BI 1015697 organisms twice daily from day 7 until discharge	MM or DM	Necrotising enterocolitis
Manzoni (2006)[27]	<1500 gm	LDC (discloflor)	6×10^9 CFU once daily from third day of life to 6 weeks or discharge from neonatal intensive care unit	MM or DM	Gut colonization by candida species
Mohan (2006)[28]	<37 weeks[a]	BBL	1.6×10^9 CFU once daily from day 1 to day 3; $4.8 10^9$ CFU once daily from day 4 to day 21	FM	Gut colonization by BBL and enteric pathogens

BB = Bifidobacterium breve. LBG = Lactobacillus GG. SB = Saccharomyces boulardii. BI = Bifidobacteria infantis. ST = Streptococcus thermophilus, BBB = Bifidobacterium bifidus. LBA = Lactobacillus bifidus. LBC = Lactobacillus casei. BBL = Bifidobacterium lactis. CFU = colony-forming units. UTI = urinary tract infection. MM = mothers' milk. DM = donor milk. FM = formula milk.

[a]Data for less than 33 weeks obtained by contacting authors.

reduced risk of NEC in the probiotic group (Fig. 9.1). Individually, only two of the studies had reported a significantly higher risk of NEC in the control group [25,26]. The number needed to treat with probiotics to prevent one case of NEC was 25.

Meta-analysis of available data from six of the seven trials ($n = 1355$) estimated no significant difference in the risk of blood culture-positive sepsis between neonates in the probiotic group and the control groups (Fig. 9.2). Furthermore, pooling of available data from five trials demonstrated a reduced risk of all-cause mortality in the probiotic group compared with the control subjects (Fig. 9.3). The number needed to treat to prevent one death due to all causes by treatment was 20. Surprisingly, there was a significantly higher risk of death due to all causes in the control group in one study [24]. Available data pooling from four trials showed no significant difference in the mortality risk due to definite NEC between the two groups.

In addition, analysis of data available from three of the studies demonstrated a significant reduction in the time to reach full feeds in the probiotic group compared to controls (Fig. 9.4).

The authors of this comprehensive meta-analysis state that their results should be interpreted carefully in view of the wide variations in patient age, demographics, and the type, dosing, and duration of the probiotic supplementation. Therefore, these results need to be validated with large-scale well-designed future studies before adopting probiotic supplementation for the routine use in the prevention of NEC in premature infants.

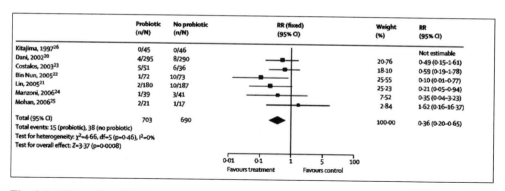

Fig. 9.1. Effect of probiotics on NEC of stage 2 or greater (Reproduced from (19)).

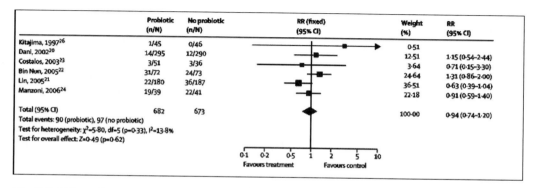

Fig. 9.2. Effect of probiotics on blood-culture-positive sepsis (Reproduced from (19))

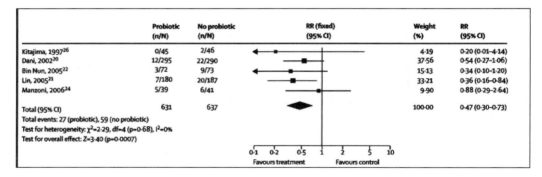

Fig. 9.3. Effect of probiotics on all-cause mortality (Reproduced from (19)).

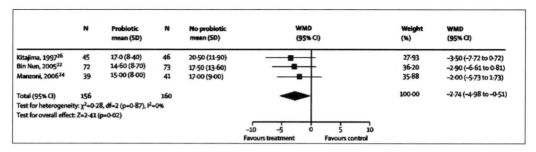

Fig. 9.4. Effect of probiotics on time to reach full feeds WMD = weighted mean difference. (Reproduced from (19)).

The issue of safety is also discussed, as premature infants are immunocompromised hosts, and rare cases of bacteremia and fungemia following probiotic use have been reported [35–37]. However, there are no reports of sepsis caused by probiotic microorganisms in any of the trials included in this meta-analysis.

SUMMARY AND CONCLUSION

It is clear that probiotics present a remarkable clinical potential in preventing NEC in premature infants. The results of the most comprehensive meta-analysis so far show that probiotic supplementation might reduce the risk of NEC and the rate of all-cause mortality, but does not have a similar effect on death due to definite NEC, in preterm neonates.

Nevertheless, in spite of the encouraging results of past research, many key issues are left unanswered. These include optimal strains of microorganisms, effectiveness of using sole strains versus a combination, optimal dosing and duration, short-term and long-term safety issues, effect of heat-killed rather than live microorganisms, efficacy of prebiotics and synbiotics, molecular genetic control of specific strains, basic research on mechanisms, evaluation of cost-effectiveness, and standard criteria for quality control.

All these aspects should be addressed in future well-designed large-scale clinical trials, before the adoption of this mode of therapy as a routine tool in the prevention of NEC.

REFERENCES

1. Kafetzis DA, Skevaki C, Costalos C. Neonatal necrotizing enterocolitis: an overview. *Curr Opin Infect Dis* 2003; 16:349–55.
2. Lin PW, Stoll BJ. Necrotising enterocolitis. *Lancet* 2006; 368:1271–83.
3. Holman RC, Stoll BJ, Curns AT, Yorita KL, Steiner CA, Schonberger LB. Necrotising enterocolitis hospitalisations among neonates in the United States. *Paediatr Perinat Epidemiol* 2006; 20:498–506.
4. Guthrie SO, Gordon PV, Thomas V, Thorp JA, Peabody J, Clark RH. Necrotizing enterocolitis among neonates in the United States. *J Perinatol* 2003; 23:278–85.
5. Henry MC, Moss RL. Current issues in the management of necrotizing enterocolitis. *Semin Perinatol* 2004; 28:221–33.
6. Caplan MS, Jilling T. Neonatal necrotizing enterocolitis: possible role of probiotic supplementation. *J Pediatr Gastroenterol Nutr* 2000; 30(Suppl 2):S18–22.
7. Berseth CL. Feeding strategies and necrotizing enterocolitis. *Curr Opin Pediatr* 2005; 17:170–3.
8. Rumbo M, Schiffrin EJ. Ontogeny of intestinal epithelium immune functions: developmental and environmental regulation. *Cell Mol Life Sci* 2005; 62:1288–96.
9. Neu J. Neonatal necrotizing enterocolitis: an update. *Acta Paediatr Suppl* 2005; 94:100–5.
10. McClure RJ. Trophic feeding of the preterm infant. *Acta Paediatr Suppl* 2001; 90:19–21.
11. Kosloske AM. Pathogenesis and prevention of necrotizing enterocolitis: a hypothesis based on personal observation and a review of the literature. *Pediatrics* 1984; 74:1086–92.
12. Barlow B, Santulli TV, Heird WC, Pitt J, Blanc WA, Schullinger JN. An experimental study of acute neonatal enterocolitis – the importance of breast milk. *J Pediatr Surg* 1974; 9:587–95.
13. Reber KM, Nankervis CA, Nowicki PT. Newborn intestinal circulation. Physiology and pathophysiology. *Clin Perinatol* 2002; 29:23–39.
14. Pietzak M. Bacterial colonization of the neonatal gut. *J Pediatr Gastroenterol Nutr* 2004; 38:389–91.
15. Weizman Z, Asli G, Alsheikh A. Effect of a probiotic infant formula on infections in child care centers: comparison of two probiotic agents. *Pediatrics* 2005; 115:5–9.
16. Saavedra JM. Use of probiotics in pediatrics: rationale, mechanisms of action, and practical aspects. *Nutr Clin Pract* 2007; 22:351–65.
17. Weizman Z, Alsheikh A. Safety and tolerance of a probiotic formula in early infancy comparing two probiotic agents: a pilot study. *J Am Coll Nutr* 2006; 25:415–9.
18. Caffarelli C, Bernasconi S. Preventing necrotising enterocolitis with probiotics. *Lancet* 2007; 369:1578–80.
19. Hallstrom M, Eerola E, Vuento R, Janas M, Tammela O. Effects of mode of delivery and necrotising enterocolitis on the intestinal microflora in preterm infants. *Eur J Clin Microbiol Infect Dis* 2004; 23:463–70.
20. Caplan MS, Miller-Catchpole R, Kaup S, et-al.. Bifidobacterial supplementation reduces the incidence of necrotizing enterocolitis in a neonatal rat model. *Gastroenterology* 1999; 117:577–83.
21. Deshpande G, Rao S, Patole S. Probiotics for prevention of necrotising enterocolitis in preterm neonates with very low birthweight: a systematic review of randomised controlled trials. *Lancet* 2007; 369:1614–20.
22. Bell MJ, Ternberg JL, Feigin RD, et-al.. Neonatal necrotizing enterocolitis. Therapeutic decisions based upon clinical staging. *Ann Surg* 1978; 187:1–7.
23. Dani C, Biadaioli R, Bertini G, Martelli E, Rubaltelli FF. Probiotics feeding in prevention of urinary tract infection, bacterial sepsis and necrotizing enterocolitis in preterm infants. A prospective double-blind study. *Biol Neonate* 2002; 82:103–8.
24. Lin HC, Su BH, Chen AC, et-al.. Oral probiotics reduce the incidence and severity of necrotizing enterocolitis in very low birth weight infants. *Pediatrics* 2005; 115:1–4.
25. Bin-Nun A, Bromiker R, Wilschanski M, et-al.. Oral probiotics prevent necrotizing enterocolitis in very low birth weight neonates. *J Pediatr* 2005; 147:192–6.
26. Costalos C, Skouteri V, Gounaris A, et-al.. Enteral feeding of premature infants with *Saccharomyces boulardii*. *Early Hum Dev* 2003; 74:89–96.
27. Manzoni P, Mostert M, Leonessa ML, et-al.. Oral supplementation with *Lactobacillus casei* subspecies *rhamnosus* prevents enteric colonization by Candida species in preterm neonates: a randomized study. *Clin Infect Dis* 2006; 42:1735–42.

28. Mohan R, Koebnick C, Schildt J, et-al.. Effects of *Bifidobacterium lactis Bb12* supplementation on intestinal microbiota of preterm infants: a double-blind, placebo-controlled, randomized study. *J Clin Microbiol* 2006; 44:4025–31.

29. Kitajima H, Sumida Y, Tanaka R, Yuki N, Takayama H, Fujimura M. Early administration of *Bifidobacterium breve* to preterm infants: randomised controlled trial. *Arch Dis Child Fetal Neonatal Ed* 1997; 76:F101–7.

30. Agarwal R, Sharma N, Chaudhry R, et-al.. Effects of oral Lactobacillus GG on enteric microflora in low-birth-weight neonates. *J Pediatr Gastroenterol Nutr* 2003; 36:397–402.

31. Reuman PD, Duckworth DH, Smith KL, Kagan R, Bucciarelli RL, Ayoub EM. Lack of effect of Lactobacillus on gastrointestinal bacterial colonization in premature infants. *Pediatr Infect Dis* 1986; 5:663–8.

32. Millar MR, Bacon C, Smith SL, Walker V, Hall MA. Enteral feeding of premature infants with Lactobacillus GG. *Arch Dis Child* 1993; 69:483–7.

33. Stansbridge EM, Walker V, Hall MA, et-al.. Effects of feeding premature infants with Lactobacillus GG on gut fermentation. *Arch Dis Child* 1993; 69:488–92.

34. Uhlemann M, Heine W, Mohr C, Plath C, Pap S. Effects of oral administration of bifidobacteria on intestinal microflora in premature and newborn infants. *Z Geburtshilfe Neonatol* 1999; 203:213–7.

35. Thompson C, McCarter YS, Krause PJ, Herson VC. *Lactobacillus acidophilus* sepsis in a neonate. *J Perinatol* 2001; 21:258–60.

36. Broughton RA, Gruber WC, Haffar AA, Baker CJ. Neonatal meningitis due to Lactobacillus. *Pediatr Infect Dis* 1983; 2:382–4.

37. Perapoch J, Planes AM, Querol A, et-al.. Fungemia with *Saccharomyces cerevisiae* in two newborns, only one of whom had been treated with ultra-levura. *Eur J Clin Microbiol Infect Dis* 2000; 19:468–70.

Section C
Probiotics and the Gut

10 Irritable Bowel Syndrome

Sonia Michail

Key Points

- Irritable bowel syndrome (IBS) is common in children.
- Gut flora and intestinal mucosal immunity can be altered in IBS.
- Probiotic therapies can influence gut flora and gut mucosal immunity.
- Several adult studies, but not all, show efficacy of probiotic preparations in relieving specific symptoms of IBS.
- Pediatric data to support the use of probiotics in IBS are scarce and less compelling.

Key Words: Pain, probiotics, irritable bowel syndrome, children, bacteria.

INTRODUCTION

Chronic abdominal pain is a common ailment that has been afflicting children for many decades. In 1958, more than 10% of all school-aged children reported having recurrent abdominal pain severe enough to interfere with their daily functioning [1]. In a more recent community-based survey, one-third of eighth and tenth graders noted abdominal pain at least six times over the previous year. The pain affected daily activities in 17–24% of these children [2]. It is estimated that irritable bowel syndrome (IBS) affects up to 25% of school-age children and adolescents, accounts for a significant number (2–4%) of office visits to primary care physicians, and represents about 25–50% of all patients who visit a gastroenterologist's clinic [3]. The prevalence of IBS increases with age. Equal gender ratio is seen in early childhood but female predominance is noted in older children and adolescents [3].

IBS is characterized by the presence of abdominal pain or discomfort in association with disturbed defecation [4]. Symptoms of IBS can be sporadically severe or can manifest as nagging abdominal pain. It can be associated with altered bowel habits with specific symptoms of diarrhea, constipation, abdominal distension, bloating, and urgency to defecate [5]. Children with functional gastrointestinal disorders display a tremendous amount of variability in degrees of severity. The challenging task of defining pediatric functional gastrointestinal disorders has been assigned to a working team,

From: *Nutrition and Health: Probiotics in Pediatric Medicine*
Edited by: S. Michail and P.M. Sherman © Humana Press, Totowa, NJ

Table 10.1

Diagnostic criteria for pediatric irritable bowel syndrome in children

Pediatric Rome III criteria (symptoms must occur at least weekly for two or more months)

Abdominal discomfort or pain associated with two or more of the following symptoms,
    which should be present at least 25% of the time:
  a. Relief with defecation
  b. Change in frequency of stools
  c. Change in form of stools

No evidence of organic etiology to explain symptoms such as inflammatory, metabolic,
anatomic, or neoplastic processes.

which met in Rome in 1997 and established the pediatric Rome II criteria [6]. This working group has recently reconvened to revise the criteria in keeping with the establishment of the Rome III criteria. The new diagnostic criteria are summarized in Table 10.1. The group also established alarming signs and symptoms to suggest an organic etiology for the pain. Those signs and symptoms include the persistence of right-sided upper or lower abdominal pain, pain awakening the child from sleep, gastrointestinal blood loss, family history of celiac, inflammatory bowel, or peptic ulcer disease, arthritis, peri-rectal disease, weight loss, delayed puberty, or unexplained fevers.

Perhaps the most significant impact of irritable bowel syndrome lies in its effect on the child's quality of life. A report by Varni et al. revealed that IBS had a significant impact on the quality of life of those children [7]. They missed more days of school, had more days when they were "too ill to play," and had impaired health-related quality of life when measuring physical, emotional, social, and school functioning.

The therapeutic options for this common and potentially incapacitating disorder remain limited, with modest symptomatic relief without the ability to change its course or natural history [8–10].

The influence of the GI flora in patients with IBS has been reported in a few studies. In twenty IBS patients, Balsari et al. was able to show a great homogeneity in the fecal flora with a decrease in coliforms, lactobacilli, and bifidobacteria in IBS patients, compared to healthy individuals [11]. Recent studies also imply that several factors implicated in IBS pathogenesis have the capacity to induce changes in the intestinal ecosystem [12]. Moreover, abnormal motility is considered an important component of functional abdominal pain [13]. There is a close interaction between small intestinal motility and endogenous digestive microflora, and normal motility patterns have a role in the regulation of the bacterial flora of the gut. This has been demonstrated by the observation that disorders of intestinal motility may lead to bacterial colonization of the jejunum and, conversely, there is good evidence that bacteria may contribute to the development of abnormal intestinal motility patterns, which in turn may lead to the development of gastrointestinal symptoms [14]. The influence of the intestinal microflora on the gastrointestinal motility appears to be mediated by a modulatory effect on the enteric nervous system rather than a direct stimulatory effect on the intestinal smooth muscle. Therefore, one may speculate that oral bacteriotherapy with probiotic strains could have a potential impact on the motility patterns of the gastrointestinal system, especially in subjects with irritable bowel syndrome.

MECHANISM OF ACTION OF PROBIOTICS; GENERAL OVERVIEW

Probiotics act favorably in the host through several different mechanisms (see chapter five for more details). They have an antimicrobial effect through modifying the microflora [15], secreting antibacterial substances [16], competing with pathogens to prevent their adhesion to the intestine [17], competing for nutrients necessary for pathogen survival [18], producing an antitoxin effect [19], and reversing some of the consequences of infection on the intestinal epithelium [20,21]. Probiotics are also capable of modulating the immune system [22], regulating allergic response of the body [23], and reducing proliferation in cancer [24]. It is interesting to note that it may not be necessary to administer the intact probiotic organism to achieve benefits. Products of the organisms such as secreted proteins and DNA can block inflammation and stop the death of epithelial cells [25,26]. As an example, DNA from VSL#3 can suppress experimental colitis in animal models [27]. The probiotic bacteria can also be genetically modified for use as a carrier for antigen delivery directly to the affected disease location in the bowel [28]. A recent study by Rousseaux and colleagues [29], found that consumption of specific Lactobacillus strains induced the expression of mu-opioid and cannabinoid receptors in the gut causing an analgesic effect similar to morphine. The authors suggested that the bacteria within the intestinal tract could affect visceral perception, which can offer new therapeutic options for treatment of abdominal pain and irritable bowel syndrome.

IBS AND INTESTINAL BACTERIA

It is estimated that the human colon contains up to 10^{14} bacteria [30]. Although this diverse flora is largely beneficial, it has been postulated that altered bacterial populations or products of bacterial metabolism may contribute to human disease. Patients with IBS have altered bacterial flora and a subset of IBS patients have small bowel bacterial overgrowth. The mechanisms by which altered fecal flora induce disease are poorly understood. Fecal short-chain fatty acids produced by microflora are critical for colonic epithelial maintenance, yet they are clearly different in children with IBS [31]. Maximal gas production and hydrogen excretion after an oral lactulose load is increased in IBS as colonic-gas production, particularly of hydrogen, is greater in patients with IBS than in controls, and both symptoms and gas production are reduced by an exclusion diet. This reduction may be associated with alterations in the activity of hydrogen-consuming bacteria further emphasizing the importance of fermentation in the pathogenesis of IBS [12]. Placing IBS patients on a carbohydrate-restricted diet reduces gas production and symptoms, suggesting a possible pathogenic role for bacterial fermentation. Moreover, increased bacterial methane production was related to constipation in IBS [32]. In such individuals, postprandial serotonin release was blunted, suggesting a possible neurochemical basis for impaired motor function in this subset of IBS patients [33].

Lactose breath testing in IBS subjects does not seem to reflect malabsorption but the pattern of hydrogen excretion is suggestive of bacterial overgrowth [34]. In a double-blinded, randomized, placebo-controlled study, improvement and resolution of symptoms of IBS, correlated with normalization of lactulose breath testing [35]. Another study suggested that IBS might be associated with rapid excretion of gaseous products of fermentation.

The reduction of these products may improve symptoms [36]. Furthermore, studies suggest that there are specific changes in the gut microflora that contribute to IBS pathophysiology, which could aid in the development of new therapeutic strategies [37,38]. The analysis of the feces microbiota using the GCMS shows a substantial portion of eubacteria among other bowel microorganisms (27% in the jejunum and 16% in the colon) and specific changes of their species in case of IBS. The concentration of streptomycetes, rhodococci, and other members of the Actinomycetales order become dozen folds higher in quantities [39]. Finally, reports of amelioration of symptoms of bloating and flatulence in patients with IBS when treated with a poorly absorbed antibiotic, rifaximin, suggest a major role for intestinal bacteria as a contributor to symptoms of IBS [40,41], and the poorly absorbed antibiotic Neomycin has been effective in reducing symptoms and decreasing hydrogen and methane production in IBS [35]. PCR analyses demonstrated a reduction of *Lactobacilli* in diarrhea-predominant IBS and a reduction of *Clostridium coccoides* and *Bifidobacterium catenulatem* counts compared with healthy individuals [42]. The number of fecal *Bifidobacterium* was significantly decreased and that of *Enterobacteriaceae* was significantly increased compared with that in healthy controls, and the microbial colonization resistance of the bowel in IBS patients was lower [43]. Recently, the use of *B. infantis* resulted in symptom reduction in IBS, which correlated with normalization of proinflammatory cytokines, suggesting an immune modulating effect of probiotics [44].The study by Bazzocchi et al. is the first observation showing a clinical improvement related to changes in the composition of the fecal bacterial flora, fecal biochemistry, and colonic motility pattern, all of which was induced by administration of probiotics, in patients with functional diarrhea [45]. While such studies mostly rely on traditional culture techniques to identify the flora, the use of molecular technology in identifying stool microflora may prove useful in further investigating the role of these bacteria in gastrointestinal symptomatology and disease.

IBS AND INFECTION

There are substantial grounds to support the association of infection with IBS. Initially reported by McKendrick and Read [46], several subsequent publications now document the occurrence of IBS following bacteriologically confirmed gastroenteritis [47–55]. The risk of developing IBS following an episode of gastroenteritis can be as high as 23%, especially in females, with severe initial symptoms, and in the presence of premorbid psychopathology [47–55]. Gwee et al. proceeded to confirm a direct association between prior exposure to an infectious agent, persisting low-grade inflammation, and IBS [51]. The study demonstrated a persistent increase in chronic inflammatory cells of the rectum only among those patients who went on to develop IBS. Other investigators demonstrated a persisting increase in rectal mucosal enteroendocrine cells, T-lymphocytes, and gut permeability in patients who developed IBS after dysentery.

IBS AND INFLAMMATION

The study by Chadwick et al. pioneered the first concept that IBS is associated with inflammation. In their study, 77 IBS patients were evaluated. Fifty-five percent were diarrhea predominant; and none had a confirmed infectious origin for IBS [56].

All patients underwent colonic biopsies for histology and immunohistology. Thirty-eight had normal histology, 31 demonstrated microscopic inflammation, and eight fulfilled the criteria for lymphocytic colitis. However, in the group with normal histology, immunohistology revealed evidence of inflammation with increased intraepithelial lymphocytes, as well as, an increase in CD3+ and CD25+ cells in the lamina propria. Therefore, all patients had evidence of immune activation. These features were more pronounced in the group already identified with microscopic inflammation, which, in addition, had increased neutrophils, mast cells, and natural killer cells. Other studies further support the role of inflammation in IBS. Gonsalkorale and colleagues showed a reduction in the antiinflammatory cytokine interleukin-10 (IL-10) [57]. Barbara et al., who showed an increase in mast cell degranulation in the colon of patients with IBS, were able to demonstrate a direct correlation between the location and proximity of mast cells in the mucosa and severity of clinical pain [58].

In ten patients with severe IBS, Tornblom and colleagues examined full-thickness jejunal biopsies obtained by laparoscopy [59]. All patients had low-grade infiltration of lymphocytes in the myenteric plexus; four of these had an increase in intraepithelial lymphocytes and six had evidence of neuronal degeneration. Nine patients had longitudinal muscle hypertrophy and seven had abnormalities in the number and size of interstitial cells of Cajal. This further provides evidence for the extension of the inflammatory process beyond the intestinal mucosa. In this study, intraepithelial lymphocytosis was noted consistent with the reports of Chadwick and colleagues [56] as described earlier. A study enrolling 78 IBS patients demonstrated an alteration in the ratio between the cytokines IL10 and IL12, which suggested a Th1 response similar to what is seen in peripheral blood mononuclear cells [44]. Spiller proposed that the inflammatory changes represent a response to an initial enteric infection affecting individuals who become susceptible by a relative deficiency of antiinflammatory cytokines [60].

RATIONALE FOR THE USE OF PROBIOTICS IN IBS

The understanding of the relationship of enteric infection and intestinal inflammation with IBS highlights the need to further explore gut flora–mucosa interactions [61]. Several studies document the new onset of IBS following infectious, bacterial gastroenteritis [52,54,62,63] and other studies confirm low-grade mucosal inflammation [56,59,64] and immune activation [49,65,66]. In addition, studies support a role for inflammatory and immune processes in contributing to enteric neuromuscular dysfunction [67], which in turn can contribute to the development of IBS.

Probiotics, defined as live or attenuated bacteria or bacterial products that confer a significant health benefit to the host [68], have the potential to provide a clinical tool to explore gut microbial and intestinal interactions. There are several reasons why probiotics would have therapeutic potential in IBS. Probiotic organisms exhibit antibacterial and antiviral effects and could potentially prevent or ameliorate postinfectious IBS [69,70]. Probiotics have also been shown to possess antiinflammatory characteristics relative to the intestinal mucosa [71,72], with an increase in mucus [17] production and reduction of the migration of neutrophils to the intestinal epithelium [20]. By reducing mucosal inflammation, probiotics could ameliorate the consequences of inflammation and reduce the neurochemical and impaired motor function found in many subjects with

IBS. In addition, probiotics are also capable of changing the composition of the gut flora. Since gut flora in IBS is different from flora of healthy subjects [9,73,74], probiotic-related changes in the enteric flora could reduce the nondesirable effects of bacteria in the gut [12] and favorably influence gut function. Finally, probiotics could change the quantity and quality of stool and gas [75–77] or increase intestinal mucus secretion [78,79], which could potentially modify symptoms such as constipation and diarrhea.

A small number of studies have evaluated the response of IBS to probiotic preparations. While results between studies are difficult to compare because of differences in study design, probiotic dose, and strain, there has been evidence of symptom improvement [80–85]. The overall impact of probiotics in IBS is becoming more evident. Several of these studies have involved either *Lactobacilli* or *Bifidobacteria* [86].

SUMMARY OF PRIOR PROBIOTIC STUDIES IN IRRITABLE BOWEL SYNDROME

Probiotic preparations have different bioavailability, composition, effective doses, and biological activities. Furthermore, it is important to acknowledge that in vitro effects of a probiotic may be different in vivo [87]. An example to further highlight this concept is the presence of good supporting evidence of the anti-inflammatory effect of Lactobacillus GG in vitro, with lack of efficacy in a controlled-double blind pediatric Crohn's disease studies [88–90].

A number of studies have evaluated the response of irritable bowel syndrome to different probiotic preparations. There are a number of shortfalls to be considered:

1. Most probiotic products have not been adequately tested for reproducibility of the claimed bacterial content or the stability and survival in the gastrointestinal tract.
2. Most adult studies were underpowered with no documentation of probiotic recovery or colonization.
3. Some studies employed single probiotic isolates while others employed multiple probiotic preparations, thus creating a significant heterogeneity among the different studies making it difficult to analyze data.
4. Majority of the studies were too short to draw firm conclusions regarding a chronic disease with variable course such as IBS.
5. Different probiotic strains have been employed in different efficacy studies and not all probiotic bacteria or strains are alike. There are also some inconsistencies between studies employing the same probiotic strains.
6. The effect of probiotic supplementation in IBS is modest.
7. Probiotic products are usually not covered by insurance carriers.

Several adult studies addressing the efficacy of probiotics in IBS have been published. A recent metanalysis, McFarland [107], suggests improvement of IBS symptoms with the use of probiotics. Zeng [110] demonstrated clinical efficacy and short term improvement of intestinal barrier function using probiotic fermented milk, while Drouault-Holowacz [106] could not demonstrate efficacy of a probiotic combination. Sinn [109] and Plassmann's [108] work suggest efficacy of *L. acidophilus* and *E-coli* Nissle, respectively. Niedzielin et al. described resolution of abdominal pain in all of the 20 patients treated for 4 weeks with *Lactobacillus plantarum* 299 V, while only 11 of 20 patients responded to placebo [91]. Halpern et al. noted a significant reduction in an IBS symptom index with 5×10^9 heat-killed *L. acidophilus*.[85] O'Sullivan and O'Morain could not demonstrate an effect of *L. casei* GG on overall symptomatology, but did show a trend towards reduction in bloating.[101] Nobaek et al., described a similar benefit in relieving bloating using *L. plantarum* (DSM 9843)[81] as did Kim et al. when employing VSL#3.[83]

Whorwell and colleagues described a multicenter European study, which is the largest published study to date [92]. The study recruited patients from 20 centers across the United Kingdom for investigating the efficacy of three different concentrations of *B. infantis* 35,624 in 362 women who met Rome II criteria for IBS. After four weeks of administering 1×10^8 CFU, significant improvement in abdominal pain was noted compared to placebo ($p = 0.023$)—a therapeutic gain of 0.31. The global symptom assessment, bloating and distention, sense of incomplete evacuation, passage of gas, straining, and bowel habit satisfaction were also significantly improved using the same dose. Surprisingly, the 1×10^{10} dosage was ineffective, which had shown efficacy in a prior study [44]. There were problems with the ability of the capsule contents to dissolve at such a high dose. The investigators suggested that formulation problems observed with the larger dose highlights the importance of rigorous clinical data on the final dose and form of a probiotic product before use in clinical practice.

A recent study by Guyonnet et al. describes the efficacy of six weeks of administering fermented milk containing *B. animalis* DN-173 010 and yoghurt strains in 274 adults with constipation-predominant IBS in a multicenter, double-blind, controlled trial. The study suggests a beneficial role for this formulation in reducing discomfort and bloating in this subgroup of IBS patients [93].

In a double-blind study, Bittner et al. report efficacy of a combined probiotic–prebiotic treatment with Prescript-Assist in reducing IBS symptomatology. This was followed by publishing data suggesting efficacy in a one-year open trial extension study [94,95]. Furthermore, in an open Chinese trial conducted by Fan et al., administration of live, combined Bifidobacterium, Lactobacillus, and Enterococcus improved symptoms of irritable bowel syndrome [96].

While studies vary in design, especially in probiotic dose (from 5 to 13 logs), probiotic strain, and duration of therapy, most studies warrant further investigation. Nevertheless, the role of probiotics in children with irritable bowel syndrome remains to be defined. Table 10.2 summarizes the results of studies describing the role of probiotics in adults and children with IBS.

Pediatric studies are far fewer than the adult counterparts. A study published by Bausserman and Michail was designed to determine whether oral administration of the probiotic *Lactobacillus GG* under randomized, placebo-controlled, double-blinded conditions would improve symptoms of irritable bowel syndrome in children. Fifty children fulfilling the Rome II criteria completed the study. *Lactobacillus GG* administration for six weeks was not superior to placebo in relieving abdominal pain (40% response rate in the placebo group versus 44% in the *Lactobacillus GG* group ($p = 0.774$). Except for a lower incidence of perceived abdominal distension ($p = 0.02$ favoring *Lactobacillus GG*), no difference in the other gastrointestinal symptoms according to the Gastrointestinal Symptom Rating Scale (GSRS) was observed. It was therefore concluded that *Lactobacillus GG* was not superior to placebo in therapy targeting a reduction in abdominal pain in children with IBS but may be helpful with bloating.

Table 10.2.
Summary of published reports of probiotic role in irritable bowel syndrome

Author	Year	Type of probiotic	Duration weeks	Population	Type of trial	Outcome of study	Level of evidence
Bausserman, Michail [80]	2005	L. GG	6	Pediatric (n = 50)	R, DB, PC	Reduced abdominal distension.	I
Gawronska [97]	2007	L. GG	4	Pediatric (n = 104)	R, DB, PC	Effective	I
Zeng [110]	2008	Probiotic fermented milk	4	Adults (n=30)	R, SB, PC	Short-term improvement of barrier function	I
Drouault-Holowacz [106]	2008	Probiotic Mix	4	Adults (n=100)	R, DB, PC	No effect	I
Sinn [109]	2008	L. acidophilus - SDC 2012, 2013	4	Adults (n=40)	R, DB, PC	Effective	I
Plassmann [108]	2007	E-coli Nissle 1917		Variable Adutls (n=150)	Open, Retro-spective	Effective	II
Bittner [94]	2007	Prescript assist	60	Adults (n = 22)	Open trial	Effective	II
Fan [96]	2006	Mix of probiotics	4	Adults (n = 74)	Open trial	Effective	II
Whorwell [92]	2006	B. infantis	4	Adult women (n = 362)	R, DB, PC	Effective	I
Kim [83]	2005	VSL#3	4 and 8	Adults (n = 48)	R, DB, PC	Reduced flatulence and slowed colonic transit	I
O'Mahoney [44]	2005	L. salivaris and B infantis	8	Adults (n = 77)	R, DB, PC	Effective	I
Saggioro [98]	2004	LP0 1 and B. breve	4	Adults (n = 70)	R, PC	Effective	I
Tsuchiya [84]	2004	Symbiotic (SCM-III)	12	Adults (n = 68)	Single-blinded	Effective	II
Kim [82]	2003	VSL#3	8	Adults (n = 25)	R, DB, PC	Reduced bloating otherwise negative	I
Sen [99]	2002	Low dose LP299v	4	Adults (n = 12)[a]	DB, PC, crossover	No effect	I

Author	Year	Product		Population	Study design	Result	Class
Sen [99]	2002	Low dose LP299v	4	Adults (n = 12)[a]	DB, PC, crossover	No effect	I
Niedzielin [91]	2001	LP299v	4	Adults (n = 40)	Open trial	Effective	II
Brigidi [100]	2001	VSL#3	3	Adults (n = 10)[a]	Open, no placebo	Effective	II
O'Sullivan [101]	2000	LGG	4	Adults (n = 19)[a]	DB, PC crossover	No effect	I
Nobaek [81]	2000	LP299v	4	Adults (n = 60)	R, PC	Effective	I
Halpern [85]	1996	Lacteol Fort	6	Adults (n = 14)[a]	DB, PC, crossover	Effective	II

[a]Very small number of subjects studied. R = randomized, PC = placebo controlled, DB = double-blinded, SB = single blinded.

A more recent double-blinded, randomized controlled trial by Gawronska et al. was designed to determine the efficacy of a four-week therapy with *L. rhamnosus GG* (LGG) in treating functional abdominal pain disorders (FAPD) in children. Twenty children with functional dyspepsia (FD), 37 children with irritable bowel syndrome (IBS), and 47 children with functional abdominal pain (FAP) were enrolled in this study. There were no statistically significant differences in any of the study outcomes except for a higher incidence of treatment success (no pain) in children with IBS receiving LGG (six children in probiotic group versus one in the placebo group, $p = 0.04$, effect size 6.3 with a 95% CI of 1.2–38). The wide confidence interval prompted the authors to ask readers to interpret evidence with caution.

The quality of the evidence is rated according to the following categories [102]:

- I, Evidence obtained from at least one properly designed randomized controlled study.
- II-1, Evidence obtained from well-designed cohort or case-controlled trials without randomization.
- II-2, Evidence obtained from well-designed cohort or case-control analytic studies, preferably from more than one center or research group.
- II-3, Evidence obtained from multiple time series with or without the intervention.
- III, Evidence obtained from opinions of respected authorities on the basis of clinical experience, descriptive studies, or reports of expert committees.

SUMMARY

The mechanism of action of probiotic bacteria remains incompletely defined, yet the information gathered over the last several years starts to depict how immunological factors may influence intestinal homeostasis and highlights the importance of the microflora in the delicate and dynamic balanced interaction between the host and microbial ecology.

Probiotics play an important role in preventing overgrowth of potentially pathogenic bacteria and in maintaining the integrity of the gut mucosal barrier [103]. Probiotic agents have been used for therapy of different gastrointestinal conditions including inflammatory bowel disease [104,105]. The beneficial effects of probiotics, albeit modest, have been previously established in adult patients with irritable bowel syndrome. However, pediatric data appear to be less compelling and more studies are necessary to address the efficacy of different types of probiotic products and to establish appropriate pediatric dosing in this common disorder.

REFERENCES

1. Apley, J.N.N., Recurrent abdominal pain, a field survey of a 1000 school children. *Arch Dis Child*, 1958; 33: 165–170.
2. Hyams, J.S. et al., Abdominal pain and irritable bowel syndrome in adolescents: a community-based study. *J Pediatr*, 1996; 129(2): 220–6.
3. Everhart, JE, Renault, PF. Irritable bowel syndrome in office-based practice in the United States. *Gastroenterology*, 1991; 100(4): 998–10005.
4. Drossman, D.A., The Rome criteria process: diagnosis and legitimization of irritable bowel syndrome. *Am J Gastroenterol*, 1999; 94(10): 2803–7.

5. Hamm, L.R., et-al., Additional investigations fail to alter the diagnosis of irritable bowel syndrome in subjects fulfilling the Rome criteria. *Am J Gastroenterol*, 1999; 94(5): 1279–82.

6. Rasquin-Weber, A., et-al., Childhood functional gastrointestinal disorders. *Gut*, 1999; 45(Suppl. 2): II60–8.

7. Varni, J.W., et-al., Health-related quality of life in pediatric patients with irritable bowel syndrome: a comparative analysis. *J Dev Behav Pediatr*, 2006; 27(6): 451–8.

8. Talley, N.J., Pharmacologic therapy for the irritable bowel syndrome. *Am J Gastroenterol*, 2003; 98(4): 750–8.

9. Drossman, D.A., et-al., AGA technical review on irritable bowel syndrome. *Gastroenterology*, 2002; 123(6): 2108–31.

10. Brandt, L.J., et-al., Systematic review on the management of irritable bowel syndrome in North America. *Am J Gastroenterol*, 2002; 97(11 Suppl.): S7–26.

11. Balsari, A., et-al., The fecal microbial population in the irritable bowel syndrome. *Microbiologica*, 1982; 5(3): 185–94.

12. King, T.S., M. Elia, and J.O. Hunter, Abnormal colonic fermentation in irritable bowel syndrome. *Lancet*, 1998; 352(9135): 1187–9.

13. Quigley, E.M. Disturbances of motility and visceral hypersensitivity in irritable bowel syndrome: biological markers or epiphenomenon. *Gastroenterol Clin North Am*, 2005; 34(2): 221–33, vi.

14. Lin, H.C., Small intestinal bacterial overgrowth: a framework for understanding irritable bowel syndrome. *JAMA*, 2004; 292(7): 852–8.

15. Agarwal, R., et-al., Effects of oral Lactobacillus GG on enteric microflora in low-birth-weight neonates. *J Pediatr Gastroenterol Nutr*, 2003; 36(3): 397–402.

16. Rossland, E., et-al., Production of antimicrobial metabolites by strains of Lactobacillus or Lactococcus co-cultured with Bacillus cereus in milk. *Int J Food Microbiol*, 2005; 98(2): 193–200.

17. Mack, D.R., et-al., Probiotics inhibit enteropathogenic *E. coli* adherence *in vitro* by inducing intestinal *mucin gene expression. Am J Physiol*, 1999; 276(4 Pt 1): G941–50.

18. Wilson, K.H. and F. Perini, Role of competition for nutrients in suppression of *Clostridium difficile* by the colonic microflora. *Infect Immun*, 1988; 56(10): 2610–4.

19. Pothoulakis, C., et-al., Saccharomyces boulardii inhibits *Clostridium difficile* toxin A binding and enterotoxicity in rat ileum. *Gastroenterology*, 1993; 104(4): 1108–15.

20. Michail, S. and F. Abernathy *Lactobacillus plantarum* inhibits the intestinal epithelial migration of neutrophils induced by enteropathogenic Escherichia coli. *J Pediatr Gastroenterol Nutr*, 2003; 36(3): 385–91.

21. Michail, S. and F. Abernathy *Lactobacillus plantarum* reduces the in vitro secretory response of intestinal epithelial cells to enteropathogenic *Escherichia coli* infection. *J Pediatr Gastroenterol Nutr*, 2002; 35(3): 350–5.

22. Dahan, S., et-al., Saccharomyces boulardii interferes with enterohemorrhagic *Escherichia coli*-induced signaling pathways in T84 cells. *Infect Immun*, 2003; 71(2): 766–73.

23. Kalliomaki, M.A. and E. Isolauri Probiotics and down-regulation of the allergic response. *Immunol Allergy Clin North Am*, 2004; 24(4): 739–52, viii.

24. Lee, J.W., et-al., Immunomodulatory and antitumor effects in vivo by the cytoplasmic fraction of *Lactobacillus casei* and *Bifidobacterium longum. J Vet Sci*, 2004; 5(1): 41–8.

25. Jijon, H., et-al., DNA from probiotic bacteria modulates murine and human epithelial and immune function. *Gastroenterology*, 2004; 126(5): 1358–73.

26. Yan, F. and D.B. Polk Probiotic bacterium prevents cytokine-induced apoptosis in intestinal epithelial cells. *J Biol Chem*, 2002; 277(52): 50959–65.

27. Rachmilewitz, D., et-al., Toll-like receptor 9 signaling mediates the anti-inflammatory effects of probiotics in murine experimental colitis. *Gastroenterology*, 2004; 126(2): 520–8.

28. Westendorf, A.M., et-al., Intestinal immunity of *Escherichia coli* NISSLE 1917: a safe carrier for therapeutic molecules. *FEMS Immunol Med Microbiol*, 2005; 43(3): 373–84.

29. Rousseaux, C., et-al., *Lactobacillus acidophilus* modulates intestinal pain and induces opioid and cannabinoid receptors. *Nat Med*, 2007; 13(1): 35–7.

30. Suau, A., Molecular tools to investigate intestinal bacterial communities. *J Pediatr Gastroenterol Nutr*, 2003; 37(3): 222–4.

31. Treem, W.R., et-al., Fecal short-chain fatty acids in patients with diarrhea-predominant irritable bowel syndrome: in vitro studies of carbohydrate fermentation. *J Pediatr Gastroenterol Nutr*, 1996; 23(3): 280–6.

32. Pimentel, M., et-al., Methane production during lactulose breath test is associated with gastrointestinal disease presentation. *Dig Dis Sci*, 2003; 48(1): 86–92.

33. Pimentel, M., Y. Kong, and S. Park IBS subjects with methane on lactulose breath test have lower postprandial serotonin levels than subjects with hydrogen. *Dig Dis Sci*, 2004; 49(1): 84–7.

34. Pimentel, M., Y. Kong, and S. Park Breath testing to evaluate lactose intolerance in irritable bowel syndrome correlates with lactulose testing and may not reflect true lactose malabsorption. *Am J Gastroenterol*, 2003; 98(12): 2700–4.

35. Pimentel, M., E.J. Chow, and H.C. Lin, Normalization of lactulose breath testing correlates with symptom improvement in irritable bowel syndrome. a double-blind, randomized, placebo-controlled study. *Am J Gastroenterol*, 2003; 98(2): 412–9.

36. Dear, K.L., M. Elia, and J.O. Hunter, Do interventions which reduce colonic bacterial fermentation improve symptoms of irritable bowel syndrome? *Dig Dis Sci*, 2005; 50(4): 758–66.

37. Quigley, E.M. Bacterial flora in irritable bowel syndrome: role in pathophysiology, implications for management. *J Dig Dis*, 2007; 8(1): 2–7.

38. Barbara, G., et-al., New pathophysiological mechanisms in irritable bowel syndrome. *Aliment Pharmacol Ther*, 2004; 20 (Suppl. 2): 1–9.

39. Osipov, G.A., et-al., [Clinical significance of studies of microorganisms of the intestinal mucosa by culture biochemical methods and mass fragmentography]. *Eksp Klin Gastroenterol*, 2003(4): 59–67, 115.

40. Sharara, A.I., et-al., A randomized double-blind placebo-controlled trial of rifaximin in patients with abdominal bloating and flatulence. *Am J Gastroenterol*, 2006; 101(2): 326–33.

41. Frissora, C.L. and B.D. Cash Review article: the role of antibiotics vs. conventional pharmacotherapy in treating symptoms of irritable bowel syndrome. *Aliment Pharmacol Ther*, 2007; 25(11): 1271–81.

42. Malinen, E., et-al., Analysis of the fecal microbiota of irritable bowel syndrome patients and healthy controls with real-time PCR. *Am J Gastroenterol*, 2005; 100(2): 373–82.

43. Si, J.M., et-al., Intestinal microecology and quality of life in irritable bowel syndrome patients. *World J Gastroenterol*, 2004; 10(12): 1802–5.

44. O'Mahony, L., et-al., Lactobacillus and bifidobacterium in irritable bowel syndrome: symptom responses and relationship to cytokine profiles. *Gastroenterology*, 2005; 128(3): 541–51.

45. Bazzocchi, G., et-al., Intestinal microflora and oral bacteriotherapy in irritable bowel syndrome. *Dig Liver Dis*, 2002; 34 (Suppl. 2): S48–53.

46. McKendrick, M.W. and N.W. Read Irritable bowel syndrome – post salmonella infection. *J Infect*, 1994; 29(1): 1–3.

47. Neal, K.R., J. Hebden, and R. Spiller Prevalence of gastrointestinal symptoms six months after bacterial gastroenteritis and risk factors for development of the irritable bowel syndrome: postal survey of patients. *BMJ*, 1997; 314(7083): 779–82.

48. Rodriguez, L.A. and A. Ruigomez Increased risk of irritable bowel syndrome after bacterial gastroenteritis: cohort study. *BMJ*, 1999; 318(7183): 565–6.

49. Gwee, K.A., et-al., Increased rectal mucosal expression of interleukin 1beta in recently acquired postinfectious irritable bowel syndrome. *Gut*, 2003; 52(4): 523–6.

50. Gwee, K.A., et-al., Psychometric scores and persistence of irritable bowel after infectious diarrhoea. *Lancet*, 1996; 347(8995): 150–3.

51. Gwee, K.A., et-al., The role of psychological and biological factors in postinfective gut dysfunction. *Gut*, 1999; 44(3): 400–6.

52. Spiller, R. and E. CampbellPost-infectious irritable bowel syndrome. *Curr Opin Gastroenterol*, 2006; 22(1): 13–7.

53. Dunlop, S.P., D. Jenkins, and R.C. Spiller Distinctive clinical, psychological, and histological features of postinfective irritable bowel syndrome. *Am J Gastroenterol*, 2003; 98(7): 1578–83.

54. Spiller, R.C., et-al., Increased rectal mucosal enteroendocrine cells, T lymphocytes, and increased gut permeability following acute Campylobacter enteritis and in post-dysenteric irritable bowel syndrome. *Gut*, 2000; 47(6): 804–11.

55. Thornley, J.P., et-al., Relationship of Campylobacter toxigenicity in vitro to the development of postinfectious irritable bowel syndrome. *J Infect Dis*, 2001; 184(5): 606–9.

56. Chadwick, V.S., et-al., Activation of the mucosal immune system in irritable bowel syndrome. *Gastroenterology*, 2002; 122(7): 1778–83.

57. Cremonini, F., et-al. Effect of CCK-1 antagonist, dexloxiglumide, in female patients with irritable bowel syndrome: a pharmacodynamic and pharmacogenomic study. *Am J Gastroenterol*, 2005; 100(3): 652–63.

58. Barbara, G., et-al., Activated mast cells in proximity to colonic nerves correlate with abdominal pain in irritable bowel syndrome. *Gastroenterology*, 2004; 126(3): 693–702.

59. Tornblom, H., et-al., Full-thickness biopsy of the jejunum reveals inflammation and enteric neuropathy in irritable bowel syndrome. *Gastroenterology*, 2002; 123(6): 1972–9.

60. Spiller, R.C., Role of nerves in enteric infection. *Gut*, 2002; 51(6): 759–62.

61. Shanahan, F., Immunology. *Therapeutic manipulation of gut flora. Science*, 2000; 289(5483): 1311–2.

62. Dunlop, S.P., et-al., Relative importance of enterochromaffin cell hyperplasia, anxiety, and depression in postinfectious IBS. *Gastroenterology*, 2003; 125(6): 1651–9.

63. Spiller, R.C., Estimating the importance of infection in IBS. *Am J Gastroenterol*, 2003; 98(2): 238–41.

64. Bercik, P., E.F. Verdu, and S.M. Collins Is irritable bowel syndrome a low-grade inflammatory bowel disease? *Gastroenterol Clin North Am*, 2005; 34(2): 235–45, vi-vii.

65. Gonsalkorale, W.M., et-al., Interleukin 10 genotypes in irritable bowel syndrome: evidence for an inflammatory component? *Gut*, 2003; 52(1): 91–3.

66. O'Sullivan, M., et-al., Increased mast cells in the irritable bowel syndrome. *Neurogastroenterol Motil*, 2000; 12(5): 449–57.

67. Collins, S.M., The immunomodulation of enteric neuromuscular function: implications for motility and inflammatory disorders. *Gastroenterology*, 1996; 111(6): 1683–99.

68. Gorbach, S.L., Probiotics in the third millennium. *Dig Liver Dis*, 2002; 34 (Suppl. 2): S2–7.

69. von Wright, A. and S. Salminen Probiotics: established effects and open questions. *Eur J Gastroenterol Hepatol*, 1999; 11(11): 1195–8.

70. Isolauri, E., P.V. Kirjavainen, and S. Salminen Probiotics: a role in the treatment of intestinal infection and inflammation? *Gut*, 2002; 50(Suppl. 3): III54–9.

71. McCarthy, J., et-al., Double blind, placebo controlled trial of two probiotic strains in interleukin 10 knockout mice and mechanistic link with cytokine balance. *Gut*, 2003; 52(7): 975–80.

72. O'Mahony, L., et-al., Probiotic impact on microbial flora, inflammation and tumour development in IL-10 knockout mice. *Aliment Pharmacol Ther*, 2001; 15(8): 1219–25.

73. Quigley, E.M., Current concepts of the irritable bowel syndrome. *Scand J Gastroenterol Suppl.*, 2003(237): 1–8.

74. Bradley, H.K., et-al., Instability in the faecal flora of a patient suffering from food-related irritable bowel syndrome. *J Med Microbiol*, 1987; 23(1): 29–32.

75. Jiang, T. and D.A. Savaiano In vitro lactose fermentation by human colonic bacteria is modified by Lactobacillus acidophilus supplementation. *J Nutr*, 1997; 127(8): 1489–95.

76. Jiang, T.A. Mustapha, and D.A. Savaiano Improvement of lactose digestion in humans by ingestion of unfermented milk containing Bifidobacterium longum. *J Dairy Sci*, 1996; 79(5): 750–7.

77. Jiang, T. and D.A. Savaiano Modification of colonic fermentation by bifidobacteria and pH in vitro. Impact on lactose metabolism, short-chain fatty acid, and lactate production. *Dig Dis Sci*, 1997; 42(11): 2370–7.

78. Ouwehand, A.C., et-al., The mucus binding of *Bifidobacterium lactis* Bb12 is enhanced in the presence of Lactobacillus GG and Lact. *delbrueckii subsp. bulgaricus. Lett Appl Microbiol*, 2000; 30(1): 10–3.

79. Ouwehand, A.C., et-al., Effect of probiotics on constipation, fecal azoreductase activity and fecal mucin content in the elderly. *Ann Nutr Metab*, 2002; 46(3–4): 159–62.

80. Bausserman, M. and S. Michail The use of Lactobacillus GG in irritable bowel syndrome in children: a double-blind randomized control trial. *J Pediatr*, 2005; 147(2): 197–201.

81. Nobaek, S., et-al., Alteration of intestinal microflora is associated with reduction in abdominal bloating and pain in patients with irritable bowel syndrome. *Am J Gastroenterol*, 2000; 95(5): 1231–8.

82. Kim, H.J., et-al., A randomized controlled trial of a probiotic, VSL#3, on gut transit and symptoms in diarrhoea-predominant irritable bowel syndrome. *Aliment Pharmacol Ther*, 2003; 17(7): 895–904.

83. Kim, H.J., et-al., A randomized controlled trial of a probiotic combination VSL# 3 and placebo in irritable bowel syndrome with bloating. *Neurogastroenterol Motil*, 2005; 17(5): 687–96.

84. Tsuchiya, J., et-al., Single-blind follow-up study on the effectiveness of a symbiotic preparation in irritable bowel syndrome. *Chin J Dig Dis*, 2004; 5(4): 169–74.

85. Halpern, G.M., et-al., Treatment of irritable bowel syndrome with Lacteol Fort: a randomized, double-blind, cross-over trial. *Am J Gastroenterol*, 1996; 91(8): 1579–85.

86. Hamilton-Miller., J. Probiotics in the management of irritable bowel syndrome: a review of clinical trials. *Microb Ecol Health Dis*, 2001; 13: 212–216.

87. Ibnou-Zekri, N., et-al., Divergent patterns of colonization and immune response elicited from two intestinal Lactobacillus strains that display similar properties in vitro. *Infect Immun*, 2003; 71(1): 428–36.

88. Bousvaros, A., et-al., A randomized, double-blind trial of Lactobacillus GG versus placebo in addition to standard maintenance therapy for children with Crohn's disease. *Inflamm Bowel Dis*, 2005; 11(9): 833–9.

89. Gupta, P., et-al., Is lactobacillus GG helpful in children with Crohn's disease? Results of a preliminary, open-label study. *J Pediatr Gastroenterol Nutr*, 2000; 31(4): 453–7.

90. Michail, S., et-al., Clinical efficacy of probiotics: review of the evidence with focus on children. *J Pediatr Gastroenterol Nutr*, 2006; 43(4): 550–7.

91. Niedzielin, K., H. Kordecki, and B. Birkenfeld A controlled, double-blind, randomized study on the efficacy of *Lactobacillus plantarum* 299 V in patients with irritable bowel syndrome. *Eur J Gastroenterol Hepatol*, 2001; 13(10): 1143–7.

92. Whorwell, P.J., et-al., Efficacy of an encapsulated probiotic *Bifidobacterium infantis* 35624 in women with irritable bowel syndrome. *Am J Gastroenterol*, 2006; 101(7): 1581–90.

93. Guyonnet, D., et-al., Effect of a fermented milk containing *Bifidobacterium animalis* DN-173 010 on the health-related quality of life and symptoms in irritable bowel syndrome in adults in primary care: a multicentre, randomized, double-blind, controlled trial. *Aliment Pharmacol Ther*, 2007; 26(3): 475–86.

94. Bittner, A.C., et-al., Prescript-assist probiotic-prebiotic treatment for irritable bowel syndrome: an open-label, partially controlled, 1-year extension of a previously published controlled clinical trial. *Clin Ther*, 2007; 29(6): 1153–60.

95. Bittner, A.C., R.M. Croffut, and M.C. Stranahan Prescript-Assist probiotic-prebiotic treatment for irritable bowel syndrome: a methodologically oriented, 2-week, randomized, placebo-controlled, double-blind clinical study. *Clin Ther*, 2005; 27(6): 755–61.

96. Fan, Y.J., et-al., A probiotic treatment containing Lactobacillus, Bifidobacterium and Enterococcus improves IBS symptoms in an open label trial. *J Zhejiang Univ Sci B*, 2006; 7(12): 987–91.

97. Gawronska, A., et-al., A randomized double-blind placebo-controlled trial of Lactobacillus GG for abdominal pain disorders in children. *Aliment Pharmacol Ther*, 2007; 25(2): 177–84.

98. Saggioro, A., Probiotics in the treatment of irritable bowel syndrome. *J Clin Gastroenterol*, 2004; 38(6 Suppl.): S104–6.

99. Sen, S., et-al., Effect of *Lactobacillus plantarum* 299v on colonic fermentation and symptoms of irritable bowel syndrome. *Dig Dis Sci*, 2002; 47(11): 2615–20.

100. Brigidi, P., et-al., Effects of probiotic administration upon the composition and enzymatic activity of human fecal microbiota in patients with irritable bowel syndrome or functional diarrhea. *Res Microbiol*, 2001; 152(8): 735–41.

101. O'Sullivan, M.A. and C.A. O'Morain Bacterial supplementation in the irritable bowel syndrome. A randomised double-blind placebo-controlled crossover study. *Dig Liver Dis*, 2000; 32(4): 294–301.

102. The periodic health examination. Canadian Task Force on the Periodic Health Examination. Can Med Assoc J, 1979; 121(9): 1193–254.

103. Bengmark, S., Ecological control of the gastrointestinal tract. *The role of probiotic flora. Gut*, 1998; 42(1): 2–7.

104. Mimura, T., et-al., Once daily high dose probiotic therapy (VSL#3) for maintaining remission in recurrent or refractory pouchitis. *Gut*, 2004; 53(1): 108–14.

105. Gionchetti, P. et-al., Prophylaxis of pouchitis onset with probiotic therapy: a double-blind, placebo-controlled trial. *Gastroenterology*, 2003; 124(5): 1202–9.

106. Drouault-Holowacz S, Bieuvelet S, Burckel A, Cazaubiel M, Dray X, Marteau P. A double blind randomized controlled trial of a probiotic combination in 100 patients with irritable bowel syndrome. *Gastroenterol Clin Biol,* 2008; 32(2):147–52.
107. McFarland LV, Dublin S. Meta-analysis of probiotics for the treatment of irritable bowel syndrome. *World J Gastroenterol,* 2008; 14(17):2650–61.
108. Plassmann D, Schulte-Witte H. [Treatment of irritable bowel syndrome with Escherichia coli strain Nissle 1917 (EcN): a retrospective survey]. *Med Klin (Munich),* 2007;102(11):888-92.
109. Sinn DH, Song JH, Kim HJ, Lee JH, Son HJ, Chang DK, et al. Therapeutic Effect of Lactobacillus acidophilus-SDC 2012, 2013 in Patients with Irritable Bowel Syndrome. *Dig Dis Sci,* 2008;53(10): 2714–8.
110. Zeng J, Li YQ, Zuo XL, Zhen YB, Yang J, Liu CH. Clinical trial: effect of active lactic acid bacteria on mucosal barrier function in patients with diarrhea-predominant irritable bowel syndrome. Aliment Pharmacol Ther 2008.

11 The Role of Probiotics in the Treatment and Prevention of Infectious Diarrhea in Children

Shafiqul A. Sarker and George J. Fuchs

Key Points

- It has been hypothesized that probiotics might be efficacious in the prevention and treatment of acute diarrhea in adults and children.
- Evidence of efficacy in the prevention of community-acquired and nosocomial diarrhea exists.
- This review summarizes the evidence of the role of probiotic agents in infectious diarrhea in children and reviews the mechanism of action and safety in their clinical application.

Key Words: Probiotics, children, diarrhoea, lactobacillus, bifidobacterium, infectious diarrhea.

INTRODUCTION

Diarrheal disease continues to place a major burden on child health. In the early 1980s, diarrheal diseases accounted for about 4.6 million deaths from around 1 billion episodes of illness annually in children younger than 5 years of age[1]. A decade later, even without significant change in incidence, the number of deaths attributable to diarrheal diseases decreased to 3.3 million per year,[2] the reduction attributed to the implementation of oral rehydration therapy (ORT) coordinated by the World Health Organization (WHO)[3]. The most recent estimates indicate that diarrheal deaths further decreased to 2.5 million[4] per year. Despite these impressive gains, diarrheal disease remains a leading killer of young children and is estimated to account for 15% of cause-specific mortality among children below 5 years of age, a rate exceeded only by acute lower respiratory infections (18%)[5] The major burden of diarrheal illness is currently experienced by the developing world, where children suffer from 6–7 episodes per year compared to only one episode in the developed countries[6] Poor water supply and sanitation, lack of education and personal hygiene, malnutrition, and HIV-associated

From: *Nutrition and Health: Probiotics in Pediatric Medicine*
Edited by: S. Michail and P.M. Sherman © Humana Press, Totowa, NJ

impaired immunity are factors behind the high incidence of diarrheal diseases in the developing countries. In contrast, deaths due to diarrheal illness are rare in developed countries, and the effects of these illnesses are often measured in financial terms. In the United States, approximately 25 million episodes of diarrheal illness occur among children below 5 years of age annually leading to 200,000 hospital admissions each year[6]. This accounts for 2% of the outpatient visits costing US$50 per visits and 4% of all hospital admissions costing an estimated US$2307 per admission[7]. Despite the successes in the control of diarrheal diseases, developed countries remain under genuine threat of enteric pathogens that emerge and reemerge in the developing countries primarily due to the dramatic increase in global travel.

Current management of diarrheal illness involves prevention and management of dehydration using oral or intravenous rehydration, as appropriate, and continued feeding including breast-feeding for young infants. Additionally, therapy with effective antimicrobial agents is required for the management of shigellosis and severe cholera. Recently, the WHO and UNICEF have recommended routine use of zinc for 10–14 days in the management of diarrhea in young children irrespective of etiology[8]. However, its successful widespread programmatic implementation in the developing countries remains a challenge. Recently, orally administrable cholera vaccine has been marketed in the United States primarily for travelers; however, its prohibitive current costs and the need for multiple doses for optimal protective efficacy, particularly among young children, are barriers to its routine use in public health programs of developing countries. An oral rotavirus vaccine, determined to be effective and safe in controlled trials, was withdrawn within a year of its marketing due to increased risk of intussusceptions among the vaccines[9–11]. Two new rotavirus vaccine candidates are currently licensed and have been demonstrated to be safe, well tolerated, and highly efficacious. Several other vaccines are in the late stages of development [90]. In the developing world, clinical trials are still needed to ensure that the vaccines being licensed will work as expected in children living in poor settings. In these settings, other enteric flora, micronutrient malnutrition, higher titers of maternal antibody and other factors still poorly defined have compromised other live oral vaccines and have required the developers to alter vaccine formulation, dose, or schedule [91]. Antimicrobial therapy, while useful, requires continuous monitoring of susceptibility of the pathogens and dissemination of such information to health care providers—not an easy task and therefore not practical in developing countries. More importantly, emergence of resistant strains is common, which leads to therapy with ineffective agents and associated problems. Even in cases where measures are effective, quite often the treatment regime is economically and logistically impossible to administer, particularly in developing countries. There is consequently a clear need to define other, cost-effective and affordable interventions for the prevention and management of infectious diarrhea including that caused by rotavirus.

For over a century researchers have suggested that live bacterial cultures, such as those found in yoghurt, might help to treat and to prevent diarrhea. The concept of using bacterial culture was established only in the last century at the Pasteur Institute by the work of a Russian Scientist, Metchnikoff, who hypothesized that the ingestion of fermented milk products had potential beneficial impact on the health and lifespan of Bulgarian peasants[12]. The formal term of probiotic (meaning "for life") was referenced first in 1954 by Ferdinand Vergin[13] followed by Lilly and Stillwell[14] in 1965 in their article discussing the effects of antibiotics on beneficial intestinal bacteria. Fuller often is credited for establishing the term "probiotics" as bacterial products conferring benefit based on his work with animals[15]. According to him, a probiotic is a live microbial feed supplement, which beneficially affects the host animal by improving its intestinal microbial balance. One of the most recent definitions proposed by a group of experts convened by the Food and Agriculture Organization of the United Nations defined probiotics as "live microorganisms administered in adequate amounts which confer a beneficial health effect on the host"[16].

Most probiotics are strains of *Bifidobacterium* or *Lactobacillus* species belonging to the normal commensal bacterial flora of the human intestine, and are currently extensively investigated as probiotics[17,18]. Their antidiarrheal properties have been investigated since the 1960s[19]. These organisms have a historical track record of safety. Because of their widespread acceptance and general lack of side effects, probiotics are increasingly popular among the community and consequently are now used widely for various indications. Nearly 25% children attending a general gastroenterology outpatient clinic in Australia had taken or were currently taking probiotics[20]; over 75% of children with chronic inflammatory bowel diseases in the same setting reported using probiotics[21]. However, evidence to support the use of probiotics in childhood infectious diarrheal disease exists for only a few, specific conditions.

MECHANISMS OF ACTION

One of the difficulties in assessing the role of probiotics in clinical practice is a limited understanding of their mechanisms of action. However, some of the biological effects of probiotics have recently been characterized. The numbers of dose-related efficacy studies are minimal and more pharmacodynamic and pharmacokinetic aspects data are needed. Two possible methods of action, microbiologic and immunologic, are hypothesized for the beneficial action of probiotics in clinical practice.

Microbiologic Mechanisms

In general, probiotics help to improve the balance of the intestinal microbiota. The human intestinal microbiota contains hundreds of different species of bacteria. Newborns are rapidly and extensively colonized in their passage through the birth canal, and the intestinal bacterial density rapidly rises to 10^{11} CFU/g, reaching 10^{14} microorganisms during adulthood[22]. The administration of probiotic bacteria to healthy neonates can significantly influence the composition of the healthy intestinal microbiota[23]; in this regard, the intestinal microbiota of infants is more amenable to manipulation by probiotic supplementation than that of adults[23, 24].

In disease states, probiotics can also affect the intestinal microbiota. Some of the protective mechanisms by which they inhibit the actions of pathogenic microbes have been elucidated. In disease states associated with impaired intestinal integrity as manifested by increased intestinal mucosal permeability, the administration of *Lactobacillus* probiotics can improve intestinal mucosal permeability[25]. Certain probiotics exhibit an antimicrobial effect through modification of the microflora, secretion of antibacterial substances, hydrogen peroxide, and biosurfactant to aid their survival in the gastrointestinal tract. Certain probiotics also have the capacity to competitively inhibit adherence of more pathogenic bacteria to the intestinal epithelium, compete with nutrients essential for pathogen survival, produce an antitoxin effect, and reverse selected consequences of infection on the gut epithelium such as secretory changes and neutrophil migration[26]. Many probiotic species induce mucin production by intestinal epithelial cells in vitro and some also induce the production of defensin-β2, antibacterial peptide [27], and maintenance of normal crypt and epithelial cell architecture[28,29].

Immunologic Mechanisms

The most important methods of action of probiotics relate to the development, maturation, and regulation of mucosal-associated immune defense[30], Elmer & McFarland[31,32]. The primary immunological effects of probiotics are likely to take place in the gut-associated lymphoid tissue, including Peyer's patches in the small intestine[33]. A range of probiotic immune effects has been described, although direct evidence for the basic mechanisms by which they achieve beneficial effects is limited. Some murine studies indicate these immune effects enhance the function of the intestinal epithelial barrier. Hooper et al., discovered that intestinal commensals upregulate the expression of mucin-encoding genes in the host intestinal epithelium, which stimulates the production of mucus to form a protective barrier[34]. Other investigators have shown that Toll-like receptor (TLR) signaling by the commensal intestinal microbiota is essential for homeostasis of the intestinal epithelium and protection from epithelial injury; this is likely a key mechanism of action of probiotics[35]. Through pattern-recognizing molecules on the commensal microorganism, TLRs stimulate the production of epithelial repair factors. Activation of TLR by molecules, such as lipopolysaccharides flagellin, and lipotechoic acid, generate the production of cytokines through intracellular signaling pathways, which activate transcription factors including nuclear factor κB (NF-κB). Some nonpathogenic enteric bacteria exert an effect on the intestinal epithelia cells by directly inhibiting the NF-κB pathway[36] while others inhibit the same pathway by promoting the nuclear export of an NF-κB subunit, thus limiting the duration of NF-κB activation[37] These inhibitory effects on the proinflammatory NF-κB pathway may be an important mechanism by which probiotics regulate intestinal inflammation.

Clinical studies have shown particular probiotics to exert specific immunologic actions, e.g., increases in the concentrations of the antiinflammatory cytokine IL-10 in association with the administration of LGG to infants[38]. The enhanced in vivo generation of IL-10 substantiates the antiinflammatory properties of specific strains of probiotic bacteria, which may be particularly relevant for their use in the treatment of patients with intestinal inflammation. LGG has also been observed to upregulate markers of phagocyte activation in healthy individuals and to downregulate the same markers in adults allergic to cow milk undergoing cow milk challenge[39]. *Lactobacillus* GG have also been shown to promote local antigen-specific immune responses (particularly of the IgA class) and to prevent permeability defects, thus conferring controlled antigen absorption in allergic disorders[40]. It has also been suggested that specific probiotics have the potential to preferentially stimulate different subsets of T helper cells (Th1 or Th2) and in this way modify intestinal inflammatory or allergic responses[41].

Other proposed probiotics mechanisms include enhancement of host defense by strengthening tight junction, stimulation of cytokine production, and the production of substances thought to secondarily act as protective nutrients (short-chain fatty acid, arginine) for the gut[42,43], *S. boulardii* also induce production of polyamines in humans that promote maturation of brush border disaccharidase and other enzymes (lactase, sucrase, maltase, and aminopeptidase) and an increase in the number of glucose carriers in the enterocyte membrane[44].

PREVENTION OF ACUTE INFECTIOUS GASTROENTERITIS AND NOSOCOMIAL DIARRHEA-POTENTIALS FOR PROBIOTIC USE

The proposed health benefits of probiotics have undergone increasingly rigorous scientific evaluation in recent years, and there is now strong evidence for their use in treatment and prevention of some human diseases. Several well-designed studies have demonstrated a prophylactic effect of certain probiotics to decrease the incidence of acute diarrhea (Table 11.1). More than 10 years ago, in a double-blind, placebo-controlled trial, Saavedra et al. observed that supplementation of an infant formula with *bifidobacteria* and *S. thermophilus* resulted in a decreased incidence of diarrheal diseases (7% cases with probiotics vs. 31% in the control group) in a population of chronically hospitalized children over 17 months. The prevalence of rotavirus shedding was also significantly lower in the infants receiving probiotic-supplemented formula (10% shedding with probiotic versus 39% with the control group)[45].

Thibault et al. assessed the prevalence of acute diarrhea in more than 900 French infants (4–6 months of age, regularly exposed to childcare or living at home) fed a formula fermented with *B. breve* c50 and *S. thermophillus* 065 for a prolonged period. The study formula was well accepted and enabled normal growth of infants; however, there was no significant difference in the incidence and duration of diarrhea episodes or the number of hospital admissions compared to the nonprobiotic control formula fed infants. However, episodes were less severe in the fermented formula group with fewer cases of dehydration, fewer medical consultations, and fewer prescriptions of oral rehydration solutions (ORS)[46]. In contrast, a more recent multicenter study in 90 infants living in residential nurseries or foster care centers in France failed to demonstrate a reduction in the prevalence of diarrhea, with a formula supplemented with a different probiotic, viable *B. lactis* strain BB12, when compared to placebo (28.3% vs., 38.7%, $P = NS$). However, the number of days with diarrhea and the daily probability of diarrhea were significantly reduced in the probiotic group (1.2 ± 2.5 and 0.8 days) versus the conventional formula group (2.3 ± 4.5 and 1.6 days) ($p = 0.0002$ and 0.0014)[47]. The *B. lactis*-fed infants also had a reduced risk of contracting diarrhea by 1.9-fold (range 1.3–2.6), suggesting that viable *Bifidobacterium lactis* strain Bb 12 added to an acidified infant formula has some protective effect against acute diarrhea in healthy children. The efficacy of *Lactobacillus casei* in preventing acute diarrhea has been evaluated by Pedone and colleagues in a randomized control trial involving 779 children (6–24 months)[48]. The healthy children who received milk fermented by yogurt cultures and *L. casei* had a significantly reduced incidence of diarrhea compared to children who received traditional yogurt (15.9% vs. 22%). Notably, the difference observed during the supplementation period was not durable and no longer significant 6 weeks after the end of supplementation, suggesting that regular intake of probiotics may be required to achieve a beneficial effect.

Table 11.1
Probiotics in the prevention of infectious or nosocomial diarrhea in children

Authors	Population studied	No (Age)	Probiotic agent	Dose	Duration of therapy	Results
Saavedra et al., 1994	Chronic care hospitalized children in the United States	55 (5–24 months)	B. breve S. thermophilus	Bb 1.9×10^9 CFU/g + St 0.14×10^8 CFU/g of powdered formula	For the duration of hospital stay	Decreased incidence of nosocomial diarrheal disease associated with decreased rotaviral shedding
Oberhelman et al., 1999	Malnourished community children in Peru	204 (18–29 months)	LGG	7×10^{10} once daily, 6 day/week	15 month	Fewer diarrhea episodes in LGG-supplemented group
Pedone et al., 2000	Childcare or residential children in France	779 (6–24 months)	L. casei	10^8 CFU/mL once daily	1 month	Reduced incidence as well as frequency of diarrhea
Hatakka et al., 2001	Finish children attending daycare center	571 (1–6 year)	LGG	$5–10 \times 10^5$ CFU/mL $\times$ 3 times a day $\times$ 5 day/week	7 month	No effect on incidence of diarrhea; 16% reduction in the number of days of absence due to GI infection
Szajewska et al., 2001	Polish children hospitalized with nondiarrheal illness	81 (1–36 mo)	LGG	6×10^9 CFU twice daily	Hospitalization period	Reduced risk of Nosocomial diarrhea, particularly nosocomial rotavirus gastroenteritis, in LGG-supplemented group
Mastretta et al., 2002	Italian children admitted with nondiarrheal illness	220 (1–18 months)	LGG	10^{10} CFU/mL	Hospitalization period	GG was ineffective in preventing nosocomial rotavirus infection; however, it reduced the risk of symptomatic rotavirus gastroenteritis
Thibault et al., 2004	Residential children in France	971 (4–6 months)	B. breve S. thermophilus	Not mentioned	5 months	No effect on incidence, duration of diarrhea episodes, or number of hospital admissions; might reduce the severity of acute diarrhea

CFU, colony forming units.

There are few randomized, controlled trials in children investigating the potential of LGG to prevent nosocomial diarrhea; limited studies of young children hospitalized for relatively short stays for nondiarrheal illness have yielded conflicting results. One double-blind study conducted on Polish children (1–36 months) showed that LGG administered twice daily significantly reduced the risk of nosocomial diarrhea compared to the placebo (6.7% vs. 33.3%, $p = 0.002$)[49]. However, the prevalence of rotavirus infection did not differ in the probiotic-treated and control groups. Another large, double-blind randomized study in 220 Italian children did not show a statistically significant protective effect of *Lactobacillus* GG administered once daily for the prevention of nosocomial rotaviral infection[50]. Further studies to define the optimal dose are needed before routine use of LGG to prevent nosocomial diarrhea in infants and toddlers can be advocated.

In a recent, prospective, 12-week, double-blind trial, Weizman et al. evaluated the preventive effects of either *B. lactis* (BB-12) or *L. reuteri* (American Type Culture Collection 55,730) supplemented formula compared with placebo in 210 healthy term infants of ages 4 to 10 months attending 14 childcare centers in Israel[51]. Infants fed *B. lactis* or *L. reuteri* supplemented formula had fewer diarrheal episodes and episodes of shorter duration than the placebo group infants; the effects were greater with *L. reuteri*. The *L. reuteri* group, compared to BB-12 or controls, had a significant fewer numbers of days with fever, clinic visits, childcare absences, and antibiotic prescriptions. The preventive beneficial effects of probiotic supplementation are therefore less obvious and conflicting in the developed world. While most trials show a positive trend, the latter is not consistent[52].

Oberhelman et al.[53] evaluated the effect of *Lactobacillus* GG in preventing community-acquired diarrhea in Peru, an area with a high burden of diarrheal diseases. In this randomized control trial with undernourished infants ($n = 204$), regular administration of a daily dose of *Lactobacillus* GG, 6 days per week for 15 months, resulted significantly in fewer diarrheal episodes in LGG compared to children in the placebo group (5.02 vs. 6.02 per child per year, $p < 0.03$). The decreased incidence of diarrhea in the L-GG group was greatest in the 18- to 29-month age group (P = 0.004) and was largely limited to nonbreastfed children (Breastfed: 6. 59 ecy L-GG, 6.32 ecy placebo, P = 0.7; Nonbreastfed: 4.69 ecy L-GG, 5. 86 ecy placebo, P = 0.005). The effect was not observed in breast-fed. The overall protective effect in this study, therefore, was modest and restricted to a relatively narrow group of children. No preventive effect was observed in a similar trial in Finland[54]. In this double-blind, randomized, long-term study of 571 healthy children of ages 1–6 years from 18 day care centers, milk containing *Lactobacillus* GG conferred no significant protection against diarrhea, as measured by the number of days with diarrheal symptoms or the proportion of children without diarrhea during the 7-month study period. However, the group treated with *Lactobacillus* GG seemed to have less severe disease, with a 16% (95% CI 2–27) reduction in the number of days absence caused by gastrointestinal and respiratory illness during the study (4.9 vs. 5.8 days; $p = 0.03$). After adjusting the age, however, none of these differences was statistically significant. In poor Indian communities, Saran et al. showed that supplementation with a probiotic agent influenced the growth and morbidity of children (aged 2–5 years). In this study, feeding a probiotic supplement (50 mL curd containing *L. acidophilus)* over a period of 6 months resulted in a significantly better weight gain and a 50% reduction in infectious diarrhea[55]. Confirmation of the clinical effects by further investigation with same or other probiotic strains is necessary because the effects appear to be strain-specific and cannot be extrapolated from strain to strain. Further, the dose amount (number of viable bacteria) needs to be considered to enable comparison and accurate interpretation.

In conclusion, available data from randomized controlled trials suggest only a modest effect of some probiotic agents (*Lactobacillus* GG, *L. reuteri. B. lactis*) in the prevention of community-acquired diarrhea. Notably, none of the studies have indicated any adverse effects of probiotic formula in healthy infants. Although there is some suggestion that probiotics may be efficacious in preventing acute diarrhea, there is a lack of data from community-based or effectiveness (in contrast to efficacy) trials and from developing countries in the context of acute diarrhea prevention unrelated to antibiotic treatment.

TREATMENT OF INFECTIOUS GASTROENTERITIS: POTENTIAL FOR PROBIOTIC USE

The most well-established benefit of probiotic agents is the antidiarrheal properties that have been investigated beginning in the 1960s[19]. Several recent, large and well-controlled studies showed a significant decrease in the duration of diarrhea in children who received *Lactobacillus* [60] GG either as a supplement or in fermented milk early in the course of the illness[56–59]. In a large multicentre trial in which *Lactobacillus* GG was added to an ORS and given to children during a diarrheal episode [60], a significant reduction in the duration of illness was observed; similar results have been reported with *L. reuteri*[59], and *L. acidophilus*[61]. The efficacy of *Lactobacillus* GG was confirmed in a study of 40 Pakistani children admitted for severe diarrhea and malnutrition, compared to controls, in reducing duration of nonbloody diarrhea (31% vs. 75% at 48 h)[57]. Comparable results have been recently obtained in a double-blind RCT involving 87 Polish children with infectious diarrhea using a combination of three *L. ramnosus* strains (573L/1, 573L/2, 573L/3)[62]. *L. rhamnosus* strains significantly shortened the duration of diarrhea due to rotavirus (76 vs. 115 h, $p = 0.04$), but not diarrhea caused by other pathogens. *S. boulardii* was introduced in France for the treatment of diarrhea in 1950. The first double-blind, randomized trials of *S. boulardii* were conducted more than 15 years ago by Höchter and Hagenhoff[63] who found persistence of diarrhea for more than 7 days in 12% in the placebo-treated group compared to 3% in the *S. boulardii* group. Subsequently, a few other clinical trials of *S. boulardii* in children with acute diarrhea have demonstrated significant improvement in diarrheal outcomes in comparison to placebo. Cetina-Sauri et al. investigated *S. boulardii* added to ORS compared to ORS alone for 5 days in 130 Mexican children (3–36 months) with acute infectious diarrhea. A significant decrease in the number of stools was apparent from day 2 onward. After day 2, diarrhea resolved in 5% in the *S. boulardii* group compared to only 8% in the placebo group. After day 4, up to 95% children had diarrhea resolution in the intervention group compared to 50% in the placebo group. The stool frequency after the second day of treatment was significantly lower in the *S. boulardii* group than the placebo group ($p = 0.003$)[64]. Kurugol et al. assessed the effect of *S. boulardii* in 200 children, 3 months to 7 years of age, hospitalized with acute diarrhea in Turkey[65].

The duration of diarrhea was significantly less in the *S. boulardii* compared to the placebo group (4.7 vs. 5.5 days, *p* = 0.03); this led to a shorter hospital stay in the *S. boulardii* group (2.9 vs. 3.9 days, *p* < 0.001). In another recently conducted study, Villaruel demonstrated *S. boulardii* as an adjuvant to ORS, in an Argentine ambulatory care with children less than 2 years old, to shorten the duration of diarrhea, accelerate recovery, and reduce the risk of prolonged diarrhea[66].

Although data from well-conducted, randomized, control trials on the efficacy of probiotics in children with diarrhea are encouraging and show modest clinical benefit, certain recent trials conducted in the developing countries have yielded disappointing results. At least three randomized controlled trials in developing countries have shown limited benefit of probiotic therapy in the treatment of children with acute diarrhea. A study from Brazil examined the effect of LGG in 124 male children (1–24 months) hospitalized with moderate to severe diarrhea; there was no significant reduction in the duration of diarrhea or stool output in children given LGG compared to the controls[67]. The lack of efficacy of LGG in this study is in contrast to the previously discussed trials and could be related to increased severity and shorter duration of illness in controls in this study than that reported by most other studies. Similarly, no beneficial effect of LGG in terms of stool output and duration of illness was observed in a second randomized controlled clinical trial by Salazar-Lindo et al.[68] in Peruvian children of ages 3–36 months with acute watery diarrhea of less than 48 h duration. Nor was there any demonstrable benefit of tyndalized (heat-killed) *L. acidophilus* in 98 Indian children of ages 6 months to 12 years with acute diarrhea[69]. The absence of clinical benefit was also reported for a combination of *L. acidophilus*, *B. lactis*, and *L. bulgaricus*[70]. A different combination product of *L. acidophilus*, *S. thermophillus*, and *L. bulgaricus* was also not beneficial in the controlled trial in the treatment of infantile diarrhea by Pearce et al. in Canada[71].

L. paracasei strain ST11 (ST11), a new probiotic strain, was tested in a double-blind, placebo-controlled RCT in Bangladesh[72] using criteria recommended by the WHO. Two hundred and thirty boys (ages, 4–24 months), with diarrhea of less than 2 days duration, received *L. paracasei* ST11 (dose, 10^{10} CFUs/day) or placebo for 5 days. No effect was observed on severe rotavirus diarrhea; however, the probiotic treatment significantly reduced 6-day cumulative stool output (225 ± 218 vs. 381 ± 240 mL/kg) (Fig. 11.1), 6-day stool frequency (27.9 ± 17 vs. 42.5 ± 26), and ORS use (180 ± 207 vs. 331 ± 236 mL/kg) in children with less severe, non-rotavirus diarrhea compared to placebo. Compared to placebo, a significantly higher proportion of non-rotavirus children receiving ST11 had resolution of diarrhea within 6 days of therapy (76% vs. 49%; p = 0.004). It was concluded that ST11 has a clinically significant benefit in the management of children with non-rotavirus-induced (probably *Escherichia coli* induced) diarrhea, but it is ineffective in rotavirus diarrhea. The discrepancy between findings of this study and those of previous studies in rotaviral gastroenteritis may relate to the severity of the illness (more severely affected children were included in the Bangladesh study) or to the slightly longer duration of illness (and closer to spontaneous improvement) after intervention in the previously conducted studies. Less rigorous diarrhea outcome variables including stool frequency rather than volume and assessment of stool form are methodological limitations of the former studies. On the contrary, more stringent assessment criteria for diarrhea (i.e., measurement of stool volume) in the Bangladesh study may also

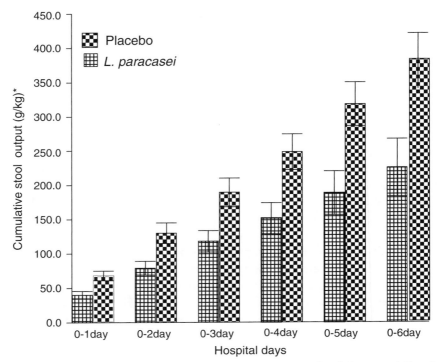

Fig. 11.1 Cumulative stool output (g/kg) of nonrotavirus children during hospitalization with diarrhea

explain less uniformly favorable results. The findings of the Bangladesh study, however, are consistent with those of Costa-Ribeiro et al.[67] with a lack of efficacy of *Lactobacillus* GG in children hospitalized with severe rotavirus gastroenteritis in Brazil. As colonization must occur before benefits of probiotics can be realized, lack of benefits in both study populations might also be due to inadequate time for colonization related to the relatively short duration or accelerated intestinal transit of acute viral diarrheal illness.

More recently, five systematic reviews have been published (Table 11.2) that focus on the role of probiotics in acute infectious diarrhea, providing evidence-based support for their use. The first review by Szajewska and her group included only eight published randomized, placebo-controlled, double-blind studies of acute diarrheal illness lasting three or more days in 731 infants and children in 2001[73]. The effect of all probiotics and individual strains of probiotics were analyzed. It was estimated that the risk of diarrhea lasting three or more days was reduced by 0.40 in the probiotics group compared to the placebo group (95% CI 0.28–0.57), with only *Lactobacillus* GG showing a consistent effect. Probiotics also significantly reduced the duration of diarrhea compared to placebo by 18.2 h (95% CI, –26.9 to –9.5; $p < 0.0001$). The second meta-analysis undertaken by Van Niel and colleagues in 2002[74] was restricted to adequately randomized and blinded studies of seven strains of Lactobacillus in 675 children. Probiotics reduced the duration of diarrhea by 0.7 days (95% confidence

Table 11.2
Meta-analyses of probiotics in the treatment of infectious diarrhea in children

Author	Number of RCTs	Number of children	Probiotic strain	Effect
Szajewska and Mrukowicz 2001	8	731	Lactobacillus GG (3) L. acidiphillus(2) L. reuteri(2) S. boulardii (1)	Reduced risk of diarrhea lasting for >3 days; RR 0.43(95% CI, 0.34 -0.53). Reduced duration of diarrhea -18.2 h (95% CI, -26.9 to -9.5)
Van Niel et al., 2002	7	675	Lactobacillus GG (3) L. reuteri (2) L. acidophilus(1) L. lactis/L. bulgaricus (1)	Decreased duration of diarrhea by 0.7 days (95% CI, 0.3–1.2) Reduction in diarrhea frequency of 1.6 stools on day 2 (95% CI, interval: 0.7–2.6 fewer stools)
Huang et al., 2002	18	1178	Lactobacillus GG (9) L. reuteri (2) L. acidophilus (2) L. rhamnosus (1) Mixture of L. rhamnosus and L. reuteri (2) Mixture of S. thermophillus, L. acidophilus, and L bulgaricus (2) – one study had also different treatment arms with S. boulardii, B. subtilis an B.bifidum and enterococcus	Reduction in duration of diarrhea by –0.8 days (95% CI, -1.1 to –0.6 days)
Allen et al., 2003	23	1,449	LAB (21) S. boulardii (2)	Reduced risk of diarrhea at 3 days (RR, 0.66 days, 95% CI, 0.55–0.77) Reduced duration of diarrhea by -30.5 h (95% CI, -18.5 to 42.5 h)
Szajweska, et al. 2007	8	988	Lactobacillus GG	Reduced duration of diarrhea by 1.1 days (95% CI -1.9 to –0.3,) Reduced duration of diarrhea due to rotavirus by –2.1 days (95% CI, -3.6 to -0.6) Reduced risk of diarrhea for >7 days by 0.25 (95% CI 0.09–0.75)

interval: 0.3–1.2 days; 7 studies) and diarrhea frequency on day 2 by 1.6 stools (95% confidence interval: 0.7–2.6 fewer stools; 3 studies including 122 children). There was considerable heterogeneity between the studies preventing the analysis of the effect of individual strains of Lactobacilli. The results of this meta-analysis indicate a statistical but modest clinical benefit of Lactobacillus and that this organism is safe in children with acute infectious diarrhea. A third meta-analysis of 18 randomized controlled trial among 1,178 children less than 5 years of age with acute diarrhea showed an overall reduction of diarrheal duration by 0.8 days[75] in favor of probiotic-treated children. Further subgroup analysis of LGG and non-LGG probiotics demonstrated a reduction of diarrheal duration by 1.2 and 0.6 days, respectively. The fourth meta-analysis was a Cochrane Review that examined 23 randomized control trials with a total of 1917 patients (1,417 children) with acute diarrhea proven or presumed to be caused by an infectious agent[76] Overall, the analysis demonstrated that probiotics reduced the risk of diarrhea at 3 days (RR 0.66, 95% CI 0.55 to 0.77; 15 studies) and mean duration of diarrhea by 30.5 h (95% CI18.5 to 42.5 h; 12 studies). The most recent meta-analysis was again undertaken by Szajewska et al. in 2007 to review and update data on the effectiveness and safety of one probiotic strain—L. rhamnosus GG (LGG)—with 8 randomized control trials in 988 participants[77]. They observed that LGG had no effect on the total stool volume in 2 RCTs with 303 participants. However, meta-analysis of seven RCTs (876 participants) showed a reduction in the duration of diarrhea of 1.1 days (95% CI −1.9 to −0.5) demonstrating moderate clinical benefits of LGG in the treatment of acute diarrhea in children. On the basis of the review they also concluded that the use of LGG appears to be safe in children with acute diarrhea.

Significant statistical heterogeneity was detected across studies evaluating the effect of probiotics on the duration of diarrhea. The incompatibility of the results in the RCTs may be explained by differences in properties of probiotic strains, in dose (CFU) of probiotics administered, and the definition of diarrhea or diarrhea intensity. The variation in the dosages of the probiotics used, in particular, is likely a factor leading to heterogeneity in the results. In the meta-analysis by Van Niel et al.,[74] there was evidence of a dose–response relationship on the duration of diarrhea. Significant positive linear association exists between the log of the lactobacillus dose and the reduction in the duration of diarrhea in days ($p < 0.01$). The dose–effect relationship noted in this meta-analysis suggests that Lactobacillus is most effective above a threshold dose (10 billion colony forming units during the first 48 h) that reduces the duration of diarrhea by more than half a day. It has been shown that a similar dose of 10^{10}–10^{11} colony forming units of the species *Lactobacillus* GG results in colonization of the intestine and inhibition of attachment by pathogens[78]. Higher doses of lactobacillus may lead to shorter duration. Live lactobacillus may potentially replicate in the gut and lead to bacteraemia[79]; therefore, judicious consideration is warranted regarding application of the dose–response concept of probiotic agents in children with diarrhea, who may have associated poor nutrition, impaired immune status, or frequent exposure to infectious agents.

Examination of all of the meta-analyses indicates that the majority of studies have been conducted in the developed world and that there was efficacy for *L. rhamnosus* GG, *L. acidophilus*, and *bulgaricus*. In particular, the duration of diarrhea (viral) was significantly reduced by about 0.7 days; RR 0.40. Furthermore, with *S. boulardii*, a 24-h reduction in hospital stay has been documented. A meta-analysis of RCTs conducted in the developing countries has not, to date, been done.

SAFETY ASPECTS

Regarding safety, *Lactobacillus* and Bifidobacteria raise little concern because these organisms reside in abundance as normal flora in the gastrointestinal tract of healthy individuals and are ubiquitous in the human diet. They have been consumed sometimes in large doses for several years in many countries and have a long history of safety[80]. Lactobacillaemia may thus occur naturally, without exogenous administration. Large-scale epidemiological studies in countries where probiotic-use rates are high demonstrates (in adults) very low rate of systemic infection, i.e., between 0.05 and 0.40%[43]. Widespread screening of a large population in Finland taking *Lactobacillus* GG failed to find a single case of *Lactobacillus* GG infection[81]. A Medline search of "*Bifidobacterium*" and "sepsis" that reviewed 15 years yielded one case report of sepsis caused by *B. longum* in a 19-year-old man after acupuncture; he had not ingested probiotics and completely recovered within 10 days[82].

Invasive infections in infants and children have been extremely rare[83]. In preterm infants, *Lactobacillus* GG administration resulted in no evidence of adverse effects[84]. However, two sporadic cases of bacteremia attributable to Lactobacillus administration were recently reported in infants who had no inherent gastrointestinal diseases and were not immunocompromised, although they did have other complex health problems[85]. Fungemia with *S. boulardii* has been reported in about 50 patients with invasive candidiasis or with intravascular catheter and antibiotic therapy[86]; indwelling central venous catheter was the main risk factor identified in this study. These case reports emphasize that probiotic supplementation should be used with caution in children with indwelling venous catheter, prolonged or complicated hospitalization, or a recognized or potential compromise of intestinal mucosal integrity[85]. Only limited number of cases have been reported in which the organism was thought to be related to the use or consumption of a commensal probiotic product, *L. rhamnosus*[87] or *Bacillus subtlis*[88]. The benefits of probiotics seem to outweigh the potential danger of sepsis. No data on safety reports are available from the developing countries and there is a need for controlled evaluation.

Between September 2000 and the end of January 2001, a workshop of recognized experts was convened[83] to critically review the current scientific and medical literature. On the basis of existing data, it was concluded that *Lactobacilli* and *bifidobacteria* probiotics are safe, even in immunocompromised populations such as premature neonates. The workshop concluded "Current evidence suggests that the risk of infection with probiotic lactobacilli or bifidobacterium is similar to that of infection with commensal strains, and that consumption of such products presents a negligible risk to consumers, including immunocompromised hosts." At present in the European Union, microorganisms intended for human use are regulated only within the context of the Novel Food Regulation EU 258/97[89]. In early 2002, the United States Food and Drug Administration accepted a "generally regarded as safe (GRAS)" notice (notice GRN 000049) from Nestlé United States for the use of *B. lactis* and *Streptococcus thermophilus* in formula milk for healthy infants aged 4 months or more.

On the basis of the evaluation of published literature it can be concluded that the risk of infection with probiotic lactobacilli or bifidobacteria is similar to that of infection with commensal bacterial strain and that the consumption of such products is of negligible risk to consumers including immunocompromised hosts[83]. The European Society of Pediatric Gastroenterology, Hepatitis, and Nutrition committee on nutrition recently summarized its approach to probiotics as follows, "probiotics so far used in clinical trials can be generally considered as safe. However, surveillance for possible side effects, such as infection in high-risk groups, is lacking and needed[52]".

SUMMARY AND CONCLUSION

Rapid rehydration and realimentation remain the cornerstones of treatment of acute infectious gastroenteritis. Probiotics administered as supplemental medicinal agents are likely to decrease the duration of acute infectious gastroenteritis in about 24 h. Literature shows a statistically significant but clinically modest benefit for some Lactobacillus strains, mainly in infants and young children, in the treatment of acute watery diarrhea, especially in rotavirus gastroenteritis. Most studies of probiotics in the management of acute diarrhea have been conducted in relatively healthy and stable populations. While a distinction between different probiotic agents is made, little emphasis thus far is given to different probiotic dosages (CFU/ml) used in studies, even among the same probiotics, and that needs to be considered in the assessment of efficacy. A role for strains found effective in developed countries needs to be evaluated in communities where diarrheal illnesses often run a protracted or severe course and are frequently complicated by immune deficiencies and malnutrition. Because most of the probiotic research has been conducted in rotaviral diarrhea, a future research agenda should include assessment of efficacy and effectiveness in diarrheal illnesses caused by other enteric pathogens, especially bacteria.

REFERENCES

1. Snyder JD, Merson MH. The magnitude of the global problem of acute diarrhoeal disease: a review of active surveillance data. *Bulletin of the World Health Organization* 1982;60(4):605–13.
2. Bern C, Martines J, de Zoysa I, Glass RI. The magnitude of the global problem of diarrhoeal disease: a ten-year update. *Bulletin of the World Health Organization* 1992;70(6):705–14.
3. Victora CG, Bryce J, Fontaine O, Monasch R. Reducing deaths from diarrhoea through oral rehydration therapy. *Bulletin of the World Health Organization* 2000;78(10):1246–55.
4. Kosek M, Bern C, Guerrant RL. The global burden of diarrhoeal disease, as estimated from studies published between 1992 and 2000. *Bulletin of the World Health Organization* 2003;81(3):197–204.
5. Thapar N, Sanderson IR. Diarrhoea in children: an interface between developing and developed countries. *Lancet* 2004;363(9409):641–53.
6. Santosham M, Keenan EM, Tulloch J, Broun D, Glass R. Oral rehydration therapy for diarrhea: an example of reverse transfer of technology. *Pediatrics* 1997;100(5):E10.
7. Zimmerman CM, Bresee JS, Parashar UD, Riggs TL, Holman RC, Glass RI. Cost of diarrhea-associated hospitalizations and outpatient visits in an insured population of young children in the United States. *Pediatr Infect Dis J* 2001;20(1):14–9.
8. Fontaine O. Zinc and treatment of diarrhoea. *Med Trop (Mars)* 2006;66(3):306–9.
9. Bines J. Intussusception and rotavirus vaccines. *Vaccine* 2006;24(18):3772–6.
10. Bines JE. Rotavirus vaccines and intussusception risk. *Curr Opin Gastroenterol* 2005;21(1):20–5.

11. Chen RT, DeStefano F. Vaccine adverse events: causal or coincidental? *Lancet* 1998;351(9103):611–2.
12. Metchnikoff E. The prolongation of life. New York: Putnam & Sons 1908.
13. Vergin F. Antibiotics and probiotics. *Hippokrates* 1954;25(4):116–9.
14. Lilly DM, Stillwell RH. Probiotics: growth-promoting factors produced by microorganisms. *Science (New York)* 1965;147:747–8.
15. Fuller R. Probiotics in man and animals. *J Appl Bacteriol* 1989;66(5):365–78.
16. FAO/WHO. Paper presented at Joint FAO/WHO Expert Consultation on Evaluation of Health and Nuritional Properties of Probiotics in Food including Powder Milk with Live Lactic Acid Bacteria, Cordoba, Arentina, 2001.
17. Reid G, Jass J, Sebulsky MT, McCormick JK. Potential uses of probiotics in clinical practice. *Clin Microbiol Rev* 2003;16(4):658–72.
18. Servin AL. Antagonistic activities of lactobacilli and bifidobacteria against microbial pathogens. *FEMS Microbiol Rev* 2004;28(4):405–40.
19. Beck C, Necheles H. Beneficial effects of administration of *Lactobacillus acidophilus* in diarrheal and other intestinal disorders. *Am J Gastroenterol* 1961;35:522–30.
20. Day AS. Use of complementary and alternative therapies and probiotic agents by children attending gastroenterology outpatient clinics. *J Paediatr Child Health* 2002;38(4):343–6.
21. Day AS, Whitten KE, Bohane TD. Use of complementary and alternative medicines by children and adolescents with inflammatory bowel disease. *J Paediatr Child Health* 2004;40(12):681–4.
22. Dai D, Walker WA. Protective nutrients and bacterial colonization in the immature human gut. *Adv Pediatr* 1999;46:353–82.
23. Vendt N, Grunberg H, Tuure T, et-al.. Growth during the first 6 months of life in infants using formula enriched with *Lactobacillus rhamnosus* GG: double-blind, randomized trial. *J Hum Nutr Diet* 2006;19(1):51–8.
24. Beno Y, He F, Hosoda M. Effect of *Lactobacillus* GG yoghurt on intestinal microecology in Japanese subjects. *Nutr Today* 1996;31(Suppl.):S9–S13.
25. Tannock GW, Munro K, Harmsen HJ, Welling GW, Smart J, Gopal PK. Analysis of the fecal microflora of human subjects consuming a probiotic product containing *Lactobacillus rhamnosus* DR20. *Appl Environ Microbiol* 2000;66(6):2578–88.
26. Michail S, Abernathy F. *Lactobacillus plantarum* reduces the in vitro secretory response of intestinal epithelial cells to enteropathogenic *Escherichia coli* infection. *J Pediatr Gastroenterol Nutr* 2002;35(3):350–5.
27. Riedel CU, Foata F, Philippe D, Adolfsson O, Eikmanns BJ, Blum S. Anti-inflammatory effects of bifidobacteria by inhibition of LPS-induced NF-kappaB activation. *World J Gastroenterol* 2006;12(23):3729–35.
28. Alam M, Midtvedt T, Uribe A. Differential cell kinetics in the ileum and colon of germfree rats. *Scand J Gastroenterol* 1994;29(5):445–51.
29. Darmoul D, Brown D, Selsted ME, Ouellette AJ. Cryptdin gene expression in developing mouse small intestine. *Am J Physiol* 1997;272(1 Pt 1):G197–206.
30. Hooper LV, Midtvedt T, Gordon JI. How host-microbial interactions shape the nutrient environment of the mammalian intestine. *Ann Rev Nutr* 2002;22:283–307.
31. Elmer GW, McFarland LV. Biotherapeutic agents in the treatment of infectious diarrhea. *Gastroenterol Clinics North Am* 2001;30(3):837–54.
32. Isolauri E. Probiotics in human disease. *Am J Clin Nutr* 2001;73(6):1142S–6S.
33. Walker WA, Goulet O, Morelli L, Antoine JM. Progress in the science of probiotics: from cellular microbiology and applied immunology to clinical nutrition. *Europ J Nutr* 2006;45 (Suppl 9):1–18.
34. Hooper LV, Wong MH, Thelin A, Hansson L, Falk PG, Gordon JI. Molecular analysis of commensal host-microbial relationships in the intestine. *Science (New York)* 2001;291(5505):881–4.
35. Rakoff-Nahoum S, Paglino J, Eslami-Varzaneh F, Edberg S, Medzhitov R. Recognition of commensal microflora by toll-like receptors is required for intestinal homeostasis. *Cell* 2004;118(2):229–41.
36. Neish AS, Gewirtz AT, Zeng H, et-al.. Prokaryotic regulation of epithelial responses by inhibition of IkappaB-alpha ubiquitination. *Science (New York)* 2000;289(5484):1560–3.
37. Kelly D, Campbell JI, King TP, et-al.. Commensal anaerobic gut bacteria attenuate inflammation by regulating nuclear-cytoplasmic shuttling of PPAR-gamma and RelA. *Nat Immunol* 2004;5(1):104–12.

38. Pessi T, Sutas Y, Hurme M, Isolauri E. Interleukin-10 generation in atopic children following oral *Lactobacillus rhamnosus* GG. *Clin Exp Allergy* 2000;30(12):1804–8.

39. Pelto L, Isolauri E, Lilius EM, Nuutila J, Salminen S. Probiotic bacteria down-regulate the milk-induced inflammatory response in milk-hypersensitive subjects but have an immunostimulatory effect in healthy subjects. *Clin Exp Allergy* 1998;28(12):1474–9.

40. Majamaa H, Isolauri E. Probiotics: a novel approach in the management of food allergy. *J Allergy Clin Immunol* 1997;99(2):179–85.

41. Sutas Y, Hurme M, Isolauri E. Down-regulation of anti-CD3 antibody-induced IL-4 production by bovine caseins hydrolysed with *Lactobacillus* GG-derived enzymes. *Scand J Immunol* 1996;43(6):687–9.

42. Duggan C, Gannon J, Walker WA. Protective nutrients and functional foods for the gastrointestinal tract. *Am J Clin Nutr* 2002;75(5):789–808.

43. Fedorak RN, Madsen KL. Probiotics and prebiotics in gastrointestinal disorders. *Curr Opin Gastroenterol* 2004;20(2):146–55.

44. Buts JP, De Keyser N. Effects of *Saccharomyces boulardii* on intestinal mucosa. *Dig Dis Sci* 2006;51(8):1485–92.

45. Saavedra JM, Bauman NA, Oung I, Perman JA, Yolken RH. Feeding of Bifidobacterium bifidum and Streptococcus thermophilus to infants in hospital for prevention of diarrhoea and shedding of rotavirus. *Lancet* 1994;344(8929):1046–9.

46. Thibault H, Aubert-Jacquin C, Goulet O. Effects of long-term consumption of a fermented infant formula (with *Bifidobacterium breve* c50 and *Streptococcus thermophilus* 065) on acute diarrhea in healthy infants. *J Pediatr Gastroenterol Nutr* 2004;39(2):147–52.

47. Chouraqui JP, Van Egroo LD, Fichot MC. Acidified milk formula supplemented with *Bifidobacterium lactis*: impact on infant diarrhea in residential care settings. *J Pediatr Gastroenterol Nutr* 2004;38(3):288–92.

48. Pedone CA, Arnaud CC, Postaire ER, Bouley CF, Reinert P. Multicentric study of the effect of milk fermented by *Lactobacillus casei* on the incidence of diarrhoea. *Int J Clin Practice* 2000;54(9):568–71.

49. Szajewska H, Kotowska M, Mrukowicz JZ, Armanska M, Mikolajczyk W. Efficacy of *Lactobacillus* GG in prevention of nosocomial diarrhea in infants. *J Pediatr* 2001;138(3):361–5.

50. Mastretta E, Longo P, Laccisaglia A, et-al.. Effect of *Lactobacillus* GG and breast-feeding in the prevention of rotavirus nosocomial infection. *J Pediatr Gastroenterol Nutr* 2002;35(4):527–31.

51. Weizman Z, Asli G, Alsheikh A. Effect of a probiotic infant formula on infections in child care centers: comparison of two probiotic agents. *Pediatrics* 2005;115(1):5–9.

52. Agostoni C, Axelsson I, Braegger C, et-al.. Probiotic bacteria in dietetic products for infants: a commentary by the ESPGHAN Committee on Nutrition. *J Pediatr Gastroenterol Nutr* 2004;38(4):365–74.

53. Oberhelman RA, Gilman RH, Sheen P, et-al.. A placebo-controlled trial of *Lactobacillus* GG to prevent diarrhea in undernourished Peruvian children. *J Pediatr* 1999;134(1):15–20.

54. Hatakka K, Savilahti E, Ponka A, et-al.. Effect of long term consumption of probiotic milk on infections in children attending day care centres: double blind, randomised trial. *BMJ (Clin Res, Ed.)* 2001;322(7298):1327.

55. Saran S, Gopalan S, Krishna TP. Use of fermented foods to combat stunting and failure to thrive. *Nutrition (Burbank, Los Angeles County, California)* 2002;18(5):393–6.

56. Isolauri E, Juntunen M, Rautanen T, Sillanaukee P, Koivula T. A human Lactobacillus strain (*Lactobacillus casei* sp strain GG) promotes recovery from acute diarrhea in children. *Pediatrics* 1991;88(1):90–7.

57. Raza S, Graham SM, Allen SJ, et-al.. *Lactobacillus* GG in acute diarrhea. *Indian Pediatr* 1995;32(10):1140–2.

58. Guarino A, Canani RB, Spagnuolo MI, Albano F, Di Benedetto L. Oral bacterial therapy reduces the duration of symptoms and of viral excretion in children with mild diarrhea. *J Pediatr Gastroenterol Nutr* 1997;25(5):516-9.

59. Shornikova AV, Casas IA, Isolauri E, Mykkanen H, Vesikari T. *Lactobacillus reuteri* as a therapeutic agent in acute diarrhea in young children. *J Pediatr Gastroenterol Nutr* 1997;24(4):399–404.

60. Guandalini S, Pensabene L, Zikri MA, et-al.. *Lactobacillus* GG administered in oral rehydration solution to children with acute diarrhea: a multicenter European trial. *J Pediatr Gastroenterol Nutr* 2000;30(1):54–60.

61. Simakachorn N, Pichaipat V, Rithipornpaisarn P, Kongkaew C, Tongpradit P, Varavithya W. Clinical evaluation of the addition of lyophilized, heat-killed *Lactobacillus acidophilus* LB to oral rehydration therapy in the treatment of acute diarrhea in children. *J Pediatr Gastroenterol Nutr* 2000;30(1):68–72.

62. Szymanski H, Pejcz J, Jawien M, Chmielarczyk A, Strus M, Heczko PB. Treatment of acute infectious diarrhoea in infants and children with a mixture of three *Lactobacillus rhamnosus* strains – a randomized, double-blind, placebo-controlled trial. *Aliment Pharmacol Therapeut* 2006;23(2):247–53.

63. Höchter WCD, Hagenhoff G. *Saccharomyces boulardii* bei akuter Erwachsenendiarrhoe. *Münch Med Wachr* 1990;132:188–92.

64. Cetina-Sauri G, Basto.G S. Therapeutic evaluation of *Saccharomyces boulardii* in children with acute diarrhea. *Ann Pediatr* 1994;41:397–400.

65. Kurugol Z, Koturoglu G. Effects of *Saccharomyces boulardii* in children with acute diarrhoea. *Acta Paediatr* 2005;94(1):44–7.

66. Villarruel G, Rubio DM, Lopez F, et-al.. *Saccharomyces boulardii* in acute childhood diarrhoea: a randomized, placebo-controlled study. *Acta Paediatr* 2007;96(4):538–41.

67. Costa-Ribeiro H, Ribeiro TC, Mattos AP, et-al.. Limitations of probiotic therapy in acute, severe dehydrating diarrhea. *J Pediatr Gastroenterol Nutr* 2003;36(1):112–5.

68. Salazar-Lindo E, Miranda-Langschwager P, Campos-Sanchez M, Chea-Woo E, Sack RB. *Lactobacillus casei* strain GG in the treatment of infants with acute watery diarrhea: a randomized, double-blind, placebo controlled clinical trial [ISRCTN67363048]. *BMC Pediatr* 2004;4:18.

69. Khanna V, Alam S, Malik A, Malik A. Efficacy of tyndalized *Lactobacillus acidophilus* in acute diarrhea. *Indian J Pediatr* 2005;72(11):935–8.

70. Kowalska-Duplaga K, Fyderek K, Szajewska H, Janiak H. Efficacy of trilack in the treatmnt of acute diarrhoea in infants and young children – a multicentre double-blind placebo-controlled study. *Pediatria Wspolczesna* 2004;3:295–9.

71. Pearce JL, Hamilton JR. Controlled trial of orally administered lactobacilli in acute infantile diarrhea. *J Pediatr* 1974;84(2):261–2.

72. Sarker SA, Sultana S, Fuchs GJ, et-al. *Lactobacillus paracasei* strain ST11 has no effect on rotavirus but ameliorates the outcome of nonrotavirus diarrhea in children from Bangladesh. *Pediatrics* 2005;116(2):e221–8.

73. Szajewska H, Mrukowicz JZ. Probiotics in the treatment and prevention of acute infectious diarrhea in infants and children: a systematic review of published randomized, double-blind, placebo-controlled trials. *J Pediatr Gastroenterol Nutr* 2001;33 (Suppl 2):S17–25.

74. Van Niel CW, Feudtner C, Garrison MM, Christakis DA. Lactobacillus therapy for acute infectious diarrhea in children: a meta-analysis. *Pediatrics* 2002;109(4):678–84.

75. Huang JS, Bousvaros A, Lee JW, Diaz A, Davidson EJ. Efficacy of probiotic use in acute diarrhea in children: a meta-analysis. *Dig Dis Sci* 2002;47(11):2625–34.

76. Allen SJ, Okoko B, Martinez B, et al. Probiotics for treating infectious diarrhoea. Cockrane Database System Rev 2003(4).

77. Szajewska H, Skorka A, Ruszczynski M, Gieruszczak-Bialek D. Meta-analysis: *Lactobacillus* GG for treating acute diarrhoea in children. *Aliment Pharmacol Therapy* 2007;25(8):871–81.

78. Saxelin ME, S. Salminen,S. Vapaatalo, M. Dose response colonization of feces after oral administration of *Lactobacillus casei* strain GG. Microbiol Ecol Health Dis 1991;4:1–8.

79. De Groote MA, Frank DN, Dowell E, Glode MP, Pace NR. *Lactobacillus rhamnosus* GG bacteremia associated with probiotic use in a child with short gut syndrome. *Pediatric Infect Dis J* 2005;24(3):278–80.

80. Simon GL, Gorbach SL. Intestinal flora in health and disease. *Gastroenterology* 1984;86(1):174–93.

81. Saxelin M, Chuang NH, Chassy B, et-al.. Lactobacilli and bacteremia in southern Finland, 1989–1992. *Clin Infect Dis* 1996;22(3):564–6.

82. Ha GY, Yang CH, Kim H, Chong Y. Case of sepsis caused by *Bifidobacterium longum. J Clin Microbiol* 1999;37(4):1227–8.

83. Borriello SP, Hammes WP, Holzapfel W, et-al.. Safety of probiotics that contain lactobacilli or bifido-bacteria. *Clin Infect Dis* 2003;36(6):775–80.

84. Stansbridge EM, Walker V, Hall MA, et-al.. Effects of feeding premature infants with *Lactobacillus* GG on gut fermentation. *Arch Dis Childhood* 1993;69(5 Spec No):488–92.

85. Cabana MD, Shane AL, Chao C, Oliva-Hemker M. Probiotics in primary care pediatrics. *Clinical Pediatr* 2006;45(5):405–10.

86. Enache-Angoulvant A, Hennequin C. Invasive Saccharomyces infection: a comprehensive review. *Clin Infect Dis* 2005;41(11):1559–68.

87. Husni RN, Gordon SM, Washington JA, Longworth DL. *Lactobacillus bacteremia* and endocarditis: review of 45 cases. *Clin Infect Dis* 1997;25(5):1048–55.

88. Oggioni MR, Pozzi G, Valensin PE, Galieni P, Bigazzi C. Recurrent septicemia in an immunocompromised patient due to probiotic strains of Bacillus subtilis. *J Clin Microbiol* 1998;36(1):325–6.

89. von Wright A. Regulating the safety of probiotics – the European approach. *Curr Pharm Design* 2005;11(1):17–23.

90. Santosham M, Nelson EA, Bresee JS. Implementing rotavirus vaccination in Asia. *Vaccine* 2007;25(44):7711–6.

91. Glass RI, Bresee J, Jiang B, Parashar U, Yee E, Gentsch J. Rotavirus and rotavirus vaccines. Advances in experimental medicine and biology 2006;582:45–54

12 Probiotics in Crohn's Disease

Esi S. N. Lamousé-Smith and Athos Bousvaros

Key Points

- The outcomes of studies utilizing probiotics to treat Crohn's disease especially in pediatrics have been disappointing.
- The use of selected probiotics has demonstrated benefits in ulcerative colitis and pouchitis.
- Future studies of probiotics in Crohn's disease will require greater scientific rigor

Key Words: IBD: inflammatory bowel disease, CD: Crohn's disease, Probiotics.

INTRODUCTION

Probiotics are defined as live nonpathogenic bacteria that confer beneficial effects on the host, after ingestion. These effects may be nutritional (enhanced metabolic or digestive functions) or non-nutritional (protection against pathogenic bacterial invasion, immune modulation). Most probiotics are bacterial species that are normal commensal inhabitants of the gastrointestinal tract. Common species utilized as probiotic species include the *Lactobacilli, Bifidobacteria*, certain nonpathogenic bacteria (i.e., *Escherichia coli*) and yeast (i.e., *Saccharomyces boulardii*). The interest in probiotic bacterial species and their mechanistic roles in modifying health and disease has become a focus of active research supported by advances in microbial genetics and mucosal immunity. This chapter will focus on the use of probiotics in the treatment of inflammatory bowel disease (IBD), with an emphasis on their use in Crohn's disease.

MICROBIOLOGY OF CROHN'S DISEASE

The main two types of idiopathic IBD in the United States are Crohn's disease (CD) and ulcerative colitis (UC). Approximately 10% of the 1–1.5 million Americans with CD and UC are children and adolescents; 20–25% patients with IBD develop the disease during childhood. During the last 5–10 years, it has been observed that the incidence in

From: *Nutrition and Health: Probiotics in Pediatric Medicine*
Edited by: S. Michail and P.M. Sherman © Humana Press, Totowa, NJ

the pediatric population appears to be increasing. A recent Finnish study documented a near-doubling in incidence from 3.9 cases/100,000 children/year in 1987 to 7.0 cases/100,000 in 2003 [1]. CD is a chronic and relapsing illness in which transmural intestinal inflammation extends from the mouth to the anus. CD is characterized by small bowel involvement (typically in the distal ileum and cecum), deep fissuring ulcers adjacent to the normal mucosa (skip areas, "cobblestone mucosa"), perianal disease, and microscopic noncaseating granulomas. Extraintestinal manifestations often accompany the gastrointestinal symptoms, and may include arthritis, uveitis, skin rashes, anemia, and growth failure. CD is rarely fatal, but is a significant cause of morbidity.

Genetic susceptibility contributes to the pathogenesis of the disease, however, the increased incidence of IBD also implicates environmental factors that contribute to this rise in incidence. The pathogenesis of IBD is thought to involve dysregulated immune responses against environmental triggers and resident intestinal microbial flora. Thus, targets of therapy can be selectively chosen to modulate the impact of environmental, bacterial, and immune effectors.

One important environmental factor and likely candidate in triggering the initiation of CD are microbial species of the intestinal flora. There is expanding evidence to support the notion that initiation and progression of mucosal inflammation in CD is due to the complex interaction of genetic and microbial factors. The identification of susceptibility genes associated with the development of IBD, particularly for CD, has illuminated the delicate interplay of interactions that occur between the host and nonpathogenic bacteria nesting within established niches throughout the intestinal tract. Current hypotheses consider that the intestinal inflammation characteristic of IBD is (1) due to an acquired imbalance in disease-inducing bacteria within the gut (dysbioisis) and (2) due to an inappropriate immune response to resident nonpathogenic bacterial species [2–4]. On the basis of these hypotheses, the clinical management of IBD has incorporated the use of antibiotics and probiotics as both treatments hold the potential to alter resident flora and possibly tip the balance back toward a noninflammatory state by inducing the emergence of "protective" bacteria.

Genetic Contributions to the Development of Crohn's Disease

Particular bacteria have been implicated as "pathogenic" in the context of inducing IBD. These bacteria normally colonize the healthy human intestine. However, only a small percentage of individuals develop CD, suggesting that common host factors determine the aggressive and dysregulated response to these bacteria. Genetic polymorphisms that seem to control innate immune responses have been identified and well described in IBD.

It is now well established that a subset of patients with CD share mutations in genes of pattern recognition receptor (PRR). Pattern recognition receptors (PRRs) are expressed on antigen presenting cells and detect conserved pathogen associated molecular patterns (PAMP) expressed on microbes (bacteria, viruses, fungi, and protozoan). PAMP engagement of PRRs expressed by antigen presenting cells activates immune responses against microbial infection and serves as a bridge between innate and adaptive immune responses. Bacterial lipopolysaccharide (LPS) is one PAMP and others include flagellin, lipotechoich acid, peptidoglycan, dsRNA, and unmethylated CpG motifs. Pattern recognition receptors may be either membrane-bound (e.g., the Toll-like receptors, TLR) or intracellular (e.g., the nucleotide oligomerization domain [NOD] family [NOD1 and NOD2]) (Fig. 12.1).

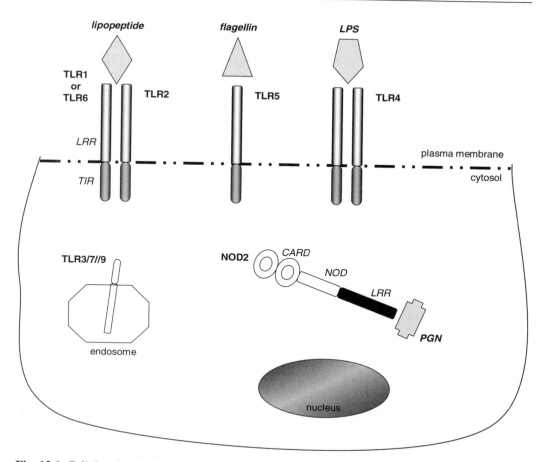

Fig. 12.1. Cellular distribution of the pattern recognition receptors, TLR and NOD. The NOD (nucleotide-binding oligomerization domain) protein NOD2 is a cytosolic molecule composed of three main domains: the carboxy-terminal leucine rich domain (LRR) domain binds peptidoglycans (PGN); the central NOD; and the caspase-recruitment domains (CARD) are involved in signaling. The Toll-like receptors (TLRs) are membrane-associated proteins that function as cell-surface (TLR2, 4, 5) or endosomal receptors (TLR3, 7, 9). TLR2 forms a heterodimer with either TLR1 or TLR6. The TLRs use Toll interleukin receptor domains (TIR) to mediated intracellular signaling events. Following ligand recognition, a cascade of intracellular signaling events (including the activation and nuclear translocation of NF-κB) results in gene transcription of inflammatory mediators. Respective ligands of the TLRs are: lipopeptide (TLR2); LPS (TLR4); flagellin (TLR5); dsRNA (TLR3); ssRNA (TLR7); bacterial DNA (TLR9).

The NOD (nucleotide-binding oligomerization domain) protein NOD2 is a cytosolic molecule composed of three main domains: the carboxy-terminal leucine-rich domain (LRR) binds peptidoglycans (PGN); the central NOD; and the caspase-recruitment domains (CARD) are involved in signaling. The TLRs are membrane-associated proteins that function as cell surface (TLR2, 4, 5) or endosomal receptors (TLR3, 7, 9). TLR2 forms a heterodimer with either TLR1 or TLR6. The TLRs use Toll interleukin receptor domains (TIR) to mediate intracellular signaling events. Following ligand recognition, a cascade of intracellular signaling events (including the activation and nuclear translocation of NF-κB) result in gene transcription of inflammatory mediators. The respective ligands of the TLRs are the lipopeptide (TLR2), LPS (TLR4), flagellin (TLR5), dsRNA (TLR3), ssRNA (TLR7), and bacterial DNA (TLR9).

Engagement of PRRs results in a cascade of events: signal activation of the transcription factor NF-κB (nuclear factor-κB), induction of inflammatory cytokines, and subsequent immune effector cell activation [5]. Altered NF-κB activation can result in abnormal (over-exuberant *or* incompetent) immune responses following PRR engagement by PAMPS [6]. Mutations identified in NOD2 (CARD15) were the first susceptibility genes identified for CD and are associated with the development of specific clinical phenotypes in some individuals [7]. Although signaling defects as a result of mutations in the NOD2/CARD15 gene clearly impacts mucosal immune regulation, the specific mechanism(s) by which defined mutations lead to the development of CD still requires further characterization.

Roughly 20% of Caucasian patients with CD carry the NOD2/CARD15 gene mutation and therefore additional host factors must also play a role in perturbations that result in the development of the disease. Additional variations in other important signaling molecules that affect immune response and regulation have also been identified. An allele of another important pattern recognition receptor, TLR4, has recently been associated with genetic susceptibility to CD and has been reconfirmed via a genome-wide association study [8,9]. TLR4 is expressed on the membranes of the intestinal mucosal epithelial cells, antigen presenting cells, neutrophils, NK-T cells, and T cells, and binds bacterial LPS. Therefore, mutations in this receptor may result in the disruption of intestinal homeostatic mechanisms required to prevent the inflammation that develops in CD.

Another recently identified genetic variation lies in the IL-23R gene, wherein a specific allele is associated with *protection* against the development of CD [10]. Engagement of the IL-23 receptor by the cytokine IL-23 is a critical step in the activation of a population of T cells (Th-17) with regulatory properties that are also implicated in some disease models of inflammation and autoimmunity [11]. Consistent with the finding that deficiency of Th-17 cells results in augmented autoimmune responses, depletion of the cytokine IL-23 is associated with decreased proinflammatory responses in the intestine [12]. Current investigations are focused on the hypothesis that alterations in the IL-23 mediated signaling results in the inability to activate important regulatory mediators required for maintaining intestinal homeostasis and therefore provides another pathway by which bacterial components of resident mucosal flora may initiate the pathogenesis in CD and UC [13,14].

In summary, the identification of gene mutations in receptors involved in innate immune response and regulation lends credence to the hypothesis that the development of CD is due to activation by specific environmental triggers (i.e., bacterial antigens) in a host genetically predisposed to respond abnormally.

Imbalanced Bacterial Flora of Crohn's Disease

There is evidence that bacterial populations are altered within the cytoadherant flora of patients with IBD, supporting the hypothesis that an imbalance in the native mucosal flora exists—a concept that can be referred to as dysbiosis. The shift in bacterial populations may be an important contributing factor in disease development, since these provide a significant source of antigens that can potentially stimulate immune responses.

Recent advances in nonculture-based techniques have provided greater sensitivity (since a large proportion of the gut flora is not identified by culture-based techniques alone) than studies that relied on culture-based techniques and that often yielded contradictory results. Sophisticated molecular and genetic techniques involve sequencing of 16S rDNA, within which taxonomic tags for bacterial groups and species can be identified. Molecular surveys of mucosal biopsies and stool specimens have characterized bacterial diversity of the intestinal tract and have identified that differences exist in the bacterial populations of normal individuals as compared to patients with CD. These differences have included identification of decreased bacterial diversity and skewing of populations as compared to normal individuals [15–17].

Metagenomics is an emerging field that is based on the genomic analysis of microbial DNA extracted from environmental samples and is not dependent on culture-based techniques. This sophisticated approach has the potential to provide a more accurate and descriptive analysis of the entire microbiome inhabiting the intestine of any one individual at a particular point in time. Applying this technique, the fecal pool of six patients in remission from CD (CDAI < 150) was found to have a reduced diversity of one of the bacterial phylotypes, the Firmicutes family. Healthy individuals maintained 43 different species within this family, whereas CD patients maintained only 13 species, and of the represented species within this family, the Clostridia were over-represented [18].

It may difficult to conclude whether the altered flora in patients with IBD leads to intestinal inflammation, or whether the bowel inflammation occurs first (and then predisposes a host to altered flora). However, growing evidence supports the notion that individuals with IBD retain a commensal flora that differs from the norm and that "microbial shift" may become implicated in the pathogenesis of the disease.

Requirements for Bacteria in the Development of IBD

Murine models of IBD have consistently demonstrated that the progression to mucosal inflammation of either a Crohn's or UC-like phenotype requires bacteria to be present to initiate disease [19–24], and supports a role for nonpathogenic bacteria in disease initiation. For example, IL-10 knockout mice derived under gnotobiotic conditions develop colitis when transferred into conventional conditions where a mixed microbial flora can associate and establish within the gastrointestinal lumen [22,25]. Similar investigations in humans have identified individual bacterial species that may be potential etiologic agents in the development of intestinal inflammation in IBD. *Mycobacterium avium paratubercolosis (MAP)* has been isolated in biopsy specimens of patients with CD and a high frequency of patients develop an anti-MAP response [26–28]. Another potential etiologic pathogen is adherent-invasive *Escherichia coli* (AIEC) [29], which also has demonstrated increased abundance in isolated tissue from patients with CD.

The particular bacterial species capable of triggering responses is not known; however, it is possible that one single bacterial species ignites an inflammatory response that broadens to include multiple bacterial targets of the native commensal flora. In a genetically susceptible host who is unable to down-modulate the response against a bacterially derived antigen, this response may broaden against additional bacterial antigens and species as chronic intestinal inflammation progresses. In support of this assertion, germ-free mice associated with a defined flora and then infected with the murine pathogen *Helicobacter bilis* developed colitis consistent with that seen in human IBD [30] and mounted serum antibody and cytokine responses against bacterial antigens specific to those of the defined flora [31,32].

Disease initiation in humans may also depend on and be reflected by the development of antigen-specific immune responses to components of the bacterial flora. B and T cells display an oligoclonal response in animal models and in humans with IBD, suggesting that responses are restricted to a limited set of antigens. Individuals with IBD develop serum antibody responses to various bacterial components [33,34], supporting the hypothesis that immune responses are elicited and directed against bacteria as part of the immunopathogenesis of IBD. Strong serologic responses to bacterial flagellin (which binds to TLR5) are noted in up to 50% of patients with CD but are not seen in patients with UC [33]. The serological analysis of bacterial-specific antibodies are utilized in the clinical setting since they can be used stratify patients and are correlated with disease severity and prognosis [35]. The identification of antibacterial antibodies in the progression of IBD has also been replicated in mouse models wherein mucosal T cells can proliferate to bacterial sonicates ex vivo, in contrast to mucosal T cells isolated from normal (non-IBD) intestinal mucosa [36], thus suggesting a loss of "tolerance" to host commensal flora.

PROBIOTIC BACTERIA IN ANIMAL MODELS OF IBD

The use of probiotics in health and disease is based on the concept that these bacteria have properties that are capable of modulating disease inducing or activating mediators. Probiotics have been extensively studied for their role in various diseases including eczema, necrotizing enterocolitis, and infectious diarrhea [37–40]. The specific mechanisms contributing to the functional role of individual probiotic species in modifying disease activity is not yet fully defined but involves both direct and indirect cellular contact (as mediated by secreted factors). Many species have been used, but those most commonly applied in clinical study are *Lactobacillus* sp., *Bifidobacterium* sp., non-pathogenic *E. coli*, and the yeast *S. boulardii*. Given the genetic diversity within each genus, it is quite likely that unique mechanisms are utilized by each to modulate inflammation, although common pathways may be shared. While the specific understanding of mechanisms employed by probiotic bacteria is still limited, antiinflammatory capacities have been observed that include the following: modulation of mucosal and peripheral host immune responses [41], direct effects on intra-epithelial and immune cells to alter production of inflammatory cytokines (i.e. TNF-alpha) [42–45], modulation of key signaling molecules (i.e., via nuclear factor-κB), and direct inhibition of pathogenic bacterial species [46–48].

In vitro and in vivo experiments in a variety of animal models of IFD have helped to expand the mechanistic understanding of how probiotics may abrogate inflammation in humans with IBD [49–51]. Many models rely on transgenic mice with specific immunodeficiences or utilize caustic agents to induce inflammation consistent with that seen in UC and CD. These models are proving useful to test the effectiveness of specific probiotic species and allow further experimental analysis to illuminate the biologic basis for the clinical effects that are observed.

As previously discussed, activation of the transcription factor NF-κB leads to downstream activation of genes involved in immune responses. A number of commensal and probiotic species can attenuate mucosal inflammation associated with inhibition of NF-κB [52–55] and presumably subsequent immune modulation [56–58]. Proinflammatory and inhibitory cytokines appear to be imbalanced in IBD and therefore restoration of a normal balance may be one approach to treatment. As one example, and also for demonstrating a role of soluble mediators produced by probiotic species, conditioned media from the nonpathogenic *Eschericia coli strain Nissle 1917* could inhibit the proliferation of blood and mucosal T cells in vitro and this was associated with decreased IFN-γ (pro-inflammatory) and increased IL-10 synthesis (inhibitory) [59]. Soluble factors from the probiotic formulation VSL#3, commonly used in patients with UC, has also been shown to inhibit TNF-mediated NF-κB activation via a common pathway that involves proteosome inhibition [56]. This in vitro observation was extended to an in vivo model, in which rats fed VSL#3 demonstrated histologic and clinical improvement of DSS-induced colitis with changes in the proinflammatory cytokine IL-1beta and the NF-κB inhibitory protein I-κB [60].

Dendritic cells (DC) in the gastrointestinal mucosa have the capacity to directly interact with bacteria and bacterial cell products by extending their dendrites from the basolateral to the apical lumen across the tight junctions of mucosal epithelial cells [61,62]. After "sampling" the intestinal lumen, these critical antigen presenting cells traffic back to the intestinal submucosa and to draining lymph nodes to interact with and influence activation of effector and regulatory cells. The capacity of DC to distinguish between pathogenic and nonpathogenic probiotic species and differentially respond has been surmised and is likely a key event in the induction of immune responses within mucosal tissues and in the maintenance of intestinal homeostasis. Contact with probiotic species can alter cell surface molecule expression, induce maturation, and cytokine production of dendritic cells, suggesting that secreted factors from commensal and probiotic species may potentially alter functional capacities [63–65]. The observation that dendritic cells cultured in the presence of Lactobacillus species can protect against TNBS-induced colitis in mice by inducing regulatory T cells [66] has been the most intriguing. This similar ability has been observed in another in vitro model via the engagement of DC-SIGN. DC-SIGN is a DC-specific cell surface molecule, member of the C-type Lectin superfamily, and a PRR that binds carbohydrates of glycoprotein molecules from fungi, bacteria, and viruses. Certain *Lactobacillus* species engage DC-SIGN and this elicits activation of a T regulatory cell population and the production of the inhibitory cytokine IL-10 [67]. The role for regulatory T cells in IBD has become a recent area of active investigation and the observation that specific probiotic species are able to induce regulatory cell populations provides one potential strategy for their use in treating IBD.

Intestinal epithelial cells (IEC) are damaged in IBD due to infiltration by inflammatory cells and mediators. Protection from this damage is another means of counteracting the pathogenic insults in IBD. Exploration of this probiotic function in *Lactobacillus GG*, an oft prescribed probiotic for infectious and antibiotic-induced diarrhea, IBS, and

IBD, has shown that a soluble factor can induce cytoprotective heat shock proteins in IEC [68]. Recently, two proteins were identified from cultures of *Lactobacillus GG* that protected IEC of mouse colon explants from TNF-induced apoptosis [69,70].

The yeast probiotic *S. boulardii* has documented clinical efficacy in diarrheal illness and has also been utilized in IBD. In a model of murine IBD, colonic inflammation was attenuated following treatment with *S. boulardii* and seems to be due to inhibition of migration of Th1 cells from draining mesenteric lymph nodes into the colon [71]. This model represents another mechanism, specifically, the regulation of adhesion molecules on epithelial and activated effector cells with resultant alterations in cellular trafficking. Thus, probiotics may impact inflammation in the intestine by modulating the activity of both the intestinal mucosal epithelium and the effector cells that traffic there.

PROBIOTICS FOR THE TREATMENT OF IBD

Studies of new treatments in CD typically involve one of three groups of patients. Trials of induction therapies are performed in ill patients, in which the goal is to induce a rapid improvement or remission, as measured by either the CD activity index (CDAI) or Pediatric CDAI (PCDAI) [72]. Trials of maintenance therapies are typically performed in patients who have already entered remission, and the goal is to prevent relapse. Trial of postoperative recurrence prevention are performed in patients who have had surgery, in which the goal is to prolong the time before the disease recurs at the surgical site. Careful clinical studies in CD are difficult to conduct, because of the high placebo response rate (approximately 30% in most studies), the large sample size of patients needed, the subjectivity of disease index scores, and the need for multicenter collaborations [73]. In the United States, such drug studies are typically performed by pharmaceutical companies under FDA supervision, and cost millions of dollars. However, probiotics are frequently marketed directly to the public as dietary supplements rather than being sold as prescription drugs. Therefore, a paucity of data on probiotic efficacy and safety in adult and pediatric IBD remains.

To date, only a few well-controlled (randomized, double blind) clinical studies performed in patients with CD that study the effectiveness of probiotics in modifying disease activity and course exist (Table 12.1). The majority of studies demonstrating a positive outcome of probiotics in IBD have been in patients with UC or with "pouchitis" (inflammation of the ileal reservoir that is created after pouch surgery). Thus far, no studies demonstrate clear efficacy of probiotics in the induction or maintenance of remission or prevention of postoperative recurrence in CD.

Major drawbacks in the comparative analysis and assessment of results of each of the studies performed to date are as follows: the variability in numbers and small sample sizes of patients studied, disease location and activity, comparison to placebo and other standard therapies, probiotic strain selection, dose, viability, and inconsistent analysis of effective colonization by utilized strains. Only two studies have focused on pediatric patients (only one a blinded randomized control trial) and three have compared the use of probiotics with placebo. The Cochrane review recently published the experience of probiotic use for the maintenance of remission in CD; only seven studies met the criterion for review [74]. Since that publication one additional placebo controlled randomized clinical trial in patients post-ileocecal resection has been published [75].

Table 12.1

Summarized clinical studies examining the effectiveness of probiotics in individuals with Crohns disease

Probiotic	Disease	Primary endpoint and outcome	Study design	Total patients	Probiotic dose	References
Lactobacillus GG	CD	Sustained remission at 6 months: No statistical difference	P/R/DB	11	2×10^9 cfu/ day	Schultz et al. (80)
	CD	Postsurgical prevention of or decreased severity of recurrence at 12 months: No statistical difference	P/R	45	12×10^9 cfu/ day	Prantera et al. [78]
	CD (peds)	Maintenance of remission: No statistical difference	P/R	75	??	Bousvaros et al. [82]
	CD (peds)	Clinical improvement at 4 weeks; decreased intestinal permeability	Open trial	4	10×10^{10} cfu/ day	Gupta (81)
Lactobacillus johnsonii (LA1)	CD	Decreased endoscopic recurrence at 12 weeks: No statistical difference	Multicenter P/R	70	10×10^{10} cfu/ day	Van Gossum et al. [75]
	CD	Postsurgical endoscopic and clinical recurrence at 6 months: No statistical difference	P/R/DB	98	4×10^9 cfu/ day	Marteau et al. [79]
E. coli Nissle	CD	Maintenance of remission	P/DB	28	5×10^{10} cfu/ day	Malchow [76]
S. boulardii	CD	Decreased relapse rate: Significant difference in treatment group ($p = 0.04$)	R/open trial	32	1 g/day	Guslandi et al. [77]

P, placebo; R, randomized; DB, double blind.

Probiotics for Treatment of CD

The first randomized double-blinded study oft cited was that performed by Malchow et al. in 1997 [76]. In this study, 28 patients with active small or large bowel CD (as defined by a CDAI > 150) were treated with E. coli Nissle or placebo following steroid-induced remission. At the end of one year, patients were compared for remission and these did not differ although a trend was seen in the time to onset of remission, which appeared to be shorter in patients receiving E. coli Nissle versus those who received placebo.

In 2000, Guslandi et al. used the nonpathogenic species S. bouldardii to study its effect on inducing remission in patients with ileocolic CD [77]. In this study, 32 patients were randomized to receive mesalamine or S. boulardii as an adjunct to mesalamine with the primary endpoint defined as rate of relapse at 6 months. At the conclusion of the study, patients randomized to the receive Saccharomyces had a statistically significant lower rate of relapse ($p = 0.04$) than the mesalamine-only group (6 vs. 38%). However, the small number of patients in this study limited its statistical power and therefore analysis with a larger number of patients is required.

Three studies have examined Lactobacillus species in patients after ileocecal resection [75,78,79]. The most recent study published in 2007 was a multicenter double-blinded study from Belgium with the primary endpoint of detecting a difference in endoscopic recurrence at 12 weeks post-ileocecal resection between patients receiving either probiotic or placebo. Seventy patients were enrolled preoperatively and then randomized to receive Lactobacillus johnsonii, LA1, Nestle or placebo postoperatively. At the end of 12 weeks of therapy, the mean endoscopic score and the clinical relapse rate (defined as a CDAI > 150 with an increase in 70 points from baseline) [75] between groups were not different. The outcome of this study was comparable to another study in which patients were given Lactobacillus GG for 12 months postoperatively [78]. Clinical and endoscopic remission rates were similar between groups (83 vs. 89% and 40% vs. 64% for the probiotic vs. placebo group respectively).

One study has tested the effectiveness of Lactobacillus GG in maintaining remission following induction therapy [80]. Both patient groups were first treated with antibiotics and a 12-week course of tapering steroids. Lactobacillus GG or placebo was introduced 2 weeks into the 3 month course of steroids. One major caveat of this study was the small sample size: only 11 patients were included and at the end of 6 months, only 5 patients had completed the study. Two patients in each treatment group (probiotic vs. placebo) maintained remission at the end of 6 months (no difference between groups). The mean time to relapse was slightly longer in the group receiving Lactobacillus GG; however, the small sample size in this study prevents interpretation of the significance of this observation.

Finally, only two published reports examining the effectiveness of probiotics in pediatric patients with IBD [81,82]I exist, and only one of these was a randomized, double-blind trial of Lactobacillus GG. The study by Bousvaros et al. compared Lactobacillus GG in addition to standard maintenance therapy (aminosalicylates, 6MP, azathioprine, corticosteroids) versus placebo in 75 patients in clinical remission. The primary endpoint was maintenance and duration of remission and patients were followed for 2 years. At the end of the observation period, the median time to relapse was 9.8 months in the probiotic treatment group versus 11 months in the placebo group with a total of 31% of patients who relapsed in the probiotic group versus 17% in the placebo group. There was no statistical difference in relapse rate (PCDAI score ≤30 points) or the length of remission between both groups.

In summary, the use of probiotics for the treatment of CD has not yet demonstrated promise in the clinical studies performed to date. Further studies that include larger numbers of patients, use of standardized doses of probiotics, and confirmation of colonization of the chosen species are required.

Probiotics in UC and Pouchitis

The use of probiotic formulations to treat UC and pouchitis has yielded more positive outcomes and are extensively reviewed in another chapter. Particularly for pouchitis, the results of studies have been promising enough to result in the use of particular probiotic formulations as part of the acceptable management approach in relapsing and recurrent pouchitis [83]. VSL#3 has demonstrated a significant benefit over placebo for maintaining remission in patients with chronic relapsing pouchitis [84]. A variety of probioitic preparations have demonstrated slight though statistically significant benefits in reducing endoscopic severity or in inducing or maintaining remission as compared to standard therapy [85–88] in UC.

SUMMARY AND CONCLUSION

The outcomes of studies utilizing probiotics to treat CD have been rather disappointing thus far. However, the initial negative results should not discourage further studies. Probiotics do have the ability to colonize the intestinal mucosa and to establish temporary short-term niches with the potential to modulate immune responses within the gastrointestinal tract. With advances in molecular and microbial genetics, the potential use for genetically engineered probiotic species in health and disease is also being realized [89,90] and may prove beneficial in IBD as demonstrated with an IL-10 secreting *Lacotcoccus lactis* that could ameliorate colitis in mice [91].

It is clear that certain probiotic species provide benefit in the treatment of diarrheal illness [40], recurrent *Clostridium difficile* [92], and IBS [93]. For IBD, the use of selected probiotics has demonstrated benefit in UC and pouchitis. Future studies of probiotics in CD will require greater scientific rigor in clinical studies with regard to blinding, measurement of outcomes, selection of species and dosing, and analysis of intestinal microflora. Complementing patient-based research by hypothesis-driven laboratory research of mechanisms utilized by probiotic species capable of modulating disease activity will offer the best promise in the applied use of probiotics in future, and in the clinical management of CD.

REFERENCES

1. Turunen P, Kolho KL, Auvinen A, et al. Incidence of inflammatory bowel disease in Finnish children, 1987–2003. *Inflamm Bowel Dis* 2006;12(8):677–83.
2. Kucharzik T, Maaser C, Lugering A, et al. Recent understanding of IBD pathogenesis: implications for future therapies. *Inflamm Bowel Dis* 2006;12(11):1068–83.
3. Baumgart DC, Carding SR. Inflammatory bowel disease: cause and immunobiology. *Lancet* 2007;369(9573):1627–40.
4. Xavier RJ, Podolsky DK. Unravelling the pathogenesis of inflammatory bowel disease. *Nature* 2007;448(7152):427–34.

5. Fritz JH, Ferrero RL, Philpott DJ, et al. Nod-like proteins in immunity, inflammation and disease. *Nat Immunol* 2006;7(12):1250–7.

6. Ben-Neriah Y, Schmidt-Supprian M. Epithelial NF-κB maintains host gut microflora homeostasis. *Nat Immunol* 2007;8(5):479–81.

7. Hugot JP, Chamaillard M, Zouali H, et al. Association of NOD2 leucine-rich repeat variants with susceptibility to Crohn's disease. *Nature* 2001;411(6837):599–603.

8. De Jager PL, Franchimont D, Waliszewska A, et al. The role of the Toll receptor pathway in susceptibility to inflammatory bowel diseases. *Genes Immun* 2007;8(5):387–97.

9. Franchimont D, Vermeire S, El Housni H, et al. Deficient host-bacteria interactions in inflammatory bowel disease? The toll-like receptor (TLR)-4 Asp299gly polymorphism is associated with Crohn's disease and ulcerative colitis. *Gut* 2004;53(7):987–92.

10. Duerr RH, Taylor KD, Brant SR, et al. A genome-wide association study identifies IL23R as an inflammatory bowel disease gene. *Science* 2006;314(5804):1461–3.

11. Weaver CT, Hatton RD, Mangan PR, et al. IL-17 family cytokines and the expanding diversity of effector T cell lineages. *Annu Rev Immunol* 2007;25:821–52.

12. Hue S, Ahern P, Buonocore S, et al. Interleukin-23 drives innate and T cell-mediated intestinal inflammation. *J Exp Med* 2006;203(11):2473–83.

13. Iwakura Y, Ishigame H. The IL-23/IL-17 axis in inflammation. *J Clin Invest* 2006;116(5):1218–22.

14. Yen D, Cheung J, Scheerens H, et al. IL-23 is essential for T cell-mediated colitis and promotes inflammation via IL-17 and IL-6. *J Clin Invest* 2006;116(5):1310–6.

15. Gophna U, Sommerfeld K, Gophna S, et al. Differences between tissue-associated intestinal microfloras of patients with Crohn's disease and ulcerative colitis. *J Clin Microbiol* 2006;44(11):4136–41.

16. Conte MP, Schippa S, Zamboni I, et al. Gut-associated bacterial microbiota in paediatric patients with inflammatory bowel disease. *Gut* 2006;55(12):1760–7.

17. Frank DN, St Amand AL, Feldman RA, et al. Molecular-phylogenetic characterization of microbial community imbalances in human inflammatory bowel diseases. *Proc Natl Acad Sci USA* 2007;104(34):13780–5.

18. Manichanh C, Rigottier-Gois L, Bonnaud E, et al. Reduced diversity of faecal microbiota in Crohn's disease revealed by a metagenomic approach. *Gut* 2006;55(2):205–11.

19. Elson CO, Cong Y, McCracken VJ, et al. Experimental models of inflammatory bowel disease reveal innate, adaptive, and regulatory mechanisms of host dialogue with the microbiota. *Immunol Rev* 2005;206:260–76.

20. Onderdonk AB, Franklin ML, Cisneros RL. Production of experimental ulcerative colitis in gnotobiotic guinea pigs with simplified microflora. *Infect Immun* 1981;32(1):225–31.

21. Duchmann R, Schmitt E, Knolle P, et al. Tolerance towards resident intestinal flora in mice is abrogated in experimental colitis and restored by treatment with interleukin-10 or antibodies to interleukin-12. *Eur J Immunol* 1996;26(4):934–8.

22. Kullberg MC, Ward JM, Gorelick PL, et al. *Helicobacter hepaticus* triggers colitis in specific-pathogen-free interleukin-10 (IL-10)-deficient mice through an IL-12- and gamma interferon-dependent mechanism. *Infect Immun* 1998;66(11):5157–66.

23. Sacco RE, Haynes JS, Harp JA, et al. *Cryptosporidium parvum* initiates inflammatory bowel disease in germfree T cell receptor-alpha-deficient mice. *Am J Pathol* 1998;153(6):1717–22.

24. Bhan AK, Mizoguchi E, Smith RN, et al. Spontaneous chronic colitis in TCR alpha-mutant mice; an experimental model of human ulcerative colitis. *Int Rev Immunol* 2000;19(1):123–38.

25. Balish E, Warner T. *Enterococcus faecalis* induces inflammatory bowel disease in interleukin-10 knockout mice. *Am J Pathol* 2002;160(6):2253–7.

26. Thayer WR Jr., Coutu JA, Chiodini RJ, et al. Possible role of mycobacteria in inflammatory bowel disease. II. Mycobacterial antibodies in Crohn's disease. *Dig Dis Sci* 1984;29(12):1080–5.

27. Singh UP, Singh S, Singh R, et al. Influence of *Mycobacterium avium* subsp. paratuberculosis on colitis development and specific immune responses during disease. *Infect Immun* 2007;75(8):3722–8.

28. Hulten K, El-Zimaity HM, Karttunen TJ, et al. Detection of *Mycobacterium avium* subspecies paratuberculosis in Crohn's diseased tissues by in situ hybridization. *Am J Gastroenterol* 2001;96(5):1529–35.

29. Darfeuille-Michaud A, Boudeau J, Bulois P, et al. High prevalence of adherent-invasive *Escherichia coli* associated with ileal mucosa in Crohn's disease. *Gastroenterology* 2004;127(2):412–21.

30. Shomer NH, Dangler CA, Schrenzel MD, et al. *Helicobacter bilis*-induced inflammatory bowel disease in scid mice with defined flora. *Infect Immun* 1997;65(11):4858–64.
31. Jergens AE, Wilson-Welder JH, Dorn A, et al. *Helicobacter bilis* triggers persistent immune reactivity to antigens derived from the commensal bacteria in gnotobiotic C3H/HeN mice. *Gut* 2007;56(7):934–40.
32. Jergens AE, Dorn A, Wilson J, et al. Induction of differential immune reactivity to members of the flora of gnotobiotic mice following colonization with *Helicobacter bilis* or *Brachyspira hyodysenteriae*. *Microbes Infect* 2006;8(6):1602–10.
33. Lodes MJ, Cong Y, Elson CO, et al. Bacterial flagellin is a dominant antigen in Crohn disease. *J Clin Invest* 2004;113(9):1296–306.
34. Devlin SM, Yang H, Ippoliti A, et al. NOD2 variants and antibody response to microbial antigens in Crohn's disease patients and their unaffected relatives. *Gastroenterology* 2007;132(2):576–86.
35. Dubinsky MC, Lin YC, Dutridge D, et al. Serum immune responses predict rapid disease progression among children with Crohn's disease: immune responses predict disease progression. *Am J Gastroenterol* 2006;101(2):360–7.
36. Duchmann R, Marker-Hermann E, Meyer zum Buschenfelde KH. Bacteria-specific T-cell clones are selective in their reactivity towards different enterobacteria or *H. pylori* and increased in inflammatory bowel disease. *Scand J Immunol* 1996;44(1):71–9.
37. Prescott SL, Bjorksten B. Probiotics for the prevention or treatment of allergic diseases. *J Allergy Clin Immunol* 2007;120(2):255–62.
38. Lin HC, Su BH, Chen AC, et al. Oral probiotics reduce the incidence and severity of necrotizing enterocolitis in very low birth weight infants. *Pediatrics* 2005;115(1):1–4.
39. Nelson R. Antibiotic treatment for *Clostridium difficile*-associated diarrhea in adults. *Cochrane Database Syst Rev* 2007;3:CD004610.
40. Johnston BC, Supina AL, Ospina M, et al. Probiotics for the prevention of pediatric antibiotic-associated diarrhea. *Cochrane Database Syst Rev* 2007M;2:CD004827.
41. Noverr MC, Huffnagle GB. *Does the microbiota regulate immune responses outside the gut? Trends Microbiol* 2004;12(12):562–8.
42. Helwig U, Lammers KM, Rizzello F, et al. Lactobacilli, bifidobacteria and *E. coli* nissle induce pro- and anti-inflammatory cytokines in peripheral blood mononuclear cells. *World J Gastroenterol* 2006;12(37):5978–86.
43. Bai AP, Ouyang Q, Zhang W, et al. Probiotics inhibit TNF-alpha-induced interleukin-8 secretion of HT29 cells. *World J Gastroenterol* 2004;10(3):455–7.
44. Sougioultzis S, Simeonidis S, Bhaskar KR, et al. *Saccharomyces boulardii* produces a soluble anti-inflammatory factor that inhibits NF-κB-mediated IL-8 gene expression. *Biochem Biophys Res Commun* 2006;343(1):69–76.
45. Ruiz PA, Hoffmann M, Szcesny S, et al. Innate mechanisms for *Bifidobacterium lactis* to activate transient pro-inflammatory host responses in intestinal epithelial cells after the colonization of germ-free rats. *Immunology* 2005;115(4):441–50.
46. Asahara T, Shimizu K, Nomoto K, et al. Probiotic bifidobacteria protect mice from lethal infection with Shiga toxin-producing *Escherichia coli* O157:H7. *Infect Immun* 2004;72(4):2240–7.
47. Corr SC, Gahan CG, Hill C. Impact of selected Lactobacillus and Bifidobacterium species on Listeria monocytogenes infection and the mucosal immune response. *FEMS Immunol Med Microbiol* 2007;50(3):380–8.
48. Corr SC, Li Y, Riedel CU, et al. Bacteriocin production as a mechanism for the antiinfective activity of *Lactobacillus salivarius* UCC118. *Proc Natl Acad Sci USA* 2007;104(18):7617–21.
49. Madsen KL, Doyle JS, Jewell LD, et al. Lactobacillus species prevents colitis in interleukin 10 gene-deficient mice. *Gastroenterology* 1999;116(5):1107–14.
50. O'Mahony L, Feeney M, O'Halloran S, et al. Probiotic impact on microbial flora, inflammation and tumour development in IL-10 knockout mice. *Aliment Pharmacol Ther* 2001;15(8):1219–25.
51. McCarthy J, O'Mahony L, O'Callaghan L, et al. Double blind, placebo controlled trial of two probiotic strains in interleukin 10 knockout mice and mechanistic link with cytokine balance. *Gut* 2003;52(7):975–80.
52. Neish AS, Gewirtz AT, Zeng H, et al. Prokaryotic regulation of epithelial responses by inhibition of IκB-alpha ubiquitination. *Science* 2000;289(5484):1560–3.

53. Kelly D, Campbell JI, King TP, et al. Commensal anaerobic gut bacteria attenuate inflammation by regulating nuclear-cytoplasmic shuttling of PPAR-gamma and RelA. *Nat Immunol* 2004;5(1):104–12.

54. Riedel CU, Foata F, Philippe D, et al. Anti-inflammatory effects of bifidobacteria by inhibition of LPS-induced NF-κB activation. *World J Gastroenterol* 2006;12(23):3729–35.

55. De Jager PL, Franchimont D, Waliszewska A, et al. The role of the Toll receptor pathway in susceptibility to inflammatory bowel diseases. *Genes Immun* 2007;8(5):387–97.

56. Petrof EO, Kojima K, Ropeleski MJ, et al. Probiotics inhibit nuclear factor-κB and induce heat shock proteins in colonic epithelial cells through proteasome inhibition. *Gastroenterology* 2004;127(5):1474–87.

57. Matsumoto S, Hara T, Hori T, et al. Probiotic Lactobacillus-induced improvement in murine chronic inflammatory bowel disease is associated with the down-regulation of pro-inflammatory cytokines in lamina propria mononuclear cells. *Clin Exp Immunol* 2005;140(3):417–26.

58. Jijon H, Backer J, Diaz H, et al. DNA from probiotic bacteria modulates murine and human epithelial and immune function. *Gastroenterology* 2004;126(5):1358–73.

59. Sturm A, Rilling K, Baumgart DC, et al. *Escherichia coli* Nissle 1917 distinctively modulates T-cell cycling and expansion via toll-like receptor 2 signaling. *Infect Immun* 2005;73(3):1452–65.

60. Fitzpatrick LR, Hertzog KL, Quatse AL, et al. Effects of the probiotic formulation VSL#3 on colitis in weanling rats. *J Pediatr Gastroenterol Nutr* 2007;44(5):561–70.

61. Niess JH, Brand S, Gu X, et al. CX3CR1-mediated dendritic cell access to the intestinal lumen and bacterial clearance. *Science* 2005;307(5707):254–8.

62. Niess JH, Reinecker HC. Lamina propria dendritic cells in the physiology and pathology of the gastrointestinal tract. *Curr Opin Gastroenterol* 2005;21(6):687–91.

63. Hoarau C, Lagaraine C, Martin L, et al. Supernatant of *Bifidobacterium breve* induces dendritic cell maturation, activation, and survival through a Toll-like receptor 2 pathway. *J Allergy Clin Immunol* 2006;117(3):696–702.

64. Drakes M, Blanchard T, Czinn S. Bacterial probiotic modulation of dendritic cells. *Infect Immun* 2004;72(6):3299–309.

65. Niers LE, Hoekstra MO, Timmerman HM, et al. Selection of probiotic bacteria for prevention of allergic diseases: immunomodulation of neonatal dendritic cells. *Clin Exp Immunol* 2007;149(2):344–52.

66. Foligne B, Zoumpopoulou G, Dewulf J, et al. A key role of dendritic cells in probiotic functionality. *PLoS ONE* 2007;2:e313.

67. Smits HH, Engering A, van der Kleij D, et al. Selective probiotic bacteria induce IL-10-producing regulatory T cells in vitro by modulating dendritic cell function through dendritic cell-specific intercellular adhesion molecule 3-grabbing nonintegrin. *J Allergy Clin Immunol* 2005;115(6):1260–7.

68. Tao Y, Drabik KA, Waypa TS, et al. Soluble factors from Lactobacillus GG activate MAPKs and induce cytoprotective heat shock proteins in intestinal epithelial cells. *Am J Physiol Cell Physiol* 2006;290(4):C1018–30.

69. Yan F, Polk DB. Probiotic bacterium prevents cytokine-induced apoptosis in intestinal epithelial cells. *J Biol Chem* 2002;277(52):50959–65.

70. Yan F, Cao H, Cover TL, et al. Soluble proteins produced by probiotic bacteria regulate intestinal epithelial cell survival and growth. *Gastroenterology* 2007;132(2):562–75.

71. Dalmasso G, Cottrez F, Imbert V, et al. *Saccharomyces boulardii* inhibits inflammatory bowel disease by trapping T cells in mesenteric lymph nodes. *Gastroenterology* 2006;131(6):1812–25.

72. Griffiths AM, Otley AR, Hyams J, et al. A review of activity indices and end points for clinical trials in children with Crohn's disease. *Inflamm Bowel Dis* 2005;11(2):185–96.

73. Su C, Lichtenstein GR, Krok K, et al. A meta-analysis of the placebo rates of remission and response in clinical trials of active Crohn's disease. *Gastroenterology* 2004;126(5):1257–69.

74. Rolfe VE, Fortun PJ, Hawkey CJ, et al. Probiotics for maintenance of remission in Crohn's disease. *Cochrane Database Syst Rev* 2006;4:CD004826.

75. Van Gossum A, Dewit O, Louis E, et al. Multicenter randomized-controlled clinical trial of probiotics (Lactobacillus johnsonii, LA1) on early endoscopic recurrence of Crohn's disease after Ileo-caecal resection. *Inflamm Bowel Dis* 2007;13(2):135–42.

76. Malchow HA. Crohn's disease and *Escherichia coli*. *A new approach in therapy to maintain remission of colonic Crohn's disease? J Clin Gastroenterol* 1997;25(4):653–8.

77. Guslandi M, Mezzi G, Sorghi M, et al. *Saccharomyces boulardii* in maintenance treatment of Crohn's disease. *Dig Dis Sci* 2000;45(7):1462–4.

78. Prantera C, Scribano ML, Falasco G, et al. Ineffectiveness of probiotics in preventing recurrence after curative resection for Crohn's disease: a randomised controlled trial with Lactobacillus GG. *Gut* 2002;51(3):405–9.

79. Marteau P, Lemann M, Seksik P, et al. Ineffectiveness of *Lactobacillus johnsonii* LA1 for prophylaxis of postoperative recurrence in Crohn's disease: a randomised, double blind, placebo controlled GETAID trial. *Gut* 2006;55(6):842–7.

80. Schultz M, Timmer A, Herfarth HH, et al. Lactobacillus GG in inducing and maintaining remission of Crohn's disease. *BMC Gastroenterol* 2004;4:5.

81. Gupta P, Andrew H, Kirschner BS, et al. Is lactobacillus GG helpful in children with Crohn's disease? Results of a preliminary, open-label study. *J Pediatr Gastroenterol Nutr* 2000;31(4):453–7.

82. Bousvaros A, Guandalini S, Baldassano RN, et al. A randomized, double-blind trial of Lactobacillus GG versus placebo in addition to standard maintenance therapy for children with Crohn's disease. *Inflamm Bowel Dis* 2005;11(9):833–9.

83. Laake KO, Bjorneklett A, Aamodt G, et al. Outcome of four weeks' intervention with probiotics on symptoms and endoscopic appearance after surgical reconstruction with a J-configurated ileal-pouch-anal-anastomosis in ulcerative colitis. *Scand J Gastroenterol* 2005;40(1):43–51.

84. Gionchetti P, Rizzello F, Venturi A, et al. Oral bacteriotherapy as maintenance treatment in patients with chronic pouchitis: a double-blind, placebo-controlled trial. *Gastroenterology* 2000;119(2):305–9.

85. Kruis W, Schutz E, Fric P, et al. Double-blind comparison of an oral *Escherichia coli* preparation and mesalazine in maintaining remission of ulcerative colitis. *Aliment Pharmacol Ther* 1997;11(5):853–8.

86. Kruis W, Fric P, Pokrotnieks J, et al. Maintaining remission of ulcerative colitis with the probiotic Escherichia coli Nissle 1917 is as effective as with standard mesalazine. *Gut* 2004;53(11):1617–23.

87. Rembacken BJ, Snelling AM, Hawkey PM, et al. Non-pathogenic *Escherichia coli* versus mesalazine for the treatment of ulcerative colitis: a randomised trial. *Lancet* 1999;354(9179):635–9.

88. Bibiloni R, Fedorak RN, Tannock GW, et al. VSL#3 probiotic-mixture induces remission in patients with active ulcerative colitis. *Am J Gastroenterol* 2005;100(7):1539–46.

89. Fu GF, Li X, Hou YY, et al. Bifidobacterium longum as an oral delivery system of endostatin for gene therapy on solid liver cancer. *Cancer Gene Ther* 2005;12(2):133–40.

90. Xu YF, Zhu LP, Hu B, et al. A new expression plasmid in *Bifidobacterium longum* as a delivery system of endostatin for cancer gene therapy. *Cancer Gene Ther* 2007;14(2):151–7.

91. Steidler L, Neirynck S, Huyghebaert N, et al. Biological containment of genetically modified Lactococcus lactis for intestinal delivery of human interleukin 10. *Nat Biotechnol* 2003;21(7):785–9.

92. McFarland LV. Meta-analysis of probiotics for the prevention of antibiotic associated diarrhea and the treatment of *Clostridium difficile* disease. *Am J Gastroenterol* 2006;101(4):812–22.

93. Quigley EM, Flourie B. Probiotics and irritable bowel syndrome: a rationale for their use and an assessment of the evidence to date. *Neurogastroenterol Motil* 2007;19(3):166–72.**Table12.1** (continued)

13 Probiotics in Ulcerative Colitis

Richard N. Fedorak

Key Points

- Ulcerative colitis (UC) is a chronic, debilitating disease, and many drugs used for therapy have undesirable side effects.
- This chapter discusses the scientific literature regarding the therapeutic role of probiotics in ulcerative colitis with a focus on the pediatric patient population.
- Evidence-based research suggests that probiotic therapy, either alone or as an adjuvant, may be an effective alternative for some UC patients
- No definitive data exist to confirm that probiotic therapy is beneficial for either active disease or maintaining remission.
- The efficacy of probiotics to achieve or maintain remission in UC pediatric patients is a topic of considerable debate.

Key Words: Probiotic, prebiotic, ulcerative colitis, inflammatory bowel disease, lactobacillus, bifidobacterium.

INTRODUCTION

Ulcerative colitis (UC) is an idiopathic chronic inflammation of the mucosa in the large intestine that may lead to loss of function and mucosal ulcerations. The disease alternates between periods of active and quiescent states, commonly referred to as flares and remission, respectively. The disease may be restricted to rectal tissues (proctitis) or may involve the majority of the colon (pancolitis). Common symptoms associated with active disease are diarrhea, rectal bleeding, abdominal pain, tachycardia, anemia, or fever (see Table 13.1). Approximately 5–10% of UC patients experience continual symptoms[1]. Extraintestinal manifestations occur in as many as 25% of UC patients and can include uveitis, arthritis, pyoderma gangrenosum, primary sclerosing cholangitis, and enteric hyperoxaluria[2,3]. UC patients are a high-risk population for developing malignancies including colon cancer[4]. During either a lengthy active period or severe flare (fulminant colitis), patients may develop toxic megacolon whereby the colon greatly expands thinning the already friable and inflamed mucosal walls. Either this state or severe, localized ulcerations may lead to intestinal wall perforation that requires lifesaving surgical intervention.

From: *Nutrition and Health: Probiotics in Pediatric Medicine*
Edited by: S. Michail and P.M. Sherman © Humana Press, Totowa, NJ

Table 13.1
Ulcerative colitis disease activity indices

Clinical index	Activity levels		
	Mild	*Moderate*	*Severe*
American College of Gastroenterology[a]	<4 stools/day ± blood, normal ESR, no sign of toxicity	≥4 stools/day ± blood, minimal signs of toxicity	>6 stools/day ± blood, evidence of toxicity (fever, tachycardia, anemia, or elevated ESR)
Truelove and Witts[b]	<5 bowel movements/day, small amounts of blood in the stool, no fever, no tachycardia, mild anemia (>75%, approximately 100 g/l), ESR < 30	Intermediate condition between mild and severe	≥6 bowel movements/day, large amounts of blood in the stool, fever (>37.5°C), pulse (>90 beats/min), anemia (haemoglobin >75%), ESR > 30
Mayo Score[c] • ≤2 indicates clinical remission if sustained for 3 days • Each of the four subcategories (stools/day, bleeding, endoscopy, and physician's global assessment) are rated 0–3 in increasing severity. The sum is the final score ranging from 0–12	Score 3–5 • 1–2 more stools/day than normal • Some blood in <50% of stools • Minimal rectal bleeding endoscopy shows erythema, mild friability, and decreased vascular pattern • Physician's global assessment is mild activity of disease	Score 6–9 • 3–4 more stools/than normal • Some blood in stools most of the time • Endoscopy shows marked erythema, lack of vascular pattern, definite friability, and mucosal erosions • Physician's global assessment is moderate disease activity	Score 10–12 • ≥5 more stools/day than normal • Rectal bleeding, passing blood-only stools • Endoscopy shows spontaneous bleeding and mucosal ulcerations • Physician's global assessment is severe disease activity
C-reactive protein (CRP)[d]	≥0 mg/l	≥3 mg/l	≥12 mg/l

ESR, erythrocyte sedimentation rate determined using the Wintrobe method.

[a]Kornbluth A, Sachar DB. Ulcerative colitis practice guidelines in adults (update): American College of Gastroenterology, Practice Parameters Committee. Am J Gastroenterol 2004; 99(7):1371–1385.

[b]Truelove SC, Witts L. Cortisone in ulcerative colitis: final report on a therapeutic trial. Br Med J 1955; 2(4947):1041–1048.

[c]Schroeder KW, Tremaine WJ, Ilstrup DM. Coated oral 5-aminosalicylic acid therapy for mildly to moderately active ulcerative colitis. A randomized study. N Engl J Med 1987; 317(26):1625–1629.

[d]Fagan EA, Dyck RF, Maton PN, et al. Serum levels of C-reactive protein in Crohn's disease and ulcerative colitis. Eur J Clin Invest 1982; 12(4):351–359.

UC is usually diagnosed between the ages of 10–30 years during which time the disease is the most active. A combination of colonoscopy and histology distinguishes UC from Crohn's disease (CD), another inflammatory bowel disease (IBD)[5]. In the western world, the UC incidence rate is 2–15 per 100,000 persons per year while prevalence ranges from 60–230 per 100,000 per year[6–10].

In pediatric patients, the prevalent symptom of UC is frequent bloody diarrhea without an underlying cause[11]. Patients diagnosed in their youth develop a more extensive disease profile compared to patients diagnosed in adulthood[12–14] and commonly have a first-degree relative with IBD[15]. The pediatric patient population represents approximately 10–15% of all UC patients[15] and the incidence rate ranges from 0.5–4.3 for 100,000[11]. Although UC is not associated with the very young, a 1-year surveillance study in the UK found that approximately 20% of all pediatric UC cases were less than 10 years old[14]. In the Greater Toronto Area, 23% of UC pediatric patients are less than 8 years while 10% are younger than 5 years of age[11].

There is no cure for UC and the exact cause(s) of the disease remains elusive. The generally accepted theory is that a combination of environmental agent(s) and a dysfunctional mucosal immune system in genetically susceptible individuals leads to the development of UC[2,16]. Environmental agents are believed to originate in the gut's plentiful commensal microflora. Thus, the focus of current treatments is to alleviate symptoms and improve the patient's quality of life. To achieve remission, drugs that have demonstrated efficacy are employed in a stepwise fashion beginning with the mildest and progressing in strength if the patient is either intolerant or refractory to it (e.g., 5-aminosalicylic acid compounds (5-ASA), corticosteroids, ciclosporin, tacrolimus, or biologic agents such as infliximab)[2]. For maintaining remission, several drugs have demonstrated effectiveness: 5-ASA formulations, azathioprine, 6-mercaptopurine, and infliximab[2]. The primary mechanism of action of these drugs is to suppress the activated immune system[17]. Without continuous medication, 70% of patients in remission are anticipated to incur flares within the year[18]. Each drug is associated with significant side effects, continuous usage may render the patient intolerant or refractory to a drug, and no single treatment identified to date is universally effective for all UC patients[17].

Pediatric UC patients face a lifetime of drug therapy and, as such, may be more susceptible to intolerance, loss of efficacy, or health issues due to side effects. Drug efficacy is routinely assessed via short-term (less than 1 year) randomized controlled trials (RCTs) with adult subjects and the results are extrapolated to the pediatric patient population. In the absence of long-term RCTs involving young pediatric patients, a drug's effect on growth and development remain unknown. In fact, the relative newness of many drugs makes it impossible to assess the impact on individuals who require a lifetime of therapy to control the symptoms of UC.

When drug therapy fails (e.g., intolerance or ineffectiveness), resection of the diseased colon tissues is an option for suitable individuals[19,20]. Advances in surgical techniques have led to the routine use of an internal storage reservoir (ileal j-pouch-anal anastomosis, IPAA), which is less obtrusive than the traditional proctocolectomy with external ileostomy bag. Although surgical intervention approximates a "cure" for UC, a variety of postoperative complications (e.g., pouchitis, high stool frequency, fecal incontinence, need for more surgeries, and risk of infertility) may reduce the patient's quality of life[19,21,22]. As IPAA is a recent surgical technique, there is debate as to the optimum patient age[19] and the robustness of the procedure to withstand a lifetime of use and aging if performed in pediatric patients. As with anything, IPAA is unsuitable for all UC patients as a recent study has demonstrated that those with extraintestinal manifestations of UC are most prone to developing repeated episodes of pouchitis[22].

Recent studies recognize that not all IBD can be diagnosed at onset. Indeterminate colitis (IC) is a clinically distinct disease subgroup of IBD and has a higher prevalence in pediatric than adult patients[23]. Patients present with either pancolitis or, in less extensive cases, this aggressive disease extends throughout the colon developing into pancolitis. Within a period of 6 years or less, approximately a third of the patients may be reclassified as either UC or CD while the majority persists as IC. Surgical outcomes for IC patients are associated with a higher rate of complications following IPAA and a 20% increase in the frequency of pouchitis than other IBD patients. As such, there is much debate regarding the appropriateness of IPAA for IC patients[19] necessitating the reliance on drug therapy to control their symptoms until their disease can be reclassified or not.

In the absence of a cure, pediatric UC (and IC) patients are in need of new treatment options to abrogate their debilitating symptoms. Additionally, adjuvant therapies are required to reduce patient intolerance to current drugs or to minimize the range of side effects that they cause. Although surgery is possible and tolerated, for many, the outcomes are associated with significant risks. Ideally, a new therapy would impart no health effects, be well tolerated by patients of all ages, and could be taken on a regular basis to induce remission in active disease and indefinitely extend periods of remission without loss of efficacy.

PROBIOTICS FOR UC

Probiotic oral and enema formulations have been demonstrated to alter the ratios of bacterial species in the gut's microflora, are well tolerated, and are nonpathogenic organisms that naturally occur in large numbers within healthy humans[16,24,25]. Although the exact cause of UC is unknown, it is likely that the gut's microflora is a contributing factor to the disease if not a causal agent. This idea is supported by outcomes of observational studies investigating the bacterial composition of the gut's microflora. For instance, biopsies from untreated, newly diagnosed UC patients differed substantially with respect to species and numbers compared to CD patients or healthy controls ($P < 0.05$ and $P < 0.01$, respectively)[26]. A second investigation found that pediatric IBD patients had more mucosa-associated aerobic and facultative-anaerobic bacteria than healthy controls[27]. As well, the authors noted an overall decrease in either certain bacterial species or groups associated with the healthy anaerobic intestinal flora of which the most notable decrease was for *Bacteroides vulgatus*.

EXPERIMENTAL MODELS

The importance of unraveling the cause of IBD is evidenced by the development of over 20 different animal models for study purposes[28]. Of these, many have been used to investigate the putative therapeutic role of probiotics and elucidate their mechanism of action in experimentally induced UC. In excess of 25 individual bacterial species and a few formulations containing multiple species (e.g., VSL#3) have been studied using experimental models. Study results can be summarized as follows: (1) probiotic strains differ greatly in their mechanisms of action; (2) it is highly unlikely that a single strain is responsible for invoking clinical effects; (3) bacterial flora are involved in a complex series of interactions between other microbes and the host's immune cells; (4) oral ingestion of purified probiotic strains can modulate the composition and metabolite levels in fecal matter; and (5) experimental colitis cannot be induced in germfree animals while UC can be induced in healthy human individuals by the direct distillation of fecal matter from an inflamed gut[16].

Of course, these initial experiments are limited to only those bacterial organisms that have been successfully cultured and are nonpathogenic. It is speculated that many more species exist within the commensal flora of the gut that have defied previous culturing attempts. Advances in metagenomics will identify genetic sequences of previously unculturable organisms which, in turn, will be cultured for identification.

HUMAN CLINICAL TRIALS

RCTs or open label studies that fulfilled the inclusion criteria and examined the therapeutic effectiveness of probiotics during active periods of UC or remission are summarized in Tables 13.2 and 13.3, respectively.

ACTIVE UC (TABLE 13.2)

In 1999, Rembacken and colleagues conducted the first RCT using 116 patients with moderate to severe disease who were failing mesalamine therapy[29]. Initially all patients were required to take a 1-week course of gentamicin to suppress their native *Escherichia coli*. Patients were then randomized to one of two treatment arms of mesalamine (1.2 g/day) or *E. coli* Nissle 1917 (1×10^{11} CFU/day). At the onset of the study, patients requiring either topical or oral steroids were permitted to continue providing that they be tapered when possible. The study found no significant difference between the study arms regarding the number of patients who achieved remission (mesalamine, 75%; *E. coli*, 68%). The authors concluded that probiotic therapy was as effective as mesalamine, yet acknowledged that the study was not powered for equivalence.

In 2003, two small open label studies were completed. Guslandi et al.[30] examined a small cohort of 25 individuals who were intolerant to corticosteroid therapy, and had been taking mesalamine (3 g/day) for maintenance purposes for a minimum of 3 months preceding their mild to moderate flares (Truelove and Witts activity index). For 4 weeks, patients received *Saccharomyces boulardii* (750 mg/day) and mesalamine therapy after which 68% achieved remission according to the multiphasic Rachmilewitz UC activity index. The results suggest that *S. boulardii* is a plausible treatment alternative to patients intolerant to corticosteroid therapy and who also wish to avoid treatment escalation with drugs such as ciclosporin or biologics such as infliximab.

The other open label study conducted in 2003 had an unconventional methodology. Borody et al.[31] included 6 patients with severe flares who were refractory to both corticosteroid and immunosuppressive treatments. On a daily basis, each person received

Table 13.2
Overview of studies using probiotics to treat active UC

First Author (Publication Date)	Trial Design	n; Mean Age ± SD	Duration (week)	Disease Activity	Probiotic	Control	Remission Rate (%)		
							Control	Probiotic	P
Matthes (2006)	R, DB	90; NR	4	Mild–moderate	E. coli N CFU > 10^8/ml 10, 20, or 40 ml Enema	Placebo	53, 40 ml 44, 20 ml 27, 10 ml	18.2	0.04
Bibilioni (2005)	OL	30; 35 ± 13	6	Mild–moderate	VSL#3 CFU > 1012	n/a	53	n/a	n/a
Kato (2004)	R, DB	20; 32 ± NR	12	Mild–moderate	BFM CFU > 10^{10}	Placebo	40	30	NS
Tursi (2004)	R, OL	90; 41 ± NR	8	Mild–moderate	Balsalazide (2.25 g) and VSL#3 CFU > 10^{11}	Balsalazide (4.5 g) Mesalamine (2.4 g)	80	77 B 53 M	0.02
Borody (2003)	OL	6 25–53 years (age range)	1	Severe	Fecal enemas from healthy donors	n/a	100	n/a	n/a
Guslandi (2003)	OL	25; 19–47 years	4	Mild–moderate	S. boulardii 750 g/day	n/a	68	n/a	n/a
Rembacken (1999)	R, DB	116; 18–80 years	12	Mild–severe	E. coli N CFU > 10^{11}	Mesalamine (2.4 g)	68	75	NS

B, balsalazide; BFM, fermented milk containing live bacteria: B. breve strain Yakult, B. bifidium strain Yakult, L. acidophilus; CFU, colony forming units; DB, double-blind; E. coli N, E. coli Nissle 1917; M, mesalamine; OL, open label; n/a, not available; NR, not reported; R, randomized; and, SD, standard deviation.

a prepared enema of saline solution and feces were collected daily from healthy donors for 5 days. Patients were prescribed a high fiber diet intended to stimulate the proliferation of donor bacteria. Over the next 4–6 weeks, each study participant withdrew completely from use of any medications including those intended for maintaining remission. During follow-up, all subjects remained in remission for 1–13 years without evidence of UC according to colonoscopies and biopsies. Although fecal bacteriotherapy is not defined as a true probiotic, the results are sufficiently dramatic to merit inclusion.

Tursi et al.[32] randomly assigned 90 patients, experiencing mild to moderate flares, to receive either balsalazide (4.5 g/day, 6 capsules), mesalamine (2.4 g/day, 3 capsules), or balsalazide (2.4 g/day, 3 capsules) and VSL#3 (CFU > 10^{11}/day), a probiotic mixture containing *Lactobacillus* (*L. casei, L. plantarum, L. acidophilus,* and *L. delbrueckii* subsp. *Bulgaricus*), *Bifidobacterium* (*B. longum, B. breve,* and *B. infantis*), and *Streptococcus salivarius* subsp. *thermophilus*. Originally, the study hypothesized that patient compliance would be superior if they had to take fewer capsules, yet there were no significant differences among the treatment arms. The authors also found a significant difference with respect to the efficacy of the balsalazide and VSL#3 to achieve remission versus either balsalazide alone or mesalamine (24/30 patients vs. 21/30 or 16/30, respectively; $P < 0.02$). Overall, the results for the balsalazide and VSL#3 treatment group indicate that this combination is a suitable choice for patients with mild to moderate disease who are intolerant to high doses of balsalazide or mesalamine.

A randomized, controlled, double-blind trial conducted by Kato et al.[33] examined the therapeutic effect of bifidobacteria-fermented milk (BFM; containing live *B. breve* Strain Yakult, *B. bifidium* Strain Yakult, *L. acidophilus*) on mild to moderate UC flares. The 20 patients were randomized to receive placebo or BFM (CFU > 10^{12}/day) for 12 weeks. The clinical activity index (CAI) was significantly lower in the experimental group than the control (3.7 ± 0.4 vs. 5.8 ± 0.8, $P < 0.05$), yet there were no significant differences in remission rates at the end of 12 weeks.

In 2005, Bibilioni and colleagues[34] completed an open label clinical trial with 30 subjects experiencing mild to moderate UC in spite of receiving corticosteroid or mesalamine treatment in excess of 2 weeks. Subjects ingested VSL#3 (CFU > 10^{12}) on a daily basis for 6 weeks after which 53% were in remission according to a score of 2 or less using the CAI for UC. Subjects on previous medications were allowed to continue taking them throughout the trial period so that any clinical effects could be attributed to the probiotic therapy. This trial supports the findings of Tursi et al.[32] and the efficacy of the VSL#3 probiotic mixture in treating active UC.

Adding to the results obtained by Rembacken et al.[29], Matthes et al.[35] conducted an RCT using *E. coli* Nissle that explored the effect of dosing on controlling mild to moderate UC flares. Ninety patients were randomized to a placebo group or one of three probiotic groups (CFU > 10^8/ml) that received enemas containing 40, 20, or 10 ml. After the 4-week trial, the remission rate for the placebo group was 18.2% (2/11 patients). In the 40, 20, and 10 ml probiotic groups, the remission rates decreased according to dosing and were 53% (9/17), 44% (8/18), and 27% (3/11), respectively ($P < 0.04$). All probiotic concentrations were well tolerated by the participants.

In summary, the evidence of the efficacy of probiotic therapy for treating mild to moderately active UC is limited to a handful of studies that are generally inconsistent with respect to the probiotic species or mixtures thereof, dosing, study length, criteria for achieving remission, and use of concurrent medicines. Overall, the trend suggests that probiotic therapy may be a viable alternative for patients intolerant or refractory to 5-ASA formulations or corticosteroid therapy. A noticeable absence is a clinical trial that has assessed the efficacy of probiotic therapy at the onset of active disease when the gut's microbiota is possibly in the most disturbed state and elicits the greatest immune response in the host.

MAINTENANCE OF REMISSION OF UC (TABLE 13.3))

In 1997, Kruis and colleagues[36] conducted a double-blind, double-dummy trial comparing the efficacy of *E. coli* Nissle 1917 to mesalamine to maintain remission for a study period of 3 months. The 120 subjects were randomized to either the probiotic study arm (CFU > 10^{10}/day) or the comparator (1.5 g/day). At the conclusion of the study, no significant difference was found between the relapse rates of the two study groups (*E. coli* Nissle, 16%; mesalamine, 11%). Although the authors concluded that the probiotic was equally as effective as the conventional therapy, the study was underpowered to demonstrate equivalence.

A second study by Kruis et al.[37] was conducted in 2004 that was similar in design and purpose as their earlier one published in 1997[36]. This larger study randomized 327 UC patients, who were in remission, to receive either *E. coli* Nissle 1917 (2.5–25 × 10^9 CFU/day) or mesalamine (1.5 g/day). During the 12-month trial, the probiotic and comparator relapse rates were similar (36% and 34%, respectively). This study was powered to assess equivalency and the authors concluded that the probiotic was as effective as mesalamine for the maintenance of remission in UC patients.

The 1999 study by Rembacken et al.[29] yielded a total of 83 patients who had achieved remission after 12 weeks. These patients were then administered a reduced dosage of *E. coli* Nissle 1917 (CFU > 10^{10}/day) and mesalamine (1.2 g/day) for maintenance purposes. During the intervening 12-month period, there was no significant difference for relapse rates between the probiotic and comparator study groups (67% vs. 73%, respectively).

To summarize, these three early studies reached the same conclusion regarding the similarity in the efficacy of *E. coli* Nissle 1917 to that of mesalamine in maintaining remission in UC patients. However, only one of the three trials was sufficiently powered to assess equivalency. A noteworthy remark is that these three studies used mesalamine dosages of either 1.2 or 1.5 g/day, which is very low[5] and may approach a placebo-effect. If this is the case, the probiotic efficacy of *E. coli* Nissle to maintain remission is questionable.

Of the five remaining studies examining the use of probiotics to maintain remission, Venturi et al.[38] were the only group to use the probiotic mixture VSL#3 even though it has been demonstrated to be effective in active disease[32,34]. UC patients that had been in remission for a minimum of 3 months were eligible for entry. Each of the 20 subjects received the probiotic mixture, VSL#3, at CFU > 10^{12}/day. After 12 months, only 4/20 patients (25%) suffered relapses.

In 2003, an RCT[39] was conducted with 21 UC patients in remission who were randomized to receive either a placebo or bifidobacteria-fermented milk (BFM; CFU > 10^{10}/day), the same product studied by Kato et al.[33]. After 12 months, 90% (9/10 sub-

Table 13.3
Overview of studies that used probiotics for the maintenance of remission in UC patients

First Author (Publication Date)	Trial Design	n; Age Range (years)	Duration (months)	Probiotic	Control	Relapse Rate (%) Probiotic	Control	P
Shanahan (2006)	R, DB	157; NR	12	*L. salivarius* (CFU = 10^9) / *B. infantis* (CFU = 10^9)	Placebo	NR / NR	NR	NSD NSD
Zocco (2006)	R, OL	180; 33 years ± 7 (Mean age ± SD)	12	LGG (CFU > 10^{10}) / LGG (CFU > 10^{10}) and mesalamine (2.4 g)	Mesalamine (2.4 g)	15, LGG / 17, LGG & M	20	0.77 NR
Cui (2004)	R, DB	30; NR	8	BIFICO (1.26 g) (CFU > 10^7)	Placebo	20	93	<0.01
Kruis (2004)	R, DB, DD	327; 19–82	12	*E. coli* N (2.5–25x10^9 CFU/day)	Mesalamine (500 mg)	36	34	0.003 SE
Ishikawa (2003)	R	21; 39–60	12	BFM (CFU > 10^{10})	Placebo	27	90	0.02
Rembacken (1999)	R, DB, DD	83; 30–60	12	*E. coli* N (CFU > 10^{10})	Mesalamine (1.2 g)	67	73	NSD
Venturi (1999)	OL	20; 30 – 65	12	VSL#3 (CFU > 10^{12})	n/a	25	n/a	n/a
Kruis (1997)	R, DB, DD	120; 19–88	3	*E. coli* N (CFU > 10^{10})	Mesalamine (1.5 g)	16	11	NSD

B, balsalazide; BFM, commercial product containing Yakult live strains of *Bifidobacterium breve*, *B. bifidum*, and *Lactobacillus acidophilus* YIT 0168; *B. infantis*, *Bifidobacterium infantis* 356234; BIFICO, commercial probiotic capsule containing *Enterococci*, *Bifidobacteria*, and *Lactobacteria*; *L. salivarius*, *Lactobacillus salivarius subsp. Salivarius* UCC118; strain; CFU, colony forming units; DB, double-blind; *E. coli* N, *E. coli* Nissle 1917; M, mesalamine; LGG, *Lactobacillus rhamnosus* GG; OL, open label; n/a, not available; NR, not reported; NSD, no significant difference; R, randomized; SD, standard deviation; SE, significant equivalence; and, VSL#3, commercial mixture containing *Bifidobacterium longum*, *B. infantis*, *B. breve*. *Lactobacillus acidophilus*, *L. casei*, *L. delbrueckii subsp bulgaricus*, *L. plantarum*, and *Streptococcus salivarius subsp thermophilus*.

jects) of those in the placebo group had relapsed compared to only 27% (3/11) in the BFM treatment group ($P < 0.02$).

In 2004, Cui and colleagues[40] conducted a randomized, double-blind trial comparing a placebo with the commercial probiotic mixture, BIFICO (containing *Enterococci, Bifidobacteria,* and *Lactobacilli* triple therapy; CFU > 10^7/day). Thirty subjects were randomized to one of the two treatment arms and followed for 8 months. The placebo group relapse rate was 93% compared to only 20% in the BIFICO group ($P < 0.01$).

The probiotic *L. rhamnosus* GG (LGG) was investigated by Zocco et al.[41] in a large-scale randomized, open label trial. The 180 subjects who were in remission, were allocated to one of three study groups: mesalamine (2.4 g/day), LGG (CFU > 10^{10}/day), or LGG (CFU > 10^{10}/day) and mesalamine (2.4 g/day). The relapse rates were less than 20% for each study arm at the conclusion of the 12-month trial and were not significantly different from one another ($P = 0.77$). However, subjects receiving the probiotic mixture alone or with mesalamine experienced a longer remission period prior to a relapse ($P = 0.01$ and $P = 0.03$, respectively). Surprisingly, the combination of the probiotic and mesalamine did not result in a synergistic therapeutic effect for the trial subjects.

In 2006, Shanahan et al.[42] randomly assigned 157 UC patients with quiescent disease to one of three study arms: placebo, *L. salivarius* subsp. *Salivarius* UCC118 (CFU = 10^9/day), or *B. infantis* 35624 (CFU = 10^9/day). After 12 months, approximately half of all subjects in each study group remained in remission and no significant difference was noted. Interestingly, these bacterial species had proven effective in previous studies with animal models[43,44].

Overall, these studies present evidence that the use of probiotics can be useful in extending the remission periods for UC patients. Comments made earlier regarding studies using probiotics to treat active disease are also applicable to these trials. The effectiveness of prolonged probiotic therapy in excess of several years is unknown but is essential if probiotic therapy is to be considered as a viable alternative or adjuvant to conventional medicines[5].

Clinical trials that focus on the use of probiotics for treating UC continue to be initiated. A phase II trial, entitled, "*Lactobacillus acidophilus* and *Bifidobacterium animalis* Subsp. Lactis, Maintenance Treatment in Ulcerative Colitis" was initiated in 2004 (NCT00268164). A second trial, "Treatment of Ulcerative Colitis with a Combination of Lactobacillus Rhamnosus and Lactobacillus Acidophilus," was completed in January 2007 (NCT00374725).

TREATMENT OF EXTRAINTESTINAL MANIFESTATIONS OF UC

Patients with IBD have an increased risk of 10 to 100 times that of the population for developing nephrolithiasis[3]. Unfortunately, there are no satisfactory treatment regimens for enteric hyperoxaluria; dietary changes is the most prevalent yet is not completely effective. The commercial probiotic mixture, Oxadrop (containing *L. acidophilus, L. brevis, S. thermophilus,* and *B. infantis* in a 1:1:4:4 ratio), was administered in increasing doses to 10 patients presenting with nephrolithiasis and enteric hyperoxlauria over a 3-month period. Calcium oxalate supersaturation was reduced during treatment with the probiotic; however, the difference was not significant. For UC patients who may be taking probiotic therapy to control active disease or maintain remission, there is an added benefit of decreasing their risk of developing stones. Even if the decrease is not significant, this preliminary study suggests that some patients may find this comforting to know.

COLORECTAL CANCER AND PROBIOTIC THERAPY

UC patients have an increased risk of developing colorectal cancer (CRC) and should undergo routine screening. Several studies have explored the use of probiotic therapy to reduce the intermediate biomarkers of CRC risk.[45] Animal studies, in which CRC is chemically induced, conclude that probiotics reduce the incidence of tumors and aberrant crypt formation[44,46–48]. Evidence of a protective effect exerted by probiotics on their intestinal environment and a possible mechanism of action have been demonstrated using in vitro studies[49,50] Although initial results are promising, the evidence is primarily anecdotal and is insufficient to support the use of probiotic therapy by either adult or pediatric UC patients to minimize the risks of developing CRC or treating early stages of the disease[45,51].

PROBIOTIC THERAPY FOR PEDIATRIC UC PATIENTS

Many probiotics have a long association with the food industry and, as such, it is not surprising that probiotic therapy is well tolerated by UC patients[16]. Although the clinical trials conducted to date have not involved any pediatric UC patients, it is still reasonable to extend their use to this subgroup. Probiotics have been demonstrated to be safely administered orally and via enemas; however, studies have been restricted to well-characterized strains[25].

As many probiotic formulations are commercially available in health food stores or via the internet, it is increasingly difficult to assume that a patient is strictly adhering to the prescribed conventional therapies. A German survey conducted with IBD patients participating in workshops concluded that 43% were self-administering probiotics[52]. The authors concluded that clinicians should better inform their patients about the benefits and limitations of probiotics in the absence of noncommerical, untrustworthy information sources. In spite of their youth, pediatric UC patients could be unknowingly consuming probiotics under the supervision of the well-meaning family who may not willingly divulge this information to the clinician. One drawback associated with probiotics is the variation in cost and that such expenses are not covered by insurance policies.

SUMMARY AND CONCLUSION

Evidence-based research suggests that probiotic therapy, either alone or as an adjuvant, may be an effective alternative for some UC patients[51]. However, the research does not definitively state that probiotic therapy is beneficial for either active disease or maintaining remission. Clinical trials suffer from small sample sizes, a noticeable lack of controls, and inconsistent results. The greatest positive that probiotics provide is that they are well tolerated by UC patients and have not been found to exacerbate symptoms nor interfere with conventional, evidence-based drug treatments. These early studies indicate that probiotic therapy may only confer small improvements in an individual's condition. Hence, it is essential to understand that, for some, subtle yet noticeable progress may translate into considerable benefits to their quality of life regardless of age. Insufficient evidence exists to support the use of probiotic therapy in either the treatment of hyperoxaluria in UC patients or in the prevention or treatment of CRC.

As the field of probiotic research matures, trial designs have also improved, although further improvements are required if the evidence-based research community will accept probiotic therapy for the treatment of UC patients. Future studies will examine the appropriate dosing, the effect of different formulations on probiotic efficacy, and a formalized safety testing strategy to assess novel bacterial strains for probiotic therapy.

REFERENCES

1. Su C, Lichtenstein GR. Ulcerative colitis. In: Feldman M, Friedman LS, Brandt LJ, Sleisenger MH., eds. Sleisenger and Fordtran's gastrointestinal and liver disease: pathophysiology, diagnosis, management. 8th ed. Philadelphia, PA: Saunders Elsevier, 2006:2499–2548.
2. Baumgart DC, Sandborn WJ. Inflammatory bowel disease: clinical aspects and established and evolving therapies. *Lancet* 2007; 369(9573):1641–1657.
3. Lieske JC, Goldfarb DS, De SC, Regnier C. Use of a probiotic to decrease enteric hyperoxaluria. *Kidney Int* 2005; 68(3):1244–1249.
4. Bernstein CN, Blanchard JF, Kliewer E, Wajda A. Cancer risk in patients with inflammatory bowel disease: a population-based study. *Cancer* 2001; 91(4):854–862.
5. Kornbluth A, Sachar DB. Ulcerative colitis practice guidelines in adults (update): American College of Gastroenterology, Practice Parameters Committee. *Am J Gastroenterol* 2004; 99(7):1371–1385.
6. Bernstein CN, Wajda A, Svenson LW, et-al. The epidemiology of inflammatory bowel disease in Canada: a population-based study. *Am J Gastroenterol* 2006; 101(7):1559–1568.
7. Berner J, Kiaer T. Ulcerative colitis and Crohn's disease on the Faroe Islands 1964–83. A retrospective epidemiological survey. *Scand J Gastroenterol* 1986; 21(2):188–192.
8. Shivananda S, Pena AS, Mayberry JF, Ruitenberg EJ, Hoedemaeker PJ. Epidemiology of proctocolitis in the region of Leiden, the Netherlands. A population study from 1979 to 1983. *Scand J Gastroenterol* 1987; 22(8):993–1002.
9. Bernstein CN, Blanchard JF, Rawsthorne P, Wajda A. Epidemiology of Crohn's disease and ulcerative colitis in a central Canadian province: a population-based study. *Am J Epidemiol* 1999; 149(10):916–924.
10. Stonnington CM, Phillips SF, Melton LJ, III, Zinsmeister AR. Chronic ulcerative colitis: incidence and prevalence in a community. *Gut* 1987; 28(4):402–409.
11. Griffiths AM. Specificities of inflammatory bowel disease in childhood. *Best Pract Res Clin Gastroenterol* 2004; 18(3):509–523.
12. Hyams J, Davis P, Lerer T, et-al.. Clinical outcome of ulcerative proctitis in children. *J Pediatr Gastroenterol Nutr* 1997; 25(2):149–152.
13. Kugathasan S, Judd RH, Hoffmann RG, et-al.. Epidemiologic and clinical characteristics of children with newly diagnosed inflammatory bowel disease in Wisconsin: a statewide population-based study. *J Pediatr 2003*; 143(4):525–531.
14. Sawczenko A, Sandhu BK.Presenting features of inflammatory bowel disease in Great Britain and Ireland. *Arch Dis Child* 2003; 88(11):995–1000.
15. Heyman MB, Kirschner BS, Gold BD, et-al.. Children with early-onset inflammatory bowel disease (IBD): analysis of a pediatric IBD consortium registry. *J Pediatr* 2005; 146(1):35–40.
16. Fedorak RN, Madsen KL.Probiotics and the management of inflammatory bowel disease. *Inflamm Bowel Dis* 2004; 10(3):286–299.
17. Hedin C, Whelan K, Lindsay JO. Evidence for the use of probiotics and prebiotics in inflammatory bowel disease: a review of clinical trials. *Proc Nutr Soc* 2007; 66(3):307–315.
18. Hanauer SB. Medical therapy for ulcerative colitis 2004. *Gastroenterology* 2004; 126(6):1582–1592.

19. Larson DW, Pemberton JH. Current concepts and controversies in surgery for IBD. *Gastroenterology* 2004; 126(6):1611–1619.

20. Itzkowitz SH, Present DH. Consensus conference: colorectal cancer screening and surveillance in inflammatory bowel disease. *Inflamm Bowel Dis* 2005; 11(3):314–321.

21. Lichtenstein GR, Cohen R, Yamashita B, Diamond RH. Quality of life after proctocolectomy with ileoanal anastomosis for patients with ulcerative colitis. *J Clin Gastroenterol* 2006; 40(8):669–677.

22. Hata K, Watanabe T, Shinozaki M, Nagawa H. Patients with extraintestinal manifestations have a higher risk of developing pouchitis in ulcerative colitis: multivariate analysis. *Scand J Gastroenterol* 2003; 38(10):1055–1058.

23. Carvalho RS, Abadom V, Dilworth HP, Thompson R, Oliva-Hemker M, Cuffari C. Indeterminate colitis: a significant subgroup of pediatric IBD. *Inflamm Bowel Dis* 2006; 12(4):258–262.

24. Ewaschuk JB, Dieleman LA. Probiotics and prebiotics in chronic inflammatory bowel diseases. *World J Gastroenterol* 2006; 12(37):5941–5950.

25. Quigley EM, Whorwell PJ, Shanahan F, et-al.. Safety and tolerability of the probiotic organism *Bifidobacterium infantis* 35624: clinical experience and molecular basis. *Gastroenterology* 2006; 4(Suppl. 2):130.

26. Bibiloni R, Mangold M, Madsen KL, Fedorak RN, Tannock GW. The bacteriology of biopsies differs between newly diagnosed, untreated, Crohn's disease and ulcerative colitis patients. *J Med Microbiol* 2006; 55(Pt 8):1141–1149.

27. Conte MP, Schippa S, Zamboni I, et-al.. Gut-associated bacterial microbiota in paediatric patients with inflammatory bowel disease. *Gut* 2006; 55(12):1760–1767.

28. Jurjus AR, Khoury NN, Reimund JM. Animal models of inflammatory bowel disease. *J Pharmacol Toxicol Methods* 2004; 50(2):81–92.

29. Rembacken BJ, Snelling AM, Hawkey PM, Chalmers DM, Axon AT. Non-pathogenic *Escherichia coli* versus mesalazine for the treatment of ulcerative colitis: a randomised trial. *Lancet* 1999; 354(9179):635–639.

30. Guslandi M, Giollo P, Testoni PA. A pilot trial of *Saccharomyces boulardii* in ulcerative colitis. *Eur J Gastroenterol Hepatol* 2003; 15(6):697–698.

31. Borody TJ, Warren EF, Leis S, Surace R, Ashman O. Treatment of ulcerative colitis using fecal bacteriotherapy. *J Clin Gastroenterol* 2003; 37(1):42–47.

32. Tursi A, Brandimarte G, Giorgetti GM, Forti G, Modeo ME, Gigliobianco A. Low-dose balsalazide plus a high-potency probiotic preparation is more effective than balsalazide alone or mesalazine in the treatment of acute mild-to-moderate ulcerative colitis. *Med Sci Monit* 2004; 10(11):I126–I131.

33. Kato K, Mizuno S, Umesaki Y, et-al.. Randomized placebo-controlled trial assessing the effect of bifidobacteria-fermented milk on active ulcerative colitis. *Aliment Pharmacol Ther* 2004; 20(10):1133–1141.

34. Bibiloni R, Fedorak RN, Tannock GW, et-al.. VSL#3 probiotic-mixture induces remission in patients with active ulcerative colitis. *Am J Gastroenterol* 2005; 100(7):1539–1546.

35. Matthes H, Krummenerl T, Giensch M, Wolff C, Schulze J. Treatment of mild to moderate acute attacks of distal ulcerative colitis with rectally-administered *E. coli* Nissle 1917: dose-dependent efficacy. *Gastroenterology* 2006; 130(Suppl. 2):A-119.

36. Kruis W, Schutz E, Fric P, Fixa B, Judmaier G, Stolte M. Double-blind comparison of an oral *Escherichia coli* preparation and mesalazine in maintaining remission of ulcerative colitis. *Aliment Pharmacol Ther* 1997; 11(5):853–858.

37. Kruis W, Fric P, Pokrotnieks J, et-al.. Maintaining remission of ulcerative colitis with the probiotic *Escherichia coli* Nissle 1917 is as effective as with standard mesalazine. *Gut* 2004; 53(11):1617–1623.

38. Venturi A, Gionchetti P, Rizzello F, et-al.. Impact on the composition of the faecal flora by a new probiotic preparation: preliminary data on maintenance treatment of patients with ulcerative colitis. *Aliment Pharmacol Ther* 1999; 13(8):1103–1108.

39. Ishikawa H, Akedo I, Umesaki Y, Tanaka R, Imaoka A, Otani T. Randomized controlled trial of the effect of Bifidobacteria-fermented milk on ulcerative colitis. *J Am Coll Nutr* 2003; 22(1):56–63.

40. Cui HH, Chen CL, Wang JD, et-al.. Effects of probiotic on intestinal mucosa of patients with ulcerative colitis. *World J Gastroenterol* 2004; 10(10):1521–1525.

41. Zocco MA, dal Verme LZ, Cremonini F, et-al.. Efficacy of Lactobacillus GG in maintaining remission of ulcerative colitis. *Aliment Pharmacol Ther* 2006; 23(11):1567–1574.

42. Shanahan F, Guaraner F, von Wright A, et-al.. A one year, double-blind, placebo controlled trial of a Lactobacillus or a *Bidfidobacterium probiotic* for maintenance of steroid-induced remission of ulcerative colitis. *Gastroenterology* 2006; 130(Suppl. 2):A-44.

43. McCarthy J, O'Mahony L, O'Callaghan L, et-al.. Double blind, placebo controlled trial of two probiotic strains in interleukin 10 knockout mice and mechanistic link with cytokine balance. *Gut* 2003; 52(7):975–980.

44. O'Mahony L, Feeney M, O'Halloran S, et-al.. Probiotic impact on microbial flora, inflammation and tumour development in IL-10 knockout mice. *Aliment Pharmacol Ther* 2001; 15(8):1219–1225.

45. Saikali J, Picard C, Freitas M, Holt P. Fermented milks, probiotic cultures, and colon cancer. *Nutr Cancer* 2004; 49(1):14–24.

46. Ohkawara S, Furuya H, Nagashima K, Asanuma N, Hino T. Oral administration of butyrivibrio fibrisolvens, a butyrate-producing bacterium, decreases the formation of aberrant crypt foci in the colon and rectum of mice. *J Nutr* 2005; 135(12):2878–2883.

47. de Moreno de LeBlanc A, Perdigon G. Reduction of beta-glucuronidase and nitroreductase activity by yoghurt in a murine colon cancer model. *Biocell* 2005; 29(1):15–24.

48. Marotta F, Naito Y, Minelli E, et-al.. Chemopreventive effect of a probiotic preparation on the development of preneoplastic and neoplastic colonic lesions: an experimental study. *Hepatogastroenterology* 2003; 50(54):1914–1918.

49. Mego M, Majek J, Koncekova R, et-al.. Intramucosal bacteria in colon cancer and their elimination by probiotic strain *Enterococcus faecium* M-74 with organic selenium. *Folia Microbiol (Praha)* 2005; 50(5):443–447.

50. Burns AJ, Rowland IR. Antigenotoxicity of probiotics and prebiotics on faecal water-induced DNA damage in human colon adenocarcinoma cells. *Mutat Res* 2004; 551(1–2):233–243.

51. Michail S, Sylvester F, Fuchs G, Issenman R. Clinical efficacy of probiotics: review of the evidence with focus on children. *J Pediatr Gastroenterol Nutr* 2006; 43(4):550–557.

52. Joos S, Rosemann T, Szecsenyi J, Hahn EG, Willich SN, Brinkhaus B. Use of complementary and alternative medicine in Germany – a survey of patients with inflammatory bowel disease. *BMC Complement Altern Med* 2006; 6:19.

14 Pouchitis

Paolo Gionchetti

Key Points:

- Pouchitis is the most frequent long-term complication following pouch surgery for ulcerative colitis.
- The etiology is unknown but an increased gut bacterial concentration is one of the main risk factors.
- The rationale for using probiotics in pouchitis is based on evidence implicating intestinal bacteria in the pathogenesis of this condition.
- Probiotics have shown efficacy in maintenance treatment of chronic pouchitis, in the prevention of pouchitis onset, and in active mild pouchitis.

INTRODUCTION

Total proctocolectomy with ileal-pouch anal anastomosis (IPAA), proposed for the first time by Parks in 1978 [1], now represents the surgical treatment of choice for the management of patients with familial adenomatous polyposis (FAP) and ulcerative colitis (UC) [2,3]. This procedure allows the removal of the whole diseased colorectal mucosal and has the great advantage of preserving anal sphincter function. Most patients undergoing IPAA for severe colitis or for chronic continuous disease will achieve excellent functional results and physical well-being. In a prospective evaluation of health-related quality of life (HRLQ) after IPAA, a significant improvement of HRQL was shown, assessed with both generic and disease-specific measures, with many patients experiencing improvements as early as 1 month postoperatively [4]. However pouchitis, a nonspecific (idiopathic) inflammation of the ileal reservoir, is the most common long-term complication after pouch surgery for UC [5].

EPIDEMIOLOGY, RISKS FACTORS, AND ETIOLOGY

Frequency

The true incidence of pouchitis is still difficult to determine; it depends on the diagnostic criteria used to define the syndrome, on the accuracy of the evaluation and, particularly, on the duration of follow-up. Reported incidence rates vary between 10 and 59%; most patients

From: *Nutrition and Health: Probiotics in Pediatric Medicine*
Edited by: S. Michail and P.M. Sherman © Humana Press, Totowa, NJ

experience their first episode of acute pouchitis within 12 months after surgery, but some may suffer their first attack only years later [6]. Recently Simchuk et al. [7] performed a retrospective review of patients who underwent IPAA, with a mean follow-up of three years; the incidence of pouchitis was 59%, but it increased with the duration of follow-up.

Risk Factors

The risk of developing pouchitis is much higher in patients with preoperative extraintestinal manifestations [8] and primary sclerosing cholangitis [9]. The predictive role of antineutrophil cytoplasmic antibody with perinuclear pattern (p-ANCA) [10–15] and the preoperative extent of UC [16,17] are more controversial. Similar to UC, smoking may be protective against the development of pouchitis [18,19]. The surgical technique (i.e., different type of reservoir) does not influence the frequency of pouchitis [20,21].

Etiology

The etiology of pouchitis is still unknown and is likely to be multifactorial; a variety of hypotheses have been suggested, including bacterial overgrowth due to fecal stasis, mucosal ischemia of the pouch, a missed diagnosis of Crohn's disease, recurrence of UC, and a novel form of IBD. Most likely, pouchitis is the bad result of the interactions of genetic and immunologic susceptibility and an ileal mucosa that has adapted from its absorptive function to a new role as a reservoir with a colon-like morphology in response to fecal stasis [22].

DIAGNOSIS

Clinical Presentation

The most frequent symptoms, which characterize this syndrome, include increased stool frequency and fluidity, rectal bleeding, abdominal cramping, urgency, malaise and tenesmus, and, in most severe cases, incontinence and fever [22]. Patients with pouchitis may also have extraintestinal manifestations, such as arthritis, ankylosing spondylitis, pyoderma gangrenosum, erythema nodosum, and uveitis [8]. These extraintestinal manifestations may develop for the first time with pouchitis, but frequently patients would have previously experienced these extraintestinal manifestations before surgery.

Endoscopic Findings

A clinical diagnosis should be confirmed by endoscopy and histology. On endoscopy, the mucosa of the neoterminal ileum above the pouch should be normal. Inflammation of the pouch mucosa, with mucosal erythema, edema, friability, petechiae, granularity, loss of vascular pattern, mucosal hemorrhages, contact bleeding, mucus exudates, erosions, and small superficial mucosal ulcerations, can be present with varying degree of severity [23–24]. Inflammation may be uniform or more severe to the distal part of the pouch.

Histologic Findings

Histologic examination shows acute inflammatory cell infiltrate with crypt abscesses and ulcerations on a background of chronic inflammatory changes with villous atrophy and crypt hyperplasia [25–26].

DISEASE ACTIVITY SCORE AND CLASSIFICATION

There is great variability in the reported incidence of pouchitis and in the assessment responses to therapy. This may be due to the lack of standardized diagnostic criteria. As a result, Sandborn and colleagues [27] developed a Pouchitis Disease Activity Index (PDAI); this 18-point index is calculated from 3 separate 6-point scales on the basis of clinical symptoms, endoscopic appearance, and histologic findings. The PDAI represents an objective and reproducible scoring system for pouchitis. Active pouchitis is defined by a total of PDAI score >7 and remission as a score <7. Once diagnosis is made, pouchitis can be further classified. Disease activity can be defined as remission, mild–moderate (increased stool frequency, urgency, infrequent incontinence), or severe (dehydration, frequent incontinence). Pouchitis can also be defined on the basis of the duration of diseaseas, either acute (<4 weeks) or chronic (>4 weeks). Another method of classifying this syndrome is to consider the following patterns: infrequent (a single or two acute episodes), relapsing (more than three acute episodes) in about 2/3 of cases, continuous or chronic disease (a treatment responsive form requiring a maintenance therapy), and a treatment-resistant form. About 15% of patients with pouchitis have a chronic disease and some of them even require surgical excision or exclusion of the pouch, because of an impairment of reservoir function and a poor quality of life [28].

The PDAI, nowadays, is the most frequently used scoring system in clinical studies to determine disease activity. The validity of the PDAI and the necessity of its application in epidemiological, pathophysiological, or clinical studies, as well as in clinical practice, in order to make a correct diagnosis of pouchitis, have been shown by Shen et al. [29] in a study evaluating the correlation between symptoms, endoscopy, and histologic findings in patients with IPAA for UC. The authors found that symptoms alone do not reliably diagnose pouchitis, while an evaluation including symptoms, endoscopy, and histology is the best way to make the diagnosis of pouchitis.

Differential Diagnosis

Before treatment is started, it is important to exclude other less frequent causes of pouch dysfunction or pouch inflammation. This is particularly necessary in the case of a refractory patient.

An anastomotic stricture, with consequent outlet obstruction and fecal stasis, is a common complication of IPAA; this increases stool frequency and makes defecation painful with an incomplete evacuation that predisposes to pouchitis. Diagnosis can be made by evacuation pouchography, while the stricture can usually be dilated with a finger or a rubber dilator.

Infectious etiologies caused by intestinal bacterial pathogens, such as *Shigellae*, *Escherichia coli*, *Salmonellae*, and *Clostridium difficile*, should be ruled out by microbiologic analysis and pouch biopsy. Multiple cases of cytomegalovirus infection have been reported [30–31], showing the need for using monoclonal immunofluorescent staining for CMV to examine pouch biopsies when the treatment with antibiotics has been proven unsuccessful. In such patients, CMV infection must be excluded before starting immune modifier therapies.

Cuffitis is the inflammation of the retained rectal mucosa (columnar cuff) above the anal transitional zone (ATZ) after stapled anastomosis between the pouch and the top of the anal canal. This kind of inflammation is usually mild and not related to the inflammation of the pouch, but can cause anal discomfort, perianal irritation, and pouch dysfunction. Clinically significant cuffitis should be defined using a triad of diagnostic criteria including clinical symptoms, endoscopic inflammation, and acute histologic inflammation [32]. This syndrome rarely reaches dramatic proportions and a clinical improvement can be obtained with topical corticosteroids, mesalazine suppositories, and the topical application of lidocaine gel. Scintigraphic pelvic pouch emptying scans can be used to evaluate patients who have inadequate pouch evacuation.

Fistulae and perianal abscesses should be suspected as an expression of undiagnosed Crohn's disease. Review of the proctocolectomy specimen and new biopsy samples are needed to make a correct diagnosis. If Crohn's disease is suspected, a small bowel with follow-through x-ray should be undertaken to rule out disease proximal to the pouch. Approximately 5–10% of IPAA surgery is performed in patients whose primary diagnosis of UC is revised at some time point after surgery to a definitive diagnosis of Crohn's disease [33]. Other disorders that can mimic pouchitis symptoms are bile acid malabsorption, irritable pouch syndrome [34], and chronic pelvic sepsis.

Medical Treatment

Until now, only a few small placebo-controlled trials and controlled comparisons of two active agents have been carried out. As a consequence, the medical treatment of pouchitis is still highly empiric. The reason for the limited number of randomized, double-blind, controlled clinical trials well relate to the lack of a general agreement about the criteria for definition, diagnosis, classification, and disease activity [35].

Antibiotics

Awareness of the crucial importance that fecal stasis and bacterial overgrowth may have in the pathogenesis of acute pouchitis has led clinicians to treat patients with antibiotics, which have become, in absence of controlled trials, the mainstay of treatment. Metronidazole generally represents the most common first therapeutic approach. Most patients with acute pouchitis respond quickly to administration of 1–1.5 gm/day [36–37]. A double-blind, randomized, placebo-controlled, crossover trial was carried out by Madden et al. [38] to assess the efficacy of 400 mg, three times a day, of metronidazole per os in 13 patients (11 completed both arms of the study) with chronic, unremitting pouchitis, defined by the presence of recurrent or persistent symptoms with almost 6 bowel movements a day and typical endoscopic findings. Patients were treated for 2 weeks, with a 7-day washout period before crossover to the second treatment. Metronidazole was significantly more effective than placebo in reducing stool frequency (73 vs 9%) ($p < 0.05$), even without improvement of endoscopic appearance and histologic grade of activity. Some patients experienced side effects of metronidazole including nausea, vomiting, abdominal discomfort, headache, skin rash, and metallic taste. Dysgeusia and peripheral neuropathy may limit long-term administration of metronidazole, while patients consuming alcohol can have a disulfiram-like reaction. Recently, Shen and colleagues [39] have compared the effectiveness and side effects of ciprofloxacin and metronidazole for treating acute pouchitis in a randomized clinical trial. Seven patients received ciprofloxacin 1 gm/day and nine patients received metronidazole 20 mg/kg/day for a period of 2 weeks. The results of this study showed that both ciprofloxacin and metronidazole are efficacious in the treatment of acute pouchitis: both reduced total PDAI scores and led to a significant improvement in clinical symptoms and both endoscopic and histologic scores. However, ciprofloxacin led to a greater degree of reduction in the total PDAI score, to a greater improvement in symptoms and endoscopic scores. Furthermore, ciprofloxacin was better tolerated than metronidazole (33% of metronidazole-treated patients reported adverse effects versus none of the ciprofloxacin-treated subjects). The authors suggested, therefore, that ciprofloxacin should be considered as first-line therapy for acute pouchitis.

Other Agents

Anecdotal reports have suggested that either oral or topical conventional corticosteroids may be of benefit to patients with pouchitis. Recently a double-blind, double-dummy, 6-week, controlled trial investigated the efficacy and tolerability of budesonide enema in the treatment of pouchitis, compared with oral metronidazole. The study showed that budesonide enemas (2 mg/100 mL at bedtime) have a similar efficacy compared to oral metronidazole (0.5 gm twice daily) in terms of disease activity, clinical, and endoscopic findings (58 and 50% of patients, respectively, improved with a decrease in PDAI score [33]), but less side effects (25 vs 57%) and better tolerability [40]. Thus budesonide enemas represent a valid therapeutic alternative for the management of active pouchitis.

While no data have been published on the efficacy of oral 5-ASA, uncontrolled studies suggest the efficacy of topical 5-ASA either as suppositories or enemas in the treatment of acute pouchitis [41]. As an immunesuppressing agent, cyclosporine enemas, in a pilot study, were reported as successful in chronic pouchitis [42]. Other anecdotal reports suggest that oral azathioprine also may be useful.

The observation, reported in some studies [43], but not all [44], that the fecal concentration of short-chain fatty acids (SCFAs) is lower in patients with pouchitis led to the hypothesis that topical administration of nutrients, such butyrate and glutamine, may produce clinical benefit. However, poor clinical results were obtained in uncontrolled trials using enemas containing SCFAs [45–46]. In a double-blind trial, glutamine and butyrate suppositories for 3 weeks were compared in a group of 19 patients with chronic pouchitis with recurrent symptoms. The end-point was clinical remission. As the relapse rate was 40% for the glutamine group and 67% for the butyrate group, and no placebo group was included, it is not clear if the two treatments were ineffective or similarly effective [47]. Taken together, nutritional therapy still cannot be considered beneficial for pouchitis.

Bismuth, effective in UC and traveller's diarrhoea because of antimicrobial and antidiarrheal effects, has also been investigated for treating pouchitis. One open-label, long-term study evaluated the efficacy and safety of bismuth-citrate carbomer enemas in achieving and maintaining remission in a group of patients with chronic, treatment-resistant pouchitis. After 45 days of nightly treatment, 83% of patients were in remission, with a significant decrease in total PDAI score from a mean of 12–6 ($p < 0.002$). Moreover, these patients entered a maintenance phase with enemas administered every third night for 12 months: 60% were able to maintain remission throughout the 12 months [48]. However, a double-blind, randomized trial in patients with active chronic pouchitis did not find a difference between bismuth enemas and placebo [49]. More recently, a 4-week open trial of treatment showed the benefits of oral bismuth subsalicylate tablets in chronic, antibiotic-resistant pouchitis [50].

Allopurinol, a scavenger of oxygen-derived free radicals through inhibition of xanthine oxidase, was evaluated as postoperative prophylaxis (100 mg twice daily) to prevent pouchitis in a randomized, placebo-controlled, double-blind study conducted at 12 centers in Sweden. However, it was not able to reduce the risk of a first attack of pouchitis [51].

Treatment of Chronic Pouchitis

Medical treatment of patients with chronic, refractory pouchitis is particularly difficult and disappointing. The usual therapeutic strategy for these patients, who either fail to respond to antibiotics or relapse once antibiotic therapy is stopped, includes: (1) a prolonged course of an antimicrobial agent, (2) a maintenance therapy with the most effective antibiotic given at the lowest clinically effective dose, and (3) cycles of multiple antibiotics given at 1-week intervals. A possible therapeutic alternative for chronic, refractory pouchitis is the use of combined antibiotics. We carried out a pilot trial to evaluate the efficacy of two antibiotics in chronic active, treatment-resistant pouchitis [52]. Eighteen patients not responding to standard therapies (metronidazole or ciprofloxacin or amoxycillin/clavulanic acid for 4 weeks) were treated orally with rifaximin 2 g/day (a nonabsorbable, broad spectrum antibiotic) and ciprofloxacin 1g/day for 15 days. Assessment of symptoms, endoscopic, and histologic evaluations were performed at baseline and after 15 days, using the PDAI. Sixteen (88.8%) out of 18 patients either improved ($n = 10$) or went into remission ($n = 6$). Median PDAI scores before and after therapy were 11 and 4, respectively ($p < 0.002$). Unfortunately, all patients relapsed within 2 months of stopping therapy.

More recently, 44 patients with refractory pouchitis received metronidazole 800 mg-1g/day and ciprofloxacin 1 g/day for 28 days. Symptomatic, endoscopic, and histological evaluations were undertaken before and after antibiotic therapy, with outcomes processed according to the PDAI score and quality of life assessed using the inflammatory bowel disease questionnaire (IBDQ). Thirty-six patients (82%) went into remission; the median PDAI scores before and after therapy were 12 and 3, respectively ($p < 0.0001$). Quality of life significantly improved for patients with the treatment. Even in the eight patients who did not go into remission the median PDAI score significantly improved from 14.5 to 9.5 and quality of life improved [53].

An alternative treatment is the controlled ileal release (CIR) formulation of oral budesonide. In an open-label study, 16 patients who did not respond after 1 month of ciprofloxacin or metronidazole were treated with budesonide CIR at 9 mg/day for 8 weeks with subsequent gradual tapering. Twelve (72%) of 16 patients went into remission [54].

Recently, infliximab (chimeric monoclonal antibody against tumor necrosis factor a) was used in 12 patients with chronic active pouchitis who did not respond after 1 month of antibiotic treatment (metronidazole or ciprofloxacin 1gm/day) and 2 months of oral budesonide CIR at 9 mg/day. Patients were treated with infliximab intravenous infusions of 5 mg/kg at 0,2 and 6 weeks; 10 (83.3%) of 12 went into remission. Median PDAI scores before and after biological therapy were 13 (range 8–18) and 2 (range 0–9), respectively ($p < 0.001$). Quality of life scores also improved significantly ($p < 0.001$) [55].

Probiotics

The term "probiotic" is defined as "living.organisms, which, on ingestion in certain numbers, exerts health benefits beyond inherent basic nutrition." Recent observations suggest a potential role for probiotics in the management of chronic Inflammatory Bowel Diseases (IBD) on the basis of evidence implicating intestinal bacteria in the pathogenesis of the disease [56]. Pouchitis has been associated with a decreased ratio of anaerobic to aerobic bacteria, reduced fecal concentrations of lactobacilli and bifidobacteria, and increased luminal pH [57].

We designed a double-blind study to compare the efficacy of VSL#3 (VSL Pharmaceuticals, Inc, Ft. Lauderdale, USA) versus placebo in the maintenance treatment of chronic pouchitis [58]. Patients ($n = 40$) who were both in clinical and endoscopic remission after 1 month of combined antibiotic treatment (2 g/day of rifaximin and 1 g/day of ciprofloxacin) were randomized to receive either VSL#3 (6 g/day, equivalent to 1800 billion bacteria) or placebo for 9 months. Patients were assessed clinically every month, assessed endoscopically and histologically at entry, and every 2 months thereafter. Stool cultures were performed before and after antibiotic treatment, and monthly during maintenance treatment. Relapse was defined as an increase of at least 2 points in the clinical section of the PDAI and was confirmed endoscopically and histologically. All 20 patients treated with placebo relapsed during the follow-up period. In contrast, 17 (85%) of the 20 patients treated with VSL#3 were still in remission after 9 months ($p < 0.001$). Interestingly, all 17 of these patients relapsed within 4 months of suspension of the active treatment. Fecal concentrations of lactobacilli, bifidobacteria, and *Streptococcus thermophilus* were significantly increased within 1 month of VSL#3 treatment and remained stable throughout the study. This increase did not affect the concentration of the other bacterial groups, suggesting that the effect was not mediated by the suppression of endogenous luminal bacteria.

A subsequent double-blind, placebo-controlled study on the effectiveness of VSL#3 (at a daily dose of 1800 billion bacteria) in the maintenance of antibiotic-induced remission in patients with refractory or recurrent pouchitis reported similar results [59]. After 1 year of treatment, 85% of those in the VSL#3 group were in remission versus only 6% in the placebo group ($p < 0.0001$). As regards the mechanism of action of VSL#3 in these patients, continuous administration of VSL#3 decreases matrix metalloproteinase activity, significantly increases tissue levels of the antiinflammatory interleukin (IL) 10, and significantly decreases tissue levels of the proinflammatory cytokines IL-1, tumor necrosis factor-a, and interferon-g [60].

A double-blind, placebo-controlled trial evaluated the efficacy of VSL#3 in the prevention of pouchitis onset in patients following IPAA for UC [57]. Within 1 week after ileostomy closure, 40 patients were randomized to receive either VSL#3 (3 gm/day, equivalent to 900 billion bacteria) or placebo for 12 months. Patients were assessed clinically, endoscopically, and histologically at 1, 3, 6, 9, and 12 months according to the PDAI score. During the first year after ileostomy closure, patients treated with VSL#3 had a significantly lower incidence of acute pouchitis, compared with those treated with placebo (10 vs 40%; $p < 0.05$). Moreover, quality of life was significantly improved only in the group treated with VSL#3 and among those who did not develop pouchitis. The median stool frequency was significantly lower in the VSL#3 group.

Recently, an open-label study evaluated the efficacy of high-dose VSL#3 in the treatment of mildly active pouchitis [61]. Twenty-three consecutive patients with mild pouchitis, defined as a score of between 7 and 12 in the PDAI, were treated with 2 sachets of VSL#3, twice daily (3600 billion bacteria/day) for 4 weeks. Symptomatic, endoscopic, and histologic evaluations were undertaken before and after treatment, according to the PDAI. Remission was defined as the combination of a PDAI clinical score of £2, endoscopic score of £1, and total PDAI score of £4. Patients in remission after treatment were treated with 1 sachet of VSL#3, orally twice daily (1800 billions bacteria), as maintenance treatment for 6 months. Sixteen (69%) of 23 patients were in remission after treatment. The median total PDAI scores before and after therapy were 10 (range 9–12) and 4 (range 2–11), respectively ($p < 0.01$). Quality of life scores also significantly improved on VSL#3 ($p < 0.001$). All 16 patients who went into remission maintained their remission during maintenance therapy. Only 1 patient experienced a transient bloating at the beginning of the treatment.

In contrast to the positive results reported using VSL#3, in a 3-month double-blind, placebo-controlled trial with *Lactobacillus rhamnosus GG* two gelatin capsule/day [(0.5–1) x 10^{10} cfu/capsule], was not superior to placebo in reducing disease activity in patients with active pouchitis [62]. These findings indicate that the efficacy of probiotics in pouchitis can be related to the presence of a high concentration of bacteria and possibly of a mixture of strains.

SUMMARY AND CONCLUSION

Pouchitis is a serious long-term complication after IPAA for UC. Many clinical and experimental observations indicate that the intestinal microflora is involved in the pathogenesis of pouchitis and broad spectrum antibiotics are the current mainstay of treatment for this condition.

Probiotics may provide a simple and attractive way of either preventing or treating pouchitis. Patients find the probiotic concept appealing because it is safe, nontoxic, and natural. VSL#3, a highly concentrated mixture of probiotics, has been shown as effective in the prevention of pouchitis onset and relapses and may be helpful in patients with mildly active pouchitis.

It is important to select a well-characterized probiotic preparation, particularly in view of the fact that the viability and survival of bacteria in many of the currently available preparations are unproven (McDermid et al., CJG 2003).

It should noted that the beneficial effect of one probiotic preparation does not imply efficacy of other preparations containing different bacterial strains, because each individual probiotic strain may well have unique biological properties.

REFERENCES

1. Parks AG, Nicholls RJ. Proctocolectomy without ileostomy for ulcerative colitis. *BMJ* 1978; 2: 85–88.
2. Pemberton JH, Kelly KA, Beart RW JR, Dozois RR, Wolff BG, Ilstrup DM. Ileal pouch-anal anastomosis for chronic ulcerative colitis. Long-term results. *Ann Surg* 1987; 206: 504–513.
3. Nicholls RJ, Moskowitz RL, Shepherd NA. Restorative proctocolectomy with ileal reservoir. *Br J Surg* 1985; 72: S76–9.
4. Muir AJ, Edwards LJ, Sanders LL Bollinger RR, Koruda MJ, Bachwich DR, et-al.. A prospective evaluation of health related quality of life after ileal pouch anal anastomosis for ulcerative colitis. *Am J Gastroenterol* 2001; 96: 1480–1485.
5. Shepherd NA, Hulten L, Tytgat GNJ, Nicholls RJ, Nasmith DG, Hill MJ, et-al.. Workshop: Pouchitis. *Int J Colorectal Dis* 1989; 4: 205–229.
6. Stahlberg D, Gullberg K, Liljeqvist L, Hellers G, Löfberg R. Pouchitis following pelvic pouch operation for ulcerative colitis. Incidence, cumulative risk and risk factors. *Dis Colon Rectum* 1996; 39: 1012–1018.
7. Simchuk EJ, Thirlby RC. Risk factors and true incidence of pouchitis in patients after ileal pouch-anal anastomosis. *World J Surg* 2000; 24: 851–856.
8. Lohmuller JL, Pemberton JH, Dozois RR, Ilstrup D, van Heerder J. Pouchitis and extraintestinal manifestations of inflammatory bowel disease after ileal pouch-anal anastomosis. *Ann Surg* 1990; 211: 622
9. Zins BJ, Sandborn WJ, Penna CR, Landers CJ, Targan SR, Tremaine WJ, et-al.. Pouchitis disease course after orthotopic liver transplantation in patients with primary sclerosing cholangitis and an ilael pouch-anal anastomosis. *Am J Gastroenterol* 1995; 90: 2177.
10. Duerr RH, Targan SR, Landers CJ, Sutherland LR, Shanahan F. Anti-neutrophil cytoplasmic antibodies in ulcerative colitis. Comparison with other colitides/diarrhea illness. *Gastroenetrology* 1991; 110: 1590.
11. Reumaux D, Colombel JF, Duclos B, Chaussade S, Belaiche J, Jacquot S, et-al.. Anti-neutrophil cytoplasmic auto-antibodies in sera from patients with ulcerative colitis after proctocolectomy with ileo-anal anastomosis. *Adv Exp Med Biol* 1993; 336: 523.
12. Vecchi M, Gionchetti P, Bianchi MB, Belluzzi A, Meucci G, Campieri M, De Franchis R P-ANCA and development of pouchitis in ulcerative colitis patients after proctocolectomy and ileal pouch-anal anastomosis. *Lancet* 1994; 344: 886.
13. Sandborn WJ, Landers CJ, Tremaine WJ, Targan SR. Antineutrophil cytoplasmic antibody correlates with chronic pouchitis after ileal pouch-anal anastomosis. *Am J Gastroenterol* 1995; 90: 740.
14. Patel RT, Stokes R, Birch D, Ibbotson J, Keighley MR. Influence of total colectomy on serum antineutrphil cytoplasmic antibody in pouchitis after proctocolectomy with ileal pouch –analanastomosis for ulcerative colitis. *Scand J Gastroeenterol* 1996; 31: 594.
15. Yang P, Oresland T, Jarnerot G, Hulten L, Danielsson D. Perinuclear antineutrophil cytoplasmic antibody in pouchitis after procolectomy with ileal pouch-anal anastomosis for ulcerative colitis. *Scand J Gastroenterol* 1996; 31: 594.
16. Samarasekera DN, Stebbing JF, Kettlewell MG, Jewell DP, Mortesen NJ. Outcome of restorative proctocolectomy with ileal reservoir for ulcerative colitis: comparison of distal colitis with more proximal disease. *Gut* 1996; 38: 574–577.
17. Schmidt CM, Lazenby AJ, Hendrickson RJ, Sitzmann JVl. Preoperatve terminal, ileal and colonic resection histopathology predicts risk of pouchitis in patients after ileo anal pull-through procedure. *Ann Surg* 1998; 227: 654–662 (discussion 663–665).

18. Merrett MN, Mortensen N, Kettlewell M, Jewell DP. Smoking may prevent pouchitis in patients with restorative proctocolectomy for ulcerative colitis. *Gut* 1996; 38: 362.

19. Fleshner P, Ippoliti A, Dubinsky M, Ognibene S, Vasiliauskas E, Chelly M, et-al.. A prospective multivariate analysis of clinical factors associated with pouchitis after ileal pouch-anal anastomosis. *Clin Gastroenterol Hepatol* 2007; 5: 952–8.

20. Oresland T, Fasth S, Nordgren S, Hallgren T, Hulten L. A prospective randomised comparison of two different pelvic pouch design. *Scand J Gastroenterol* 1990; 25: 986–996.

21. Sagar PM, Holdsworth PJ, Godwin PJ, Quirke P, Smith AN, Johnston D. Comparison of triplicated (S) and quadruplicated (W) pelvic ileal reservoirs: studies on manovolumetry, fecal bacteriology, fecal volatile fatty acids, mucosal morphology, and functional results. *Gastroenterology* 1992; 102: 520–528.

22. Sandborn WJ. Pouchitis following ileal pouch-anal anastomosis: definition, pathogenesis and treatment. *Gastroenterology* 1994; 107: 1856–1860.

23. Madden MV, Farthing MJ, Nicholls RJ. Inflammation in the ileal reservoir: Pouchitis. *Gut* 1990; 31: 247–249.

24. Di Febo G, Miglioli M, Lauri A, Biasco G, Paganelli GM, Poggioli G, et-al.. Endoscopic assessment of acute inflammation of the reservoir after restorative proctocolectomy with ileoanal reservoir. *Gastrointest Endosc* 1990; 36: 6–9.

25. Moskowitz RL, Shepherd NA, Nicholls RJ. An assessment of inflammation in the reservoir after restorative proctocolectomy with ileoanal ileal reservoir. *Int J Colorectal Dis* 1986; 1: 167–174.

26. Shepherd NA, Jass JR, Duval I, Moskowitz RL, Nicholls RJ, Morson BC. Restorative proctoclolectomy with ileal reservoir: pathological and histochemical study of mucosal biopsy. *J Clin Pathol* 1987; 40: 601–607.

27. Sandborn WJ, Tremaine WJ, Batts KP, Pemberton JH, Phillips SF. Pouchitis after ileal pouch-anal anastomosis: a pouchitis disease activity index. *Mayo Clinic Proc* 1994; 69: 409–415.

28. Pardi DS, Sandborn WJ. Systematic review: the management of pouchitis. *Aliment Pharmacol Ther* 2006; 23:1087–1096.

29. Shen B, Achkar JP, Lashner BA, Ormsby AH, Remzi FH, Bevins CL, et-al.. Endoscopic and histologic evaluation together with symptoms assessment are required to diagnose pouchitis. *Gastroenterology* 2001; 121: 261–267.

30. Moonka D, Furth EE, MacDermott RP, Lichtentein GR. Pouchitis associated with primary cytomegalovirus infection. *Am J Gastroenterol* 1998; 93: 264–266.

31. Munoz-Juarez M, Pemberton JH, Sandborn WJ, Tremaine WJ, Dozois RR. Misdiagnosis of specific cytomegalovirus infection of the ileoanal pouch as refractory idiopathic chronic pouchitis: Report of two cases. *Dis Colon Rectum* 1999; 42: 117–120.

32. Thompson-Fawcett MW; Mortensen NJ, Warren BF. "Cuffitis" and inflammatory changes in the columnar cuff, anal transitional zone and ileal reservoir after stapled pouch-anal anastomosis. *Dis Colon Rectum* 1999; 42: 348–55.

33. Shen B, Fazio VW, Remzi FH, Lashner BA. Clinical approach to disease of ileal pouch-anal anastomosis. *Am J Gastroenterol* 2005; 100: 2796–2807.

34. Shen B, Achkar JP, Lashner BA, Ormsby AH, Brzezinsky A, et-al.. Irritable pouch syndrome : a new category of diagnosis for symptomatic patients with ileal pouch-anal anastomosis. *Am J Gastroenterol* 2002; 97: 972–977.

35. Sandborn WJ, Mc Leod R, Jewell DP. Medical therapy for induction and maintenance of remission in pouchitis. A systematic review. *Inflamm Bowel Dis* 1999; 5: 33–39.

36. Hurst RD, Molinari M, Chung P, Rubin M, Michelassi F. Prospective study of the incidence, timing and treatment of pouchitis in 104 consecutive patients after restorative proctocolectomy. *Arch Surg* 1996; 131: 497–502.

37. Keighley MRB. Review article: the management of pouchitis. *Aliment Pharmacol Ther* 1996; 10: 449–457.

38. Madden M, McIntyre A, Nicholls RJ. Double- blind cross-over trial of metronidazole versus placebo in chronic unremitting pouchitis. *Dig Dis Sci* 1994; 39: 1193–96.

39. Shen B, Achkar JP, Lashner BA, Ormsby AH, Remzy FH, Brzezinsky A, et-al.. A randomized clinical trial of ciprofloxacin and metronidazole to treat acute pouchitis. *Inflamm Bowel Dis* 2001; 7: 301–5.

40. Sambuelli A, Boerr L, Negreira S, Gil A, Camartino G, Huernos S, et-al.. Budesonide enema in pouchitis. A double-blind, double-dummy, controlled trial. *Aliment Pharmacol Ther* 2002; 16: 27–34.

41. Miglioli M, Barbara L, Di Febo G, Gozzetti G, Lauri A, Paganelli GM, et-al.. Topical administration of 5-aminosalicylic acid: a therapeutic proposal for the treatment of pouchitis. *N Engl J Med* 1989; 320: 257.

42. Winter TA, Dalton HR, Merrett MN, Campbell A, Jewell DP. Cyclosporine A retention enemas in refractory distal ulcerative colitis and pouchitis. *Scand J Gastroenterol* 1993; 28: 701–704.

43. Clausen MR, Tvede M, Mortensen PB. Short chain fatty acids in pouch contents with and without pouchitis after ileal pouch-anal anastomosis. *Gastroenterology* 1992; 103: 1144–1449.

44. Sandborn WJ, Tremaine WJ, Batts KP, Pemberton JH, Rossi SS, Hofmann AF, et-al.. Faecal bile acids, short-chain fatty acids and bacteria after ilal pouch-anal anastomosis do not differ in patients with pouchitis. *Dig Dis Sci* 1995; 40: 1474–1483.

45. De Silva HJ, Ireland A, Kettlewell M, Mortensen N, Jewell DP. Short-chain fatty acids irrigation in severe pouchitis. *N Engl J Med* 1989; 321: 416–417.

46. Tremaine WJ, Sandborn WJ, Phillips SF, Wolff BG, Zinsmeister AR, Pemberton JH, et-al.. Short-chain fatty acid (SCFA) enema therapy for treatment-resistant pouchitis following ileal pouch-anal anastomosis (IPAA) for ulcerative colitis. *Gastroenterology* 1999; 106: A784.

47. Wischmeyer P, Pemberton JH, Phillips SF. Chronic pouchitis after ileal pouch-anal anastomosis: responses to butyrate and glutamine suppositories in a pilot study. *Mayo Clin Proc* 1993; 68: 978–81.

48. Gionchetti P, Rizzello F, Venturi A, Ferretti M, Brignola C, Peruzzo S, et-al.. Long-term efficacy of bismuth carbomer enemas in patients with treatment-resistant chronic pouchitis. *Aliment Pharmacol Ther* 1997; 11: 673–78.

49. Tremaine WJ, Sandborn WJ, Wolff BG, Carpenter HA, Zinsmeister AR, Metzger PP. Bismuth carbomer foam enemas for active chronic pouchitis. A randomised, double-blind, placebo- controlled trial. *Aliment Pharmacol Ther* 1997; 11: 1041–46.

50. Mahadevan U, Sandborn WJ. Diagnosis and management of pouchitis. *Gastroenterology* 2003; 124: 1636–1650.

51. Joelsson M, Andersson M, Bark T, Gullberg K, Hallgren T, Jiborn H, et-al.. Allopurinol as prophylaxis against pouchitis following ileal pouch-anal anastomosis for ulcerative colitis. A randomised placebo-controlled double-blind study. *Scand J Gastroenterol* 2001; 36: 1179–1184.

52. Gionchetti P, Rizzello F, Venturi A, Ugolini F, Rossi M, Brigidi P, et-al.. Antibiotic combination therapy in patients with chronic, treatment-resistant pouchitis. *Aliment Pharmacol Ther* 1999; 13: 713–18.

53. Mimura T, Rizzello F, Helwig U, Poggioli G, Schreiber S, Talbot IC, et-al.. Four week open-label trial of metronidazole and ciprofloxacin for the treatment of recurrent or refractory pouchitis. *Aliment Pharmacol Ther* 2002; 16: 909–917.

54. Gionchetti P, Rizzello F, Morselli C, Poggioli G, Pierangeli F, Laureti s, et-al.. Oral budesonide in the treatment of chronic refractory pouchitis. *Aliment Pharmacol Ther* 2007; 25: 1231–6.

55. Gionchetti P, Morselli C, Rizzello F, Poggioli G, Pierangeli F, Laureti S, et-al.. Infliximab in the treatment of Refractory pouchitis. *Gastroenterology* 2005; 128: A578.

56. Campieri M, Gionchetti P. *Probiotics in inflammatory bowel disease: new insight to pathogenesis or a possible therapeutic alternative? Gastroenterology* 1999; 116: 1246–1249.

57. Gionchetti P, Rizzello F, Venturi A, Brigidi P, Matteuzzi D, Bazzocchi G, et-al.. Oral bacteriotherapy as maintenance treatment in patients with chronic pouchitis: a double-blind, placebo-controlled trial. *Gastroenterology* 2000; 119: 305–309.

58. Mimura T, Rizzello F, Helwig U, et-al.. Once daily high dose probiotic therapy for maintaining remission in recurrent or refractory pouchitis. *Gut* 2004; 53: 108–14.

59. Ulisse S, Gionchetti P, D'Alò S, et-al.. Increased expression of cytokines, inducible nitric oxide synthase and matrix metalloproteinases in pouchitis: effects of probiotic treatment (VSL#3). *Gastroenterology* 2001; 96: 2691–9.

60. Gionchetti P, Rizzello F, Helvig U, Venturi A, Lammers KM, Brigidi P, et-al.. Prophylaxis of pouchitis onset with probiotic therapy: a double-blind placebo controlled trial. *Gastroenterology* 2003; 124: 1202–1209.

61. Gionchetti P, Rizzello F, Morselli C, Poggioli G, et al.. High dose probiotics in the treatment of active pouchitis. Dis Colon Rectum 2007 in press.

62. Kuisma J, Mentula S, Kahri A, et-al.. Effect of *Lactobacillus rhamnosus GG* on ileal pouch inflammation and microbial flora. *Aliment Pharmacol Ther* 2003; 17: 509–15.

15 Probiotics in Antibiotic-Associated Diarrhea and *Clostridium difficile* Infection

Hania Szajewska

Key Points

- Antibiotic-associated diarrhea (AAD) is a common pediatric disorder.
- This chapter summarizes the available evidence on the efficacy of probiotics in children in the prevention and treatment of any diarrhea associated with the use of antibiotics and that was caused by *Clostridium difficile*.
- Results emerging from pediatric trials provide evidence of a moderate beneficial effect of selected probiotic microorganisms, such as *Saccharomyces boulardii* or *Lactobacillus* GG, in the prevention of AAD in children.

Key Words: Live microbial supplements, *Lactobacilli*, *Bifidobacteria*, *Saccharomyces boulardii*, microflora.

INTRODUCTION

The field of probiotics is progressing rapidly. Probiotics, once used primarily in the context of alternative medicine, are now entering mainstream medicine. An increasing number of potential health benefits are being attributed to probiotic therapies [1,2]. However, only a few have been confirmed in well-designed and randomized controlled trials (RCTs) conducted and even less in the pediatric population [2]. This chapter summarizes the available evidence of the efficacy of probiotics in children in the prevention and treatment of any diarrhea associated with the use of antibiotics and that caused by *Clostridium difficile*. In addition to published data regarding children, adult studies are also discussed; however, the conclusions of these studies, whether positive or negative, may not be applicable to the pediatric population. To identify the published evidence, MEDLINE, EMBASE, the Cochrane Database of Systematic Reviews, and the Cochrane Controlled Trials Register (until July 2007) were searched. The search was restricted to double-blind, RCTs or their meta-analyses, using relevant keywords.

From: *Nutrition and Health: Probiotics in Pediatric Medicine*
Edited by: S. Michail and P.M. Sherman © Humana Press, Totowa, NJ

The reference lists of articles identified by these strategies were also searched. Additionally, several key review articles and book chapters were considered. Only English language papers were included.

ANTIBIOTIC-ASSOCIATED DIARRHEA AND *C. DIFFICILE* INFECTION

A common side effect of antibiotic treatment is antibiotic-associated diarrhea (AAD) defined as otherwise unexplained diarrhea that occurs in association with the administration of antibiotics [3]. In the pediatric population, AAD occurs in approximately 11–40% of children between the initiation of therapy and up to 2 months after cessation of treatment [4,5]. Virtually any antimicrobial agent may cause diarrhea and pseudomembranous colitis, but ampicillin, amoxicillin-clavulanate, cephalosporins, and clindamycin are most often incriminated [6,7]. AAD has been associated with an increased number of days of hospitalization and higher medical costs. The spectrum of clinical illness of AAD ranges from mild, self-limited diarrhea to severe, life-threatening pseudomembranous colitis. The mechanism of AAD is presumably related to alterations in the normal intestinal microflora and colonization by resistant flora. Although no infectious agent is found in most cases, the bacterial agent commonly associated with AAD, particularly in the most severe episodes (pseudomembranous colitis), is *C. difficile* [8], a spore-forming, obligately anaerobic, gram-positive bacillus, producing toxins. However, other enteropathogens may also cause AAD, including salmonella, *C. perfringens* type A, *Staphylococcus aureus*, and possibly *Candida albicans* [9].

Management of AAD includes discontinuation of the offending antimicrobial therapy as soon as possible in patients in whom clinically significant diarrhea or colitis develops. If it is necessary to treat the original infection, an antibiotic that is infrequently implicated in AAD (e.g., aminoglycosides, sulfonamides, macrolides, vancomycin, tetracycline, or possibly fluoroquinolones) should be used. Antimicrobial therapy for *C. difficile* infection is indicated for patients with severe disease or in whom diarrhea persists after antimicrobial therapy is discontinued. The optimal treatment strategy for *C. difficile* has not been identified, but like in adults, metronidazole (30 mg/kg per day in four divided doses, maximum 500 mg) is most widely recommended, even if solid evidence on its use (dose and duration) is not available. Both in adults and children, vancomycin is a second-line agent because of the potential for promoting vancomycin-resistant organisms [3,10]. The vast majority of patients who have an episode of *C. difficile* diarrhea, whether antibiotic-associated or sporadically acquired, respond to proper antibiotic treatment with eradication of the infection. However, in adults, up to 20% of them experience a recurrence of the infection, which may reflect relapse of infection due to the original infecting organism or infection by a new strain [11]. Solid data on the frequency of recurrences in children are not available, but according to some reports *C. difficile* may recur after treatment in as many as 43–67% of pediatric patients [11]. Recently, numerous investigators have reported an increase in the frequency and severity of *C. difficile* disease in institutions in the US and Canada [12], prompting interest in adjunctive strategies to optimally prevent and treat *C. difficile* disease. Preventive measures include the use of probiotics, which are live microbial food ingredients that are beneficial to health [13].

POTENTIAL FOR USE OF PROBIOTICS

The rationale for the use of probiotics is based on the assumption that the use of antibiotics leads to a disturbance in the normal intestinal microflora and that this is a key factor in the pathogenesis of AAD and *C. difficile* infection [14]. However, the exact mechanism by which probiotics might exert their activity against enteropathogens in humans remains unknown. Several possible mechanisms have been proposed, mostly based on results of in vitro and animal studies. These include the synthesis of antimicrobial substances (e.g., *Lactobacillus* GG and *Lactobacillus acidophilus* strain LB have been shown to produce inhibitory substances against some Gram-positive and Gram-negative pathogens) [15–17], competition for nutrients required for growth of pathogens [18,19], competitive inhibition of adhesion of pathogens [20–23], and modification of toxins or toxin receptors [24,25]. Additionally, studies have shown that probiotics stimulate or modify nonspecific and specific immune responses to pathogens: in fact, certain probiotics increase the number of circulating lymphocytes [26] and lymphocyte proliferation [27], stimulate phagocytosis, increase specific antibody responses to rotavirus vaccine strain [28], and increase cytokine secretion, including interferon γ [27, 29–31]. Recently, Mack et al. [32] have shown that *Lactobacillus* species (*L. rhamnosus* strain GG, as well as *L. plantarum* strain 299v) inhibit, in a dose-dependent manner, binding of *E. coli* strains to intestinal-derived epithelial cells grown in a tissue culture by stimulation of synthesis and secretion of mucins (glycoproteins known to have a protective effect in intestinal infections). Furthermore, probiotics have been shown to enhance mucosal immune defenses [33] and protect against structural and functional damage promoted by enterovirulent pathogens in the brush border of enterocytes, probably by interfering with the cross talk between the pathogen and host cells (i.e., inhibition of pathogen-induced cell signaling) [34]. It is likely that several of the above-described mechanisms operate simultaneously, and they may well differ depending on the properties of an enteric pathogen and probiotic strain.

PREVENTION OF AAD

Published Meta-Analyses in Pediatric Population

Three systematic reviews of RCTs involving only children were found [35–37]. The first review [35] (search date December 2005) identified 6 RCTs involving 766 children. The review found that the treatment with probiotics compared with placebo reduced the risk of AAD from 28.5 to 11.9% (relative risk [RR] 0.44, 95% confidence interval [CI] 0.25–0.77, random effect model). Preplanned subgroup analysis showed that the reduction in the risk of AAD was associated with the use of *Lactobacillus* GG (2 RCTs, 307 participants, RR 0.3, 95% CI 0.15–0.6), *S. boulardii* (1 RCT, 246 participants, RR 0.2, 95% CI 0.07–0.6), or *B. lactis* and *Str. thermophilus* (1 RCT, 157 participants, RR 0.5, 95% CI 0.3–0.95). It was concluded that probiotics reduce the risk of AAD in children. For every seven patients that would develop diarrhea while being treated with antibiotics, one fewer will develop AAD if also receiving probiotics. This meta-analysis, as almost all, is limited by the quantity and quality of existing data. The methodology of the included studies differed and often was suboptimal. Potential limitations included unclear or inadequate allocation concealment, and no intention-to-treat analysis (ITT). Study limitations also included a small sample size in some trials and no widely agreed upon definition of diarrhea.

A more recent systematic review [37] (search date August 2006) identified 10 RCTs (6 of them were included in the above-mentioned meta-analysis) involving 1,986 participants, of poor to moderate methodological quality, comparing treatment with either *Lactobacilli* spp., *Bifidobacterium* spp., *Streptococcus* spp., or *Saccharomyces boulardii* alone or in combination, in children up to 18 years of age treated with antibiotics. Six studies used a single strain probiotic agent and four combined two probiotic strains. While in seven trials, the intervention was compared to placebo, in two trials probiotics were compared to interventions other than placebo (i.e., diosmectite, infant formula) and in one to no treatment. The per protocol analysis for nine trials reporting on the incidence of diarrhea shows statistically significant results favoring probiotics over active and non-active controls (RR 0.49; 95% CI 0.32 to 0.74). However, ITT analysis showed nonsignificant results overall (RR 0.90; 95% CI 0.50–1.63). However, as indicated by the authors of this review, the validity of intention to treat (ITT) analysis in this review can be questioned due to high losses to follow-up. Five of ten trials were monitored for adverse events (*n* = 647); none reported a serious adverse event.

A third meta-analysis [36] (search date January 2005) covers data included in the Cochrane Review by the same authors, and therefore is not discussed here (Table 15.1).

OTHER PUBLISHED META-ANALYSES

Several other systematic reviews of RCTs that included both adults and children were found (Table 15.1). The first [38] review searched MEDLINE and the Cochrane Library (search date 2000) and identified nine trials with 1214 patients, including two trials in children [39,40]. No statistical heterogeneity or publication bias was detected among these nine trials. The pooled odds ratio (OR) showed that probiotic treatment was more effective than placebo in the prevention of diarrhea (OR 0.37, 95% CI: 0.26–0.53). The combined odds ratios for four trials that used *S. boulardii* also favored probiotic treatment (OR 0.39, 95% CI: 0.25–0.62), as did studies that used lactobacilli or enterococci (OR 0.34, 95% CI: 0.19–0.61) [38].

The second meta-analysis [41] (search date 2001) identified 7 studies with 881 patients (5 of those were also identified in the above-mentioned meta-analysis). Two studies involved children, and the rest were performed in adults. These studies showed a significant reduction in diarrhea, and the pooled RR was 0.4 (95% CI 0.3–0.6).

The scope of the third meta-analysis [42] was to evaluate the evidence for the use of probiotics in the prevention of acute diarrhea. Of 19 trials with data on AAD, 18 had positive point estimates; 6 of these attained statistical significance, with an overall reduction of 52% (95% CI 35–56%). In some of these trials, probiotics were administered together with eradication therapy for *Helicobacter pylori*. These factors need to be considered when interpreting and extrapolating overall results.

SYSTEMATIC REVIEWS LIMITED TO ONE PROBIOTIC MICROORGANISM

Critics of using a meta-analytical approach to assess the efficacy of probiotics argue that beneficial effects of probiotics seem to be strain specific; thus, pooling data on different strains may result in misleading conclusions. Given these concerns, the author of

Table 15.1
Probiotic in prevention of antibiotic-associated diarrhea: results of meta-analyses of RCTs

Study	Probiotics	Number of RCTs (n)	Measure of effect size	Effect (95% CI)	Number needed to treat (95% CI)
Children only					
Szajewska et al. [35]	Various[a]	6 (766)	RR	0.48 (0.35–0.65)	8 (7–11)
Johnston et al. [36]	Various[b]	6 (707)	RR	0.43 (0.25–0.75)	
Johnston et al. [37]	Various[e]	9 (1946)	RR	1.01 (0.64–1.61)	
				0.49 (0.32–0.74)	
Adults and children					
D'Souza et al. [38]	S. boulardii	4 (830)	OR	0.39 (0.25–0.62)	11 (8–20)
	Lactobacillus spp.[c]	5 (384)	OR	0.34 (0.19–0.61)	11 (8–18)
	Total	9 (1214)	OR	0.37 (0.26–0.53)	
Cremonini et al. [41]	Lactobacillus spp.[d]	4 (446)	RR	0.5 (0.4–0.7)	9 (7–17)
	S. boulardii	3 (435)	RR	0.6 (0.4–0.9)	14 (8–108)
	Total	7 (881)	RR	0.4 (0.3–0.6)	9 (7–14)
Szajewska et al. [43]	S. boulardii	5 (1076)	RR	0.4 (0.2–0.8)	10 (7–16)
Hawrelak et al. [48]	LGG	6 (692)	No statistical pooling		
Sazawal et al. [42]	Various	19 (no data)	RR	0.48 (0.35–0.65), NNT 8 (7–11)	
RCT		N (Exp/Cont)			
McFarland et al. [52]	Various	25 (2810)	RR	0.43 (0.31–0.58)	
Wenus et al. [49]	LGG, La-5, Bb-12	87 (46/41) FU 63/87 (72%)	RR	0.21 (0.05–0.93)	
Hickson et al. [50]	Lactobacillus casei DN-114 001, S. thermophilus, L. bulgaricus	113 (57/56) FU 113/135 (83%)	RR	0.36 (0.2–0.76)	5 (3–16)

[a] *L. acidophilus* + *L. bulgaricus* (1 RCT), *L. acidophilus* + *B. infantis* (1 RCT), *B. lactis* Bb12 + *Str. thermophilus* (1 RCT), LGG (2 RCTs), *S. boulardii* (1 RCT).
[b] *L. acidophilus* + *L. bulgaricus* (1 RCT), *L. acidophilus* + *B. infantis* (1 RCT), LGG (2 RCTs), *S. boulardii* (1 RCT), *L. sporogens* + fructooligosaccharides (1 RCT).
[c] *L. acidophilus* + *L. bulgaricus* (2 RCTs), *L. acidophilus* + *B. longum* (1 RCT), *Lactobacillus* GG (1 RCT), *E. faecium* SF68 (1 RCT)
[d] *Lactobacillus* GG (3 RCTs), *Lactobacillus* spp. (1 RCT)
[e] *Lactobacillus* GG (2 RCTs), *S. boulardii* (3 RCTs), *B. lactis* + *Str. thermophilus* (1 RCT), *L. acidophilus* + *B. infantis* (1 RCT), *L. sporogenes* + fructooligosaccharides (1 RCT), *L. acidophilus* + *L. bulgaricus* (1 RCT).

CI, confidence interval; FU, follow-up; RR, relative risk; WMD, weighted mean difference (negative values indicate that duration of diarrhea was shorter in the probiotic than control group). OR, odds ration; RCT, randomized controlled trial.

this chapter coreviewed data on the effectiveness and safety of only one probiotic microorganism—*S. boulardii* —in the prevention of AAD [43]. Of 16 potentially relevant clinical trials identified (search date – December 2004), 5 RCTs (1076 participants) met the inclusion criteria for this systematic review. Treatment with *S. boulardii* compared with placebo reduced the risk of AAD from 17.2 to 6.7% (RR 0.43, 95% CI 0.23–0.78; random effect model). The number needed to treat to prevent one case of AAD was 10 (95% CI 7-16). No side effects were reported. Thus, a meta-analysis of data from 5 RCTs showed that *S boulardii* is moderately effective in preventing AAD in children and adults treated with antibiotics for any reason (mainly respiratory tract infections). For every 10 patients receiving *S. boulardii* daily with antibiotics, one fewer will develop AAD. The mechanism by which *S. boulardii,* a nonpathogenic yeast, exerts its action in preventing AAD is unclear. Possible mechanisms, which have been demonstrated in animals, include the production of a protease that inactivates a receptor for toxin A of *C. difficile*, secretion of increased levels of secretory IgA and IgA antitoxin A, and competition for attachment sites [44–46]. *S. boulardii* has also been shown to block *C. difficile* adherence to cells in vitro [47].

Another systematic review [48] focused on the efficacy of *L. rhamnosus* GG versus placebo. MEDLINE, CINAHL, AMED, the Cochrane Controlled Trials Register and the Cochrane Database of Systematic Reviews were searched up to July 2003 using the reported search terms. The reference lists of identified primary studies were checked for further studies. Six RCTs involving 692 participants (including 307 children) met the inclusion criteria. Two of the included studies addressed treatment of *H. pylori*. Significant statistical heterogeneity of the trials precluded meta-analysis. Four of the six trials found a significant reduction in the risk of AAD with coadministration of *Lactobacillus* GG. One of the trials found a reduced number of days with antibiotic-induced diarrhea with Lactobacillus GG administration, while one trial failed to find the benefit of *Lactobacillus* GG supplementation.

PUBLISHED RCTS APPEARING AFTER THE PUBLICATION OF THE META-ANALYSES

The evidence from the above analyses is indeed very encouraging. Also, a few of some of the more recent trials, not included in the meta-analyses, showed encouraging results.

The first RCT involving adult patients found that the use of fermented milk drink containing *Lactobacillus* GG, La-5, and Bb-12 (n = 46), or placebo with heat-killed bacteria (n = 41), during a period of 14 days reduced the risk of AAD from 27.6% in the control group to 5.9% in the experimental group (RR 0.21, 95% CI 0.05–0.93) [49].

The second randomized, double-blind trial involving 113 hospital patients (mean age 74) taking antibiotics found reduced risk of diarrhea associated with antibiotic use in the group consuming a readily available probiotic drink containing *L. casei* DN-114 001, *S. thermophilus*, and *L. bulgaricus* twice daily during a course of antibiotics and for 1 week after the course was completed compared to the placebo group (19/56 (34%) versus 7/57 (12%), RR 0.36, 95% CI 0.2–0.76). The absolute risk reduction was 21.6% (6.6–36.6%), and the number needed to treat was 5 (3 to 15). No one in the probiotic group and 9 of 53 (17%) in the placebo group had diarrhea caused by *C. difficile* (P = 0.001). The absolute risk reduction was 17% (7–27%), and the number needed to treat was 5 (3 to 15). It was calculated that the cost to prevent one case of diarrhea was £50 (€74; $100) and £60 (€87.5; $120) to prevent one case of *C. difficile* [50]. The limitations of this trial include highly selective inclusion and exclusion criteria (e.g., exclusion of subjects receiving "high risk antibiotics") and quite liberal definition of diarrhea.

PROBIOTICS FOR PREVENTION AND TREATMENT OF *C. DIFFICILE* DIARRHEA

Two systematic reviews that assessed the efficacy and safety of probiotics for the prevention and treatment of *C. difficile*-associated diarrhea were found (Table 15.2). For the first review [51], PubMed, EMBASE, INAHTA, HEN, and Cochrane Collaboration databases were searched up to March 2005 for RCTs in which prevention or treatment of *C. difficile*-associated diarrhea was the primary or secondary outcome. The authors identified 4 studies in which prevention (1 RCT) or treatment (3 RCTs) of *C. difficile* diarrhea was the primary outcome. All studies were in adults. The benefit of probiotic therapy with *S. boulardii* seen in two of the studies was restricted to subgroups of patients with severe disease and increased use of vancomycin. The poor methodological quality of the remaining 2 RCTs precluded authors from drawing conclusions. Four other RCTs were identified in which *C. difficile*-associated diarrhea was the secondary outcome. These studies were limited by the small number of patients enrolled and provided no evidence of effective prevention. No statistical pooling was performed due to heterogeneity. The authors concluded that

Table 15.2

Probiotics in prevention and treatment of *C. difficile* –associated diarrhea: Results of meta-analyses of RCTs

Study	Probiotics	Number of RCTs (n)	Measure of effect size	Effect (95% CI)	Number needed to treat (95% CI)
Treatment					
Dendukuri et al. [51]	Various[a]	3 (no data)	No statistical pooling		
McFarland et al. [52]	Various[b]	6 (354)	RR	0.59 (0.4–0.85)	8 (6–22)
Prevention					
Dendukuri et al. [51]	Various[c]	5	No statistical pooling		
McFarland et al. [52]	*L. acidophilus* plus *B. Bifidum*	1 (no data)	RR	0.33 (0.07 to 1.59) NS	

[a]*S. boulardii* (2 RCTs), *L. plantarum* 299v (1 RCT).

[b]*S. boulardii* (2 RCTs), *Lactobacillus* GG (2 RCTs), *L. plantarum* 299v (1 RCT), *L. acidophilus* plus *B. bifidum* (1 RCT).

[c]*S. boulardii* (3 RCT), *Lactobacillus* GG (1 RCT), *L. acidophilus* plus *B. bifidum* (1 RCT).

available evidence (all in adults) does not support the administration of probiotics with antibiotics to prevent or treat *C. difficile* diarrhea in adults.

The second review [52] searched MEDLINE and Google Scholar (2005), Cochrane Library, metaRegister of Controlled Trials, National Institutes of Health clinical trial register, conference abstracts, and bibliographies of relevant studies. Six RCTs ($n = 354$) for *C. difficile* diarrhea were found (all in adults, five treatment and one prevention). The RR for *C. difficile* diarrhea was 0.59 (95% CI 0.4–0.85). Of the three different probiotics tested for the treatment of *C. difficile* diarrhea, only *S. boulardii* showed significant reductions in recurrences of *C. difficile* diarrhea. *Lactobacillus* GG and *L. plantarum* 299v did not show significant differences in *C. difficile* diarrhea recurrence rates in the experimental compared with the control group. The only trial testing a probiotic mixture *(L. acidophilus* and *B. bifidum)* for the prevention of *C. difficile* diarrhea did not show significant efficacy. This meta-analysis has been criticized for combining the results from one study on the prevention of *C. difficile* diarrhea with results from five studies on the treatment of *C. difficile* diarrhea, and for pooling data on different probiotics, different conditions, and different patient characteristics, as well as some methodological issues calling for caution in interpreting the conclusions [53,54].

In spite of some anecdotal evidence of the efficacy of probiotics for *C. difficile* diarrhea [55,56], no RCT investigating such possibility in children has been conducted. Well-conducted RCTs addressing the role of probiotics in *C. difficile*-associated diarrhea both in children and adults are still needed.

SAFETY

Administration of probiotics is not without risk, albeit adverse effects seem to be rare [57]. Of concern, there have been instances of fungemia caused by *S. boulardii* [58–60] and bacteremia with certain probiotic bacteria involving high-risk populations [61]. Endocarditis, pneumonia, and meningitis have very rarely been reported in association with lactobacilli [62–64]. Most complications have occurred in immunocompromised subjects or in patients with other life-threatening illnesses managed in intensive care units. While the use of probiotics in immunocompetent subjects seems to be safe, it is not clear whether they could be used in the prevention of AAD in immunocompromised patients. As recently pointed out, in these patients potential bacteremia and fungemia may outweigh the benefits in immuno-compromised and debilitated patients, who are also the ones at highest risk for *C. difficile* infection [65].

RECOMMENDATIONS FROM PROFESSIONAL PEDIATRIC SOCIETIES

The Clinical Report recently published by the NASPGHAN Nutrition Report Committee addressed the clinical efficacy of probiotics. Regarding AAD, it has been stated that efficacy has been clearly shown but not all probiotics are effective [66].

SUMMARY AND IMPLICATIONS FOR PRACTICE

Should children treated with antibiotics routinely receive probiotics? The results emerging from RCTs in children provide evidence of a moderate beneficial effect of selected probiotic microorganisms, such as for example *S. boulardii* or *Lactobacillus* GG, in the prevention of AAD in children. As the above-mentioned probiotics have been shown to be capable of providing reasonable protection against the development of AAD, their use is probably warranted whenever the physician feels that preventing this usually self-limited complication is important. However, as evidence is still limited, caution should be exercised until the results are confirmed. As of today, very few probiotics have been tested. Clearly, other microorganisms may be also effective but their efficacy needs to be confirmed in well-conducted RCTs. The available data provide evidence that selected probiotics significantly reduce the risk of diarrhea in children treated with antibiotics in general. However, not all antibiotics are likely to be equally selective for causing AAD. Currently, conclusions about the efficacy of probiotics in preventing diarrhea attributable to any single antibiotic class cannot be made. The role of probiotics in the prevention and treatment of diarrhea associated with *C. difficile* infection remains unclear, particularly in the pediatric population.

IMPLICATIONS FOR RESEARCH

The limitations discussed earlier suggest steps to improve the quality of research in this area. Further well-conducted clinical studies using validated outcomes are recommended to (1) further identify populations at high risk of AAD that would benefit most from probiotic therapy; (2) evaluate the efficacy of other probiotic strains; (3) evaluate the efficacy of probiotics in preventing AAD caused specifically by *C. difficile* or those antibiotics that are most likely to cause diarrhea; (4) determine the most effective dosing schedule; and (5) address the cost-effectiveness of using probiotics to prevent AAD in children. Given the uncertainty involved in the probiotic therapy for *C. difficile* infection, an adequately powered, placebo-controlled RCT is recommended.

REFERENCES

1. Andersson H, Asp NG, Bruce A, et al. Health effects of probiotics and prebiotics. A literature review on human studies. *Scand J Nutr* 2001;45:58–5.
2. Szajewska H, Setty M, Mrukowicz J, Guandalini S. Probiotics in gastrointestinal diseases in children: hard and not-so-hard evidence of efficacy. *J Pediatr Gastroenterol Nutr* 2006;42:454–75.
3. Bartlett JG. Antibiotic-associated diarrhea. *N Engl J Med* 2002;346:334–9.
4. Turck D, Bernet JP, Marx J, et al. Incidence and risk factors of oral antibiotic-associated diarrhea in an outpatient pediatric population. *J Pediatr Gastroenterol Nutr* 2003;37:22–6.
5. Elstner CL, Lindsay AN, Book LS, Matsen JM. Lack of relationship of *Clostridium difficile* to antibiotic-associated diarrhea in children. *Pediatr Inf Dis* 1983;2:364–6.
6. Barbut F, Meynard JL, Guiguet M, et al. *Clostridium difficile*-associated diarrhea in HIV infected patients: epidemiology and risk factors. *J Acq Immun Def Synd* 1997;16:176–81.
7. McFarland LV, Surawicz CM, Stamm WE. Risk factors for *Clostridium difficile* carriage and *C. difficile*-associated diarrhea in a cohort of hospitalized patients. *J Infect Dis* 1990;162:678–84.

8. Bartlett JG, Chang TW, Gurwith M, Gorbach SL, Onderdonk AB. Antibiotic-associated pseudomembranous colitis due to toxin producing Clostridia. *N Engl J Med* 1978;298:531–4.

9. Bartlett JG. Antibiotic-associated diarrhea. *N Engl J Med* 2002;346:334–9.

10. American Academy of Pediatrics. *Clostridium difficile*. In: Pickering LK, ed., Red book: 2006 Report of the Committee on Infectious Diseases. 26th ed. Elk Grove Village, IL: American Academy of Pediatrics, 2006:261–3.

11. McFarland LV, Brandmarker SA, Guandalini S. *Pediatric Clostridium difficile: a phantom menace or clinical reality? J Pediatr Gastroenterol Nutr* 2000;31:220–31.

12. McDonald LC, Killgore GE, Thompson A, et al. An epidemic, toxin gene-variant strain of *Clostridium difficile*. *N Engl J Med* 2005;353:2433–41.

13. Diplock AT, Aggett PJ, Ashwell M, et al. Scientific concepts of functional foods in Europe: consensus document. *Br J Nutr* 1999;81(Suppl. 1):S1–S27.

14. Surawicz CM. Probiotics, antibiotic-associated diarrhoea and *Clostridium difficile* diarrhoea in humans. *Vest Practice Res Clin Gastroenterol* 2003; 17: 775–83.

15. Goldin BR, Gorbach SL, Saxelin M, et al. Survival of *Lactobacillus* species (strain GG) in human gastrointestinal tract. *Dig Dis Sci* 1992;37:121–28.

16. Silva M, Jacobus NV, Deneke C, et al. Antimicrobial substance from a human *Lactobacillus* strain. *Antimicrob Agents Chemother* 1987;31:1231–3.

17. Coconnier MH, Lievin V, Bernet-Camard MF, et al. Antibacterial effect of the adhering human *Lactobacillus acidophilus* strain LB. *Antimicrob Agents Chemother* 1997;41:1046–52.

18. Wilson KH, Perini I. Role of competition for nutrients in suppression of *Clostridium difficile* by the colonic microflora. *Infect Immunol* 1988;56:2610–14.

19. Walker WA. Role of nutrients and bacterial colonisation in the development of intestinal host defense. *J Pediatr Gastroenterol Nutr* 2000;30(Suppl.):S2–7.

20. Bernet MF, Brassart D, Nesser JR, et al. *Lactobacillus acidophilus* LA1 binds to human intestinal cell lines and inhibits cell attachment and cell invasion by enterovirulent bacteria. *Gut* 1994;35:483–9.

21. Davidson JN, Hirsch DC. Bacterial competition as a mean of preventing diarrhea in pigs. *Infect Immun* 1976;13:1773–4.

22. Rigothier MC, Maccanio J, Gayral P. Inhibitory activity of *Saccharomyces* yeasts on the adhesion of *Entamoeba histolytica* trophozoites to human erythrocytes in vitro. *Parasitol Res* 1994;80:10–15.

23. Michail S, Abernathy F. *Lactobacillus plantarum* reduces the in vitro secretory respone of intestinal epithelial cells to enteropathogenic *Escherichia coli* infection. *J Pediatr Gastroenterol Nutr* 2002;35:350–5.

24. Pothoulakis C, Kelly CP, Joshi MA, et al. *Saccharomyces boulardii* inhibits *Clostridium difficile* toxin A binding and enterotoxicity in rat ileum. *Gastroenterology* 1993;104:1108–15.

25. Czerucka D, Roux I, Rampal P. *Saccharomyces boulardii* inhibits secretagogue-mediated adenosine 3,5 -cyclic monophosphate induction in intestinal cells. *Gastroenterology* 1994;106:65–72.

26. De Simone C, Ciardi A, Grassi A, et al. Effect of *Bifidobacterium bifidum* and *Lactobacillus acidophilus* on gut mucosa and peripheral blood B lymphocytes. *Immunopharmacol Immunotoxicol* 1992;14:331–40.

27. Aattour N, Bouras M, Tome D, et al. Oral ingestion of lactic-acid bacteria by rats increases lymphocyte proliferation and interferon-gamma production. *Br J Nutr* 2002;87:367–73.

28. Isolauri E, Joensuu J, Suomalainen H, et al. Improved immunogenicity of oral D × RRV reassortant rotavirus vaccine by *Lactobacillus casei* GG. *Vaccine* 1995;13:310–20.

29. Kaila M, Isolauri E, Soppi E, et al. Enhancement of the circulating antibody secreting cell response in human diarrhea by a human *Lactobacillus* strain. *Pediatr Res* 1992;32:141–4.

30. Majamaa H, Isolauri E, Saxelin M, et al. Lactic acid bacteria in the treatment of acute rotavirus gastroenteritis. *J Pediatr Gastroenterol Nutr* 1995;20:333–8.

31. Miettinen M, Vuopio-Varkila J, Varkila K. Production of human tumor necrosis factor alpha, interleukin-6 and interleukin-10 is induced by lactic acid bacteria. *Infect Immun* 1996;64:5403–5.

32. Mack DR, Michail S, Wei S, et al. Probiotics inhibit enteropathogenic *E. coli* adherence in vitro by inducing intestinal mucin gene expression. *Am J Physiol* 1999;276:G941–50.

33. Isolauri E, Majamaa H, Arvola T, et al. *Lactobacillus casei* strain GG reverses increased intestinal permeability induced by cow milk in suckling rats. *Gastroenterology* 1993;105:1643–50.

34. Lievin-Le Moal V, Amsellem R, Servin AL, Coconnier M-H. *Lactobacillus acidophilus* (strain LB) from the resident adult human gastrointestinal microflora exerts activity against brush border damage promoted by a diarrheagenic *Escherichia coli* in human enterocyte-like cells. *Gut* 2002;50:803–11.

35. Szajewska H, Ruszczynski M, Radzikowski A. Probiotics in the prevention of antibiotic-associated diarrhea in children: a meta-analysis of randomized controlled trials. *J Pediatr* 2006;149:367–72.

36. Johnston BC, Supina AL, Vohra S. Probiotics for pediatric antibiotic-associated diarrhea: a meta-analysis of randomized placebo-controlled trials. *CMAJ* 2006;175:377–383. Erratum in: CMAJ 2006;175:777.

37. Johnston BC, Supina AL, Ospina M, Vohra S. Probiotics for the prevention of pediatric antibiotic-associated diarrhea. Cochrane Database Syst Rev 2007 April 18;(2):CD004827.

38. D'Souza AL, Rajkumar C, Cooke J, Bulpitt CJ. Probiotics in prevention of antibiotic associated diarrhea: meta-analysis. *Br Med J* 2002;324:1361–1364.

39. Vanderhoof JA, Whitney DB, Antonson DL, Hanner TL, Lupo JV, Young RJ. *Lactobacillus* GG in the prevention of antibiotic-associated diarrhea in children. *J Pediatrics* 1999;135:564–8.

40. Tankanov RM, Ross MB, Ertel IJ, Dickinson DG, McCormick LS, Garfinkel JF. Double blind, placebo-controlled study of the efficacy of Lactinex in the prophylaxis of amoxicillin-induced diarrhea. *DICP Ann Pharm* 1990;24:382–4.

41. Cremonini F, di Caro S, Nista EC, et al. Meta-analysis: the effect of probiotic administration on antibiotic-associated diarrhea. *Aliment Pharmacol Ther* 2002;16:1461–7.

42. Sazawal S, Hiremath G, Dhingra U, Malik P, Deb S, Black RE. Efficacy of probiotics in prevention of acute diarrhoea: a meta-analysis of masked, randomised, placebo-controlled trials. *Lancet Infect Dis* 2006;6:374–82.

43. Szajewska H, Mrukowicz J. Meta-analysis: non-pathogenic yeast *Saccharomyces boulardii* in the prevention of antibiotic-associated diarrhoea. *Aliment Pharmacol Ther* 2005;22:365–72.

44. Pothoulakis C, Kelly CP, Joshi MA, et al. *Saccharomyces boulardii* inhibits *Clostridium difficile* toxin A binding and enterotoxicity in rat ileum. *Gastroenterology* 1993;104:1108–15.

45. Wilson KH, Perini I. Role of competition for nutrients in suppresion of *Clostidium difficile* by the colonic microflora. *Infect Immun* 1988;56:2610–14.

46. Qamar A, Aboudola A, Warny M, et al. *Saccharomyces boulardii* stimulates intestinal immunoglobulin A immune response to *Clostridium difficile* toxin A in mice. *Infect Immun* 2001;69:2762–5.

47. Tasteyre A, Barc MC, Karjalainen T, et al. Inhibition of in vitro cell adherence of Clostridium difficile by *Saccharomyces boulardii*. *Microbiol Pathogens* 2002;32:219–25.

48. Hawrelak JA, Whitten DL, Myers SP. Is *Lactobacillus rhamnosus* GG effective in preventing the onset of antibiotic-associated diarrhoea: a systematic review. *Digestion* 2005;72:51–6.

49. Wenus C, Goll R, Loken EB, Biong AS, Halvorsen DS, Florholmen J. Prevention of antibiotic-associated diarrhoea by a fermented probiotic milk drink. Eur J Clin Nutr 2007 Mar 14; [Epub ahead of print].

50. Hickson M, D'Souza AL, Muthu N, Rogers TR, Want S, Rajkumar C, Bulpitt CJ. Use of probiotic Lactobacillus preparation to prevent diarrhoea associated with antibiotics: randomised double blind placebo controlled trial. *Br Med J* 2007;335:80–4.

51. Dendukuri N, Costa V, McGregor M, Brophy J. Probiotic therapy for the prevention and treatment of *Clostridium difficile*-associated diarrhea: a systematic review. *CMAJ* 2005;173:167–70.

52. McFarland LV. Meta-analysis of probiotics for the prevention of antibiotic associated diarrhea and the treatment of *Clostridium difficile* disease. *Am J Gastroenterol* 2006;101:812–22.

53. Dendukuri N, Brophy J. Inappropriate use of meta-analysis to estimate efficacy of probiotics. *Am J Gastroenterol* 2007;102:201–204.

54. Lewis S. Response to the article: McFarland LV. Meta-analysis of probiotics for the prevention of antibiotic-associated diarrhea and the treatment of Clostridium difficile disease. *Am J Gastroenterol* 2006; 101:812–22. Am J Gastroenterol 2007;102:201–2.

55. Buts JP, Corthier G, Delmee M. *Saccharomyces boulardii* for *Clostridium difficile*-associated enteropathies in infants. *J Pediatr Gastroenterol Nutr* 1993;16:419–25.

56. Biller JA, Katz AJ, Flores AF, Buie TM, Gorbach SL. Treatment of recurrent *Clostridium difficile* colitis with Lactobacillus GG. *J Pediatr Gastroenterol Nutr* 1995;21:224–6.

57. Salminen MK, Rautelin H, Tynkkynen S, et al. *Lactobacillus* bacteremia, clinical significance, and patient outcome, with special focus on probiotic *L. rhamnosus* GG. *Clin Infect Dis* 2004;38:62–9.

58. Zunic P, Lacotte J, Pegoix M, et al. *S. boulardii* fungemia. Apropos of a case. *Therapie* 1991;46:498–9.

59. Bassetti S, Frei R, Zimmerli W. Fungemia with *Saccharomyces cerevisiae* after treatment with *S. boulardii*. *Am J Med* 1998;105:71–2.

60. Rijnders BJA, Van Wijngaerden E, Verwaest C, Peetermans WE. *Saccharomyces fungemia* complicating *S. boulardii* treatment in a non-immunocompromised host. *Intensive Care Med* 2000;26:825.

61. Kalima P, Masterton RG, Roddie PH, Thomas AE. *Lactobacillus rhamnosus* infection in a child following bone marrow transplant. *J Infect* 1996;32:165–7.

62. Soleman N, Laferl H, Kneifel W, Tucek G, Budschedl E, Weber H. How safe is safe? A case of *Lactobacillus paracasei* ssp. *paracasei* endocarditis and discussion of the safety of lactic acid bacteria. *Scand J Infect Dis* 2003;35:759–62.

63. Salminen MK, Tynkkynen S, Rautelin H, Saxelin M, Vaara M, Ruutu P, et al. *Lactobacillus bacteremia* during a rapid increase in probiotic use of *Lactobacillus rhamnosus* GG in Finland. *Clin Infect Dis* 2002;35:1155–60.

64. Kunz AN, Noel JM, Fairchok MP. Two cases of *Lactobacillus bacteremia* during probiotic treatment of short gut syndrome. *J Pediatr Gastroenterol Nutr* 2004;38:457–8.

65. Segarra-Newnham M. Probiotics for *Clostridium difficile*-associated diarrhea: focus on *Lactobacillus rhamnosus* GG and *Saccharomyces boulardii*. *Ann Pharmacother* 2007;41:1212–21.

66. NASPGHAN Nutrition Report Committee, Michail S, Sylvester F, Fuchs G, Issenman R. Clinical efficacy of probiotics: Review of the evidence with focus on children. J Pediatr Gastroenterol Nutr 2006;43:550–7.

16 Probiotics and the Immunocompromised Host

Yuliya Rekhtman and Stuart S. Kaufman

Key Points

- Current information concerning the use of probiotics in both the prevention and treatment of immunocompromised states associated with the breakdown of the gastrointestinal mucosal barrier is discussed in this chapter.
- Many reports support the theoretical rationale for probiotic therapy in patients with short bowel syndrome.
- Further studies are needed, but initial results are encouraging for a role of probiotics in the treatment of hepatic disease.
- Probiotic supplementation has shown some promise in reducing antiretroviral therapy induced diarrhea.

Key Words: Human immunodeficiency virus, liver, probiotics, short gut, transplant.

INTRODUCTION

Bacteria of numerous types in specific distribution are necessary for normal digestive function. Proliferation of these bacteria to a degree that results in local or systemic disease is normally prevented by an anatomic and functional gastrointestinal mucosal barrier.[1] This barrier has three major components: (1) the luminal microflora, (2) an intact surface epithelium, and (3) an intact gut-associated lymphoid mass.[2] Numerous inherited and acquired immunodeficiency states undermine the integrity of the gastrointestinal mucosal barrier. These immunodeficiency states include both systemic disorders and those that are limited to the digestive system. Irrespective of the specific cause, compromised immune function usually affects all three parts of the gastrointestinal mucosal barrier in various degrees.

Several factors have motivated consideration of probiotics for use in the management of gastrointestinal diseases that are associated with impaired local immunity, generally, and regulation of luminal bacterial flora, in particular. These

From: *Nutrition and Health: Probiotics in Pediatric Medicine*
Edited by: S. Michail and P.M. Sherman © Humana Press, Totowa, NJ

factors include recognition of the often suboptimal response to antibiotics when used to suppress potentially pathogenic gastrointestinal flora (a prime example of which is the increasing presence of antibiotic-resistant bacterial strains such as methicillin-resistant *Staphylococcus aureus*, vancomycin-resistant *Enterococcus facium*, and extended spectrum, beta-lactamase-producing coliforms), the inability of the pharmaceutical industry to stay ahead by producing new classes of antibiotics, and increasing public interest in alternative, "natural" therapies. In this chapter, current information is reviewed concerning use of probiotics in both the prevention and treatment of immunocompromised states associated with the breakdown of the gastrointestinal mucosal barrier. In particular, the seeming paradox of using living organisms to treat immunocompromised patients in whom such agents, ordinarily innocuous, may become pathogenic is addressed. Digestive-based immunological disorders are considered on the basis of structural and metabolic abnormalities in the digestive system, such as short bowel syndrome and cirrhosis, and those in which the gastrointestinal tract is altered by systemic phenomena, including the impact of stem cell and bone marrow transplantation.

SHORT BOWEL SYNDROME AND SMALL INTESTINAL BACTERIAL OVERGROWTH

Short bowel syndrome (SBS) is defined as the sum of functional impairments, including diarrhea, malabsorption, dehydration, and electrolyte and micronutrient deficiencies that result from congenital or acquired intestinal loss, usually at least 70% of standard intestinal length for age.[3] Intrinsic to this definition of short bowel syndrome is the resulting need for specialized therapies, often including parenteral nutrition.

Small bowel intestinal bacterial overgrowth occurs in short bowel syndrome for several interrelated reasons. Loss of small bowel per se places remnant proximal small bowel in much closer proximity than usual to the normally bacteria-dense colon. Furthermore, the ascending migration of colon microflora to the proximal jejunum and duodenum is abetted in short bowel syndrome by the concurrent loss of the ileocecal valve and by the altered motility of the remnant bowel.[4,5] Poor intestinal motility and the resulting stagnation of luminal contents is due, in turn, to the persistence of the original injury to the muscularis and submucosal layers, including smooth muscle atrophy, fibrosis, and strictures. The mucosa may be inherently atrophic and chronically inflamed due to the original insult resulting in short bowel syndrome and associated persistent microvascular injury with ischemia.[6] Bacterial overgrowth is more likely in the setting of vigorous attempts to establish or reestablish enteral nutrition following intestinal resection, because loss of small intestinal absorptive surface area inevitably leads to reduced nutrient uptake by the diseased intestine and an increased supply of luminal nutrients available to the microflora.

From a metabolic perspective, symptomatic intestinal bacterial overgrowth in short bowel syndrome can be considered to be a pathologically exaggerated response to massive intestinal resection, as increased number of bacteria, specifically strict anaerobes in the colon, compensate for loss of small intestinal absorptive surface area by accelerating the usual fermentation of complex nutrients, especially starches and soluble fibers, into the highly bioavailable short-chain fatty acids including acetate, propionate, and butyrate.[7] A diet rich in fiber may also contribute to the preservation of absorption in the setting of small intestinal loss, since increased succus viscosity due to fiber may slow intestinal transit enough to improve overall assimilation.8 For the most part, however, small intestinal bacterial overgrowth is deleterious to digestive function. It likely disrupts the gastrointestinal mucosal barrier by direct injury to the epithelial surface. One needs to remember that in the healthy gut the bacteria vary in numbers and oxygen requirement depending on the location (Table 16.1). The anatomical relationship changes with structural and surgical alterations, thus affecting bacterial–mucosal interactions. Additionally, excessive numbers of bacteria in the remnant upper small bowel increase the deconjugation of bile salts to a degree that contributes to excessive bile acid loss and resulting mucosal injury, thereby exacerbating reduced digestive efficiency in a vicious cycle.[5,9] Delayed intestinal adaptation that perpetuates parenteral nutrition dependence may result.[10]

Compounding the problem for infants with SBS is the frequent unavailability of breast milk, which independently contributes to an increased concentration of potentially pathogenic luminal coliform bacteria, as compared to numbers of these bacteria in breast-fed infants.[11,12] Indeed, oral antibiotic regimens intended to suppress intestinal bacterial overgrowth in short bowel syndrome specifically target these organisms. [13,14] Strict anaerobes, including *Bacteroides* spp., also probably contribute to symptomatic bacterial overgrowth in most circumstances, accounting for the historically widespread use of metronidazole in affected patients. Additional bacteria play a role in small intestinal bacterial overgrowth, producing disease by their ability to produce large quantities of bioavailable d-lactic acid in excess of the body's degradative capacity, resulting in d-lactic acidemia.[15] Clinical sequels of d-lactic acidemia include recurrent metabolic acidosis with an increased anion gap, and encephalopathy presenting as an

Table 16.1
Intestinal microflora content by location

Part of the gut	Numbers per gram of material	Types	Examples
Stomach	$0–10^3$	Aerobes	*Enterobacter, Lactobacillus, Staphylococcus, Streptococcus*
Duodenum and jejunum	$10^4–10^6$ CFU	Aerobes and facultative anaerobes	*Streptococcus, Lactobacillus, Enterobacteriaceae*
Ileum	$10^5–10^7$ CFU	Strict anaerobes	*Bacteroides*
Colon (fecal data)	$10^9–10^{11}$ CFU	**Predominant-**Anaerobes	*Bacteroides* (25%) *Eubacterium* (25%) *Peptostreptococcus* (8%) *Bifidobacterium* (12%) *Clostridium*
		Subdominant Facultative anaerobes	*Escherichia coli, Streptococcus, Lactobacillus-2, Enterococcus*

Table 16.2
Symptoms of D-lactic acidosis

Symptoms of d-lactic acidosis
Change in mental status and recurrent encephalopathy
Speech alteration
Abusive and aggressive behavior
Lack of concentration
Ataxia and gait disturbance
Nystagmus
Metabolic acidosis with increased anion gap
Serum d-lactate level > 3 mmol/l
Normal serum l-lactate levels

intoxicated-like state with somnolence and ataxia[16] (Table 16.2). L-lactic acid levels are typically normal in this condition.[15,17]

PROBIOTICS AND SHORT BOWEL SYNDROME

A primary justification for the use of probiotics in SBS is the establishment of a luminal bacterial population that displaces bacteria most likely to interfere with digestive function while retaining the capacity to support macronutrient fermentation into short-chain fatty acids, presumably most intensely in the colon but also in the remnant small bowel. Accordingly, a beneficial effect of probiotics may be most likely in patients with all, or part, of the colon in anatomic continuity with the small bowel. That probiotic agents are capable of repopulating the intestinal lumen and displacing pathogenic microflora was confirmed by Jain et al.[18] who demonstrated that the ingestion of a synbiotic mixture of *Lactobacillus* sp., *Bifidobacterium* sp., and *Streptococcus* sp. along with a preferred carbohydrate substrate, fructose oligosaccharides, significantly decreased numbers of potentially pathogenic bacteria in nasogastric aspirates of critically ill patients within 8 days. Additionally, Rinne et al.[19] showed that the addition of probiotics to formula-fed infants changes the character of stool microflora to the one very similar to that seen in breast-fed infants.

Theoretical advantages of probiotics over antibiotics for the suppression of intestinal bacterial overgrowth are numerous. First and foremost, probiotics could enhance the physiological mechanism of adaptation to massive intestinal resection by mobilization of the distal alimentary tract for participation in the digestive process through fermentation.[7,20] Second, probiotics do not promote antibiotic resistance by pathogenic bacteria. Another factor is cost: on average, a 1-month supply of probiotics can be obtained for about US$30, whereas the price of antibiotics given for the same interval ranges between hundreds to thousands of dollars.

Mechanisms by which probiotics may be beneficial in patients with SBS extend beyond preservation of an alimentary tract microflora optimizing to general, minimally toxic, bioavailable nutrients from complex substrates that would otherwise be malabsorbed. For example, Dock et al.[21] demonstrated in an animal model of malnutrition that probiotics might, at least under some circumstances, be directly trophic to the intestinal mucosa, thereby contributing to mucosal recovery. Twelve malnourished rats were randomized to receive either probiotics or placebo for 2 weeks, six in each group. Mucosa from animals treated with probiotics demonstrated both greater villi height and crypt depth compared to the placebo-treated group. A benefit to mucosal health may also explain the findings of Candy,[22] who observed a significant reduction in water and electrolyte losses in a child with a high jejunostomy following therapy with *Lactobacillus casei*. Another potentially beneficial property of probiotics, including species of *Lactobacillus*, *Bacteroides*, and *Bifidobacterium*, is a reduced capacity to deconjugate bile acids as compared to the microflora that they supplant, thus reducing the risk of bile-acid induced diarrhea and resulting mucosal injury in short bowel syndrome patients.[23]

Animal models suggest that excessive numbers of intestinal bacteria, particularly gram-negative facultative anaerobes, are a risk factor for bacteremia and sepsis, which is common in patients following massive intestinal resection. Loss of the gut-associated lymphoid mass resulting from resection per se, may contribute to this risk.[24] In addition to increasing the absorptive capacity of the remnant small bowel, the trophic effect of probiotics on the gut mucosa may contribute to their purported ability to interfere with bacterial translocation out of the alimentary tract. Eizaguirre et al.[25] provided evidence for this benefit by showing that rats fed with *Lactobacillus* spp. following subtotal small bowel resection had a relative risk reduction for bacterial translocation of 0.43.

A concern that the administration of bacteria into the gastrointestinal tract of immunologically compromised patients increases the risk of systemic infection with these agents appears not to be justified. The risk is overall rather low, just 0.05–0.4%.[26] In Finland, where uniform reporting maximizes reliability of these data, the incidence of bacteremia has not changed since the use of probiotics has increased in that country.[27] However, there are some reports of bloodstream infection with probiotic species following treatment. Kunz et al.[28] observed bacteremia in two children with short bowel syndrome treated with *Lactobacillus* spp. Similarly, Land et al.[29] reported two cases in postoperative patients and Groote et al.[30] in one patient with short bowel syndrome In addition, Patel et al.[31] reported infections in eight patients following liver transplantation, while Riqueline et al.[32] noted *Saccharomyces boulardii* fungemia in two additional patients. Overall, the low risk of infection from probiotic therapy in short bowel syndrome patients and other compromised populations suggests that their trophic effect on mucosa generally overrides the theoretical risk of bacteremia and fungemia associated with increased mucosal permeability existing at the onset of treatment.

PROBIOTICS IN THE TREATMENT OF SHORT BOWEL SYNDROME: HUMAN TRIALS

Most reports of probiotic administration in clinical short bowel syndrome represent observations in small groups of patients employing different mixes of species in empiric doses and durations rather than randomized, placebo-controlled trials. However, the findings of many of these reports support the theoretical rationale for probiotic therapy in patients with short bowel syndrome, particularly in the setting of actual or threatened small intestinal bacterial overgrowth. For example, Kanamori et al.[33] reported a 4-year-old with parenteral nutrition-dependent short bowel syndrome secondary to gastroschisis who was treated with a mixture of *Bifidobacterium breve*, *L. casei*, and galactose oligosaccharides. Prior to therapy, the child experienced monthly episodes of metabolic acidosis, fever, and ileus with intestinal dilatation. Twelve months of therapy produced a decrease in plasma d-lactic acid concentration accompanied by reduced densities of *Escherichia coli* and *Candida* species in the feces, episodic ileus improved, and parenteral nutrition was successfully ended. These investigators followed this report with a trial of the same mixture of probiotic and prebiotic agents in seven additional patients, administered three times daily for an average duration of 36 months. Success was repeated, as six of the seven patients ended parenteral nutrition in concert with diminished intestinal colonization with methicillin-resistant *S. aureus*, *Pseudomonas* species, and *Candida* species.[34] Additionally, several studies report that therapy with probiotic *Lactobacillus* sp., which predominantly produces l-lactate rather than d-lactate, reduces the occurrence of d-lactic acidosis.[14,35,36]

PROBIOTICS AND CHRONIC LIVER DISEASE

There are indications the hepatic cirrhosis favors small intestinal bacterial overgrowth, even in the absence of coexisting, structural intestinal tract abnormalities.[37] The presence of intestinal bacterial overgrowth, typically with gram-negative facultative organisms, may contribute to the well-known association between advanced liver disease and systemic infections, including sepsis and spontaneous bacterial peritonitis.[38] Reasons for the association between chronic liver disease and impaired local gastrointestinal immunity remain ill defined. Potential contributor includes inability of the cirrhotic liver to produce adequate quantities of immunogenic proteins such as complement.[39, 40] Other contributors include malnutrition in general, and fat soluble vitamin deficiencies, in particular. In the pediatric population, two major causes of cirrhosis are biliary atresia and the parenteral nutrition when given to patients with short bowel syndrome or intestinal failure of other etiology.[41] The Kasai enteric conduit, used in a surgical management of biliary atresia,[42] is a blind loop of bowel that further promotes bacterial proliferation, particularly when postoperative bile flow is poor. The porto-enterostomy brings enteric flora into close proximity with the normally sterile biliary tree, thereby favoring the occurrence of ascending bacterial cholangitis[43,44] and increases TNF-α production. [45] Prolonged antimicrobial therapy is frequently utilized in this setting.

Conceptually, probiotic therapy should be useful to patients with chronic liver disease, particularly for those with surgical manipulation of the gastrointestinal tract.[46] Whenever there is a perceived need for antibiotics to suppress microbial proliferation, as is the case of biliary atresia,[47] particularly of potentially invasive gram-negative facultative organisms, there may well be a role for probiotics. Although there are no reports of probiotic therapy in patients who have undergone the Kasai procedure for biliary atresia, probiotics have been used to prevent bacterial translocation in other cirrhotic patients, with mixed results.[48–50] More favorably, however, Logurcio et al.[51] demonstrated that one proprietary probiotic, VSL#3, positively influenced biochemical parameters of liver dysfunction in patients with cirrhosis. Finally, modification of the gut flora with probiotics may reduce bacterial production of lithocholic acid, widely recognized as a hepatotoxin, which production is increased in the presence of intestinal bacterial overgrowth.[9,52]

Hepatic encephalopathy (HE) is a well-known complication of cirrhosis. It affects the quality of life and cognitive abilities.[53] Traditionally, HE has been treated with antibiotics and lactulose with various success.[54] Indeed, lactulose can be considered the first prebiotic therapy for HE.[55] Recently, the probiotic and prebiotic therapies gained interest in HE. Stig Bengmark et al.[56] demonstrated that supplementation of cirrhotic patients with a mixture of bioactive fiber of glucan, inulin, pectin, and resistant starch, with or without lactic acid bacteria, reversed the symptoms of minimal HE in 50% of patients vs 13% in the placebo group. In addition, this synbiotic supplementation led to the decrease in *E. coli*, *Staphylococcus* spp., and *Fusobacterium* spp. counts, and the sustained increase in viable counts of *Lactobacillus* spp. Further studies are needed in this area, but initial results are encouraging.[57]

PROBIOTICS IN BONE MARROW AND STEM CELL TRANSPLANTATION

Bone marrow and stem cell transplant recipients are susceptible to opportunistic infection through direct injury to their immune systems from conditioning radiation and chemotherapy. Complications include delayed engraftment or, at the other extreme, graft vs host disease (GVHD), either of which can perpetuate an increased vulnerability to infection. Bacterial lipopolysaccharides produced by gram-negative bacteria in the native alimentary tract appear to amplify the alloresponsivness of the graft[58]; thereby increasing both the frequency and severity of GVHD both in the intestine and in the body elsewhere. The combination of mucosal injury associated with intestinal GVHD[59] and increased numbers of pathogenic microorganisms organisms may contribute to the frequent occurrence of bacteremia and sepsis in these patients.[60,61]

Gerbitz et al.[62] showed that the administration of *L. rhamnosus* GG to mice in an experimental bone marrow transplant model improves survival with reduced scores of intestinal GVHD, compared to controls. Parameters such as weight loss and skin integrity improved the most, linking probiotic therapy to improved cell regeneration and decreased apoptosis. A lower percentage of bacterial translocation from the intestinal tract to the mesenteric lymph nodes was also demonstrated, implying that probiotic therapy produces a generalized downregulation of graft lymphocyte activity that extends beyond an effect in the bowel. A similar phenomenon was described by Budagov et al.[63] who demonstrated that the probiotic *L. acidophilus* reduces systemic cytokine levels, including IL-3 and IL-6, in patients undergoing radiation and chemotherapy, apparently by reducing the proliferation of luminal gram-negative facultative organisms. The ability of probiotics to reduce the density of resident gastrointestinal microflora as well as to inhibit translocation of these organisms and their ability to produce proinflammatory cytokines is likely unique to individual species. Members of the genera *Lactobacillus* and *Bifidobacterium* show the greatest impact in animal models[64,65] and *Saccharomyces boulardii* the least.[66]

PROBIOTICS AND HUMAN IMMUNODEFICIENCY VIRUS

HIV-induced AIDS is a severe acquired immunodeficiency state. Pathologic conditions of the gastrointestinal tract associated with HIV infection are widely recognized.[67] Presentations vary from HIV enteropathy to infectious diarrhea, and diarrhea associated with antiretroviral therapy.[68] The literature regarding utilization of probiotics in HIV-related gastrointestinal injury is scant. The utilization of probiotics appears to be safe.[69] Probiotic supplementation has shown some promise in reducing antiretroviral therapy induced diarrhea. Heiser et al.[70] demonstrated complete resolution of highly active antiretroviral therapy associated diarrhea in 10 out of 28 HIV-positive men treated with a combination of probiotics and fiber. The use of antidiarrheal drugs diminished as well. The majority of the research in this field concentrated on the utilization of various probiotic strains as a therapy for HIV-associated infectious diarrhea [71,72] as well as the utilization of probiotics as a part of nutritional therapy in the developing world [69,72–74] with moderate success. The group at the university of Washington and Canadian R&D Center for probiotics performed an interesting study.[75] The researcher genetically modified *L. reuteri*, which is known to safely colonize the human vagina, to produce anti-HIV proteins, thus causing virucidal effect. This finding raises the possibility of utilizing probiotics as preventative agents for HIV transmission and potential therapeutic vectors.[76,77]

FUTURE CONSIDERATIONS IN PROBIOTIC THERAPY IN IMMUNOCOMPROMISED PATIENTS

One intriguing question is whether viability of probiotics is essential for their function, because, as the foregoing discussion indicates, questions regarding the safety of administering live organisms of any kind to immunocompromised patients remain. Recent studies indicate that viability may not be essential to probiotic function. For example, Jijon et al.[78] demonstrated that DNA derived from a probiotic mixture VSL#3 limits proinflammatory responses in both cell culture and murine models. In the same vein, Rachmilewitz et al.[79] demonstrated that immunostimulatory probiotic-derived DNA alone reduces inflammation in murine colitis. Thus, future probiotic development may profitably focus on the utilization of DNA rather than live strains. Such an approach could diminish if not eliminate the small risk of producing systemic infections with the use of these agents in immunocompromised hosts.

Another issue is utilization of probiotics as therapy for viral infections in immunocompromised states. The efficacy of probiotics in rotavirus diarrhea in otherwise healthy patients is well documented.[80,81] There is emerging evidence that *Lactobacillus* spp. has virucidal effect, thus decreasing the risk of disease transmission.[75,76] Additional patient-based research is required to determine if probiotics will be effective in the prevention and treatment of viral infections in immunocompromised hosts; for instance, rotavirus infections in the post-transplant patients.

SUMMARY

The use of probiotics in immunocompromised patients is still in its infancy; there remain many more questions than answers concerning appropriate indications, optimal types, and combinations of individual species to be administered, optimal dosing schedules, and optimal coincident nutrient regimens, in order to obtain beneficial effects to health while avoiding adverse effects.

REFERENCES

1. Rolfe RD. Interactions among microorganisms of the indigenous intestinal flora and their influence on the host. *Rev Infect Dis* 1984;6(Suppl 1):S73–9.
2. Tlaskalova-Hogenova H, Stepankova R, Hudcovic T, et al. Commensal bacteria (normal microflora), mucosal immunity and chronic inflammatory and autoimmune diseases. *Immunol Lett* 2004;93(2–3):97–108.
3. Kaufman SS. Short Bowel Syndrome, Pediatric Gastrointestinal and Liver Disease: Pathophysiology, Diagnosis, Management (Hardcover) by Robert Wyllie (Editor), Jeffrey S. Hyams (Editor), Chapter 34. 3rd edn ed: Saunders; 2005.
4. Ecker KW, Pistorius G, Harbauer G, Feifel G. [Bacterial clearance of the terminal ileum in relation to the ileocolic connection]. *Zentralblatt fur Chirurgie* 1995;120(4):336–42.
5. Mathias JR, Clench MH. Review: pathophysiology of diarrhea caused by bacterial overgrowth of the small intestine. *Am J Med Sci* 1985;289(6):243–8.
6. Madesh M, Bhaskar L, Balasubramanian KA. Enterocyte viability and mitochondrial function after graded intestinal ischemia and reperfusion in rats. *Mol Cell Biochem* 1997;167(1–2):81–7.
7. Wong JM, de Souza R, Kendall CW, Emam A, Jenkins DJ. Colonic health: fermentation and short chain fatty acids. *J Clin Gastroenterol* 2006;40(3):235–43.
8. Roberfroid M. Dietary fiber, inulin, and oligofructose: a review comparing their physiological effects. *Critl Rev Food Sci Nutr* 1993;33(2):103–48.
9. Benedetti A, Alvaro D, Bassotti C, et al. Cytotoxicity of bile salts against biliary epithelium: a study in isolated bile ductule fragments and isolated perfused rat liver. *Hepatology* 1997;26(1):9–21.
10. Kaufman SS, Loseke CA, Lupo JV, et al. Influence of bacterial overgrowth and intestinal inflammation on duration of parenteral nutrition in children with short bowel syndrome. *J Pediatr* 1997;131(3):356–61.
11. Harmsen HJ, Wildeboer-Veloo AC, Raangs GC, et al. Analysis of intestinal flora development in breast-fed and formula-fed infants by using molecular identification and detection methods. *J Pediatr Gastroenterol Nutr* 2000;30(1):61–7.
12. Rubaltelli FF, Biadaioli R, Pecile P, Nicoletti P. Intestinal flora in breast- and bottle-fed infants. *J Perinat Med* 1998;26(3):186–91.
13. Kocoshis S. Small intestinal failure in children. *Curr Treat Options Gastroenterol* 2001;4(5):423–32.
14. Vanderhoof JA, Young RJ, Murray N, Kaufman SS. Treatment strategies for small bowel bacterial overgrowth in short bowel syndrome. *J Pediatr Gastroenterol Nutr* 1998;27(2):155–60.
15. Zhang DL, Jiang ZW, Jiang J, Cao B, Li JS. D-lactic acidosis secondary to short bowel syndrome. *Postgrad Med J* 2003;79(928):110–2.
16. Oh MS, Phelps KR, Traube M, Barbosa-Saldivar JL, Boxhill C, Carroll HJ. D-lactic acidosis in a man with the short-bowel syndrome. *N Engl J Med* 1979;301(5):249–52.
17. Uribarri J, Oh MS, Carroll HJ. D-lactic acidosis. A review of clinical presentation, biochemical features, and pathophysiologic mechanisms. *Medicine* 1998;77(2):73–82.
18. Jain PK, McNaught CE, Anderson AD, MacFie J, Mitchell CJ. Influence of synbiotic containing Lactobacillus acidophilus La5, Bifidobacterium lactis Bb 12, Streptococcus thermophilus, Lactobacillus bulgaricus and oligofructose on gut barrier function and sepsis in critically ill patients: a randomised controlled trial. *Clin Nutr* 2004;23(4):467–75.
19. Rinne MM, Gueimonde M, Kalliomaki M, Hoppu U, Salminen SJ, Isolauri E. Similar bifidogenic effects of prebiotic-supplemented partially hydrolyzed infant formula and breastfeeding on infant gut microbiota. *FEMS Immunol Med Microbiol* 2005;43(1):59–65.
20. Olesen M, Gudmand-Hoyer E, Holst JJ, Jorgensen S. Importance of colonic bacterial fermentation in short bowel patients: small intestinal malabsorption of easily digestible carbohydrate. *Dig Dis Sci* 1999;44(9):1914–23.
21. Dock DB, Aguilar-Nascimento JE, Latorraca MQ. Probiotics enhance the recovery of gut atrophy in experimental malnutrition. *Biocell* 2004;28(2):143–50.
22. Candy DC, Densham L, Lamont LS, et al. Effect of administration of Lactobacillus casei shirota on sodium balance in an infant with short bowel syndrome. *J Pediatr Gastroenterol Nutr* 2001;32(4):506–8.

23. Wollowski I, Rechkemmer G, Pool-Zobel BL. Protective role of probiotics and prebiotics in colon cancer. *Am J Clin Nutr* 2001;73(2 Suppl):451S–5S.

24. Quigley EM, Quera R. Small intestinal bacterial overgrowth: roles of antibiotics, prebiotics, and probiotics. *Gastroenterology* 2006;130(2 Suppl 1):S78–90.

25. Eizaguirre I, Urkia NG, Asensio AB, et al. Probiotic supplementation reduces the risk of bacterial translocation in experimental short bowel syndrome. *J Pediatr Surg* 2002;37(5):699–702.

26. Borriello SP, Hammes WP, Holzapfel W, et al. Safety of probiotics that contain lactobacilli or bifidobacteria. *Clin Infect Dis* 2003;36(6):775–80.

27. Saxelin M, Chuang NH, Chassy B, et al. Lactobacilli and bacteremia in southern Finland, 1989–1992. *Clin Infect Dis* 1996;22(3):564–6.

28. Kunz AN, Noel JM, Fairchok MP. Two cases of Lactobacillus bacteremia during probiotic treatment of short gut syndrome. *J Pediatr Gastroenterol Nutr* 2004;38(4):457–8.

29. Land MH, Rouster-Stevens K, Woods CR, Cannon ML, Cnota J, Shetty AK. Lactobacillus sepsis associated with probiotic therapy. *Pediatrics* 2005;115(1):178–81.

30. De Groote MA, Frank DN, Dowell E, Glode MP, Pace NR. Lactobacillus rhamnosus GG bacteremia associated with probiotic use in a child with short gut syndrome. *Pediatr Infect Dis J* 2005;24(3):278–80.

31. Patel R, Cockerill FR, Porayko MK, Osmon DR, Ilstrup DM, Keating MR. Lactobacillemia in liver transplant patients. *Clin Infect Dis* 1994;18(2):207–12.

32. Riquelme AJ, Calvo MA, Guzman AM, et al. Saccharomyces cerevisiae fungemia after Saccharomyces boulardii treatment in immunocompromised patients. *J Clin Gastroenterol* 2003;36(1):41–3.

33. Kanamori Y, Hashizume K, Sugiyama M, Morotomi M, Yuki N. Combination therapy with Bifidobacterium breve, Lactobacillus casei, and galactooligosaccharides dramatically improved the intestinal function in a girl with short bowel syndrome: a novel synbiotics therapy for intestinal failure. *Dig Dis Sci* 2001;46(9):2010–6.

34. Kanamori Y, Sugiyama M, Hashizume K, Yuki N, Morotomi M, Tanaka R. Experience of long-term synbiotic therapy in seven short bowel patients with refractory enterocolitis. *J Pediatr Surg* 2004;39(11):1686–92.

35. Bongaerts GP, Tolboom JJ, Naber AH, et al. Role of bacteria in the pathogenesis of short bowel syndrome-associated D-lactic acidemia. *Microb Pathog* 1997;22(5):285–93.

36. Coronado BE, Opal SM, Yoburn DC. Antibiotic-induced D-lactic acidosis. *Ann Intern Med* 1995;122(11):839–42.

37. Almeida J, Galhenage S, Yu J, Kurtovic J, Riordan SM. Gut flora and bacterial translocation in chronic liver disease. *World J Gastroenterol* 2006;12(10):1493–502.

38. Christou L, Pappas G, Falagas ME. Bacterial infection-related morbidity and mortality in cirrhosis. *Am J Gastroenterol* 2007;102(7):1510–7.

39. Miyaike J, Iwasaki Y, Takahashi A, et al. Regulation of circulating immune complexes by complement receptor type 1 on erythrocytes in chronic viral liver diseases. *Gut* 2002;51(4):591–6.

40. Sobhonslidsuk A, Roongpisuthipong C, Nantiruj K, et al. Impact of liver cirrhosis on nutritional and immunological status. *J Med Assoc Thai* 2001;84(7):982–8.

41. 1996–2005 OSAR. 2006 Annual Report of the U.S. Organ Procurement and Transplantation Network and the Scientific Registry of Transplant Recipients: Transplant Data 1996–2005.. In: Organ Procurement and Transplantation Network; 2006.

42. Kasai M. Treatment of biliary atresia with special reference to hepatic porto-enterostomy and its modifications. *Prog Pediatr Surg* 1974;6:5–52.

43. Gardikis S, Antypas S, Kambouri K, et al. The Roux-en-Y procedure in congenital hepato-biliary disorders. *Rom J Gastroenterol* 2005;14(2):135–40.

44. Riordan SM, Williams R. The intestinal flora and bacterial infection in cirrhosis. *J Hepatol* 2006;45(5):744–57.

45. Narayanaswamy B, Gonde C, Tredger JM, Hussain M, Vergani D, Davenport M. Serial circulating markers of inflammation in biliary atresia--evolution of the post-operative inflammatory process. *Hepatology* 2007;46(1):180–7.

46. Nomura T, Tsuchiya Y, Nashimoto A, et al. Probiotics reduce infectious complications after pancreaticoduodenectomy. *Hepatogastroenterology* 2007;54(75):661–3.

47. Bu LN, Chen HL, Chang CJ, et al. Prophylactic oral antibiotics in prevention of recurrent cholangitis after the Kasai portoenterostomy. *J Pediatr Surg* 2003;38(4):590–3.

48. Adawi D, Kasravi FB, Molin G, Jeppsson B. Effect of Lactobacillus supplementation with and without arginine on liver damage and bacterial translocation in an acute liver injury model in the rat. *Hepatology* 1997;25(3):642–7.

49. Chiva M, Soriano G, Rochat I, et al. Effect of Lactobacillus johnsonii La1 and antioxidants on intestinal flora and bacterial translocation in rats with experimental cirrhosis. *J Hepatol* 2002;37(4):456–62.

50. Wiest R, Garcia-Tsao G. Bacterial translocation (BT) in cirrhosis. *Hepatology* 2005;41(3):422–33.

51. Loguercio C, Federico A, Tuccillo C, et al. Beneficial effects of a probiotic VSL#3 on parameters of liver dysfunction in chronic liver diseases. *J Clin Gastroenterol* 2005;39(6):540–3.

52. Fickert P, Fuchsbichler A, Marschall HU, et al. Lithocholic acid feeding induces segmental bile duct obstruction and destructive cholangitis in mice. *Am J Pathol* 2006;168(2):410–22.

53. Groeneweg M, Quero JC, De Bruijn I, et al. Subclinical hepatic encephalopathy impairs daily functioning. *Hepatology* 1998;28(1):45–9.

54. Rothenberg ME, Keeffe EB. Antibiotics in the management of hepatic encephalopathy: an evidence-based review. *Reviews in gastroenterological disorders* 2005;5(Suppl 3):26–35.

55. Salminen S, Salminen E. Lactulose, lactic acid bacteria, intestinal microecology and mucosal protection. *Scand J Gastroenterol* 1997;222:45–8.

56. Liu Q, Duan ZP, Ha DK, Bengmark S, Kurtovic J, Riordan SM. Synbiotic modulation of gut flora: effect on minimal hepatic encephalopathy in patients with cirrhosis. *Hepatology* 2004;39(5):1441–9.

57. Solga SF, Diehl AM. Gut flora-based therapy in liver disease? The liver cares about the gut. *Hepatology* 2004;39(5):1197–200.

58. Cooke KR, Hill GR, Crawford JM, et al. Tumor necrosis factor- alpha production to lipopolysaccharide stimulation by donor cells predicts the severity of experimental acute graft-versus-host disease. *J Clin Invest* 1998;102(10):1882–91.

59. Koltun WA, Bloomer MM, Colony P, Kauffman GL. Increased intestinal permeability in rats with graft versus host disease. *Gut* 1996;39(2):291–8.

60. Sayer HG, Longton G, Bowden R, Pepe M, Storb R. Increased risk of infection in marrow transplant patients receiving methylprednisolone for graft-versus-host disease prevention. *Blood* 1994;84(4):1328–32.

61. Busca A, Locatelli F, Barbui A, et al. Infectious complications following nonmyeloablative allogeneic hematopoietic stem cell transplantation. *Transpl Infect Dis* 2003;5(3):132–9.

62. Gerbitz A, Schultz M, Wilke A, et al. Probiotic effects on experimental graft-versus-host disease: let them eat yogurt. *Blood* 2004;103(11):4365–7.

63. Budagov RS, Ul'ianova LP, Pospelova VV. [The protective activity of a new variant of the probiotic acilact in exposure to ionizing radiation and anticancer chemotherapy under experimental conditions]. *Vestn Ross Akad Med Nauk* 2006(2):3–5.

64. Adawi D, Molin G, Jeppsson B. Inhibition of nitric oxide production and the effects of arginine and Lactobacillus administration in an acute liver injury model. *Ann Surg* 1998;228(6):748–55.

65. Garcia-Urkia N, Asensio AB, Zubillaga Azpiroz I, et al. [Beneficial effects of Bifidobacterium lactis in the prevention of bacterial translocation in experimental short bowel syndrome]. *Cir Pediatr* 2002;15(4):162–5.

66. Zaouche A, Loukil C, De Lagausie P, et al. Effects of oral Saccharomyces boulardii on bacterial overgrowth, translocation, and intestinal adaptation after small-bowel resection in rats. *Scand J Gastroenterol* 2000;35(2):160–5.

67. Grohmann GS, Glass RI, Pereira HG, et al Enteric viruses and diarrhea in HIV-infected patients. Enteric Opportunistic Infections Working Group. *N Engl J Med* 1993;329(1):14–20.

68. Mitra AK, Hernandez CD, Hernandez CA, Siddiq Z. Management of diarrhoea in HIV-infected patients. *Int J STD & AIDS* 2001;12(10):630–9.

69. Wolf BW, Wheeler KB, Ataya DG, Garleb KA. Safety and tolerance of Lactobacillus reuteri supplementation to a population infected with the human immunodeficiency virus. *Food Chem Toxicol* 1998;36(12):1085–94.

70. Heiser CR, Ernst JA, Barrett JT, French N, Schutz M, Dube MP. Probiotics, soluble fiber, and L-Glutamine (GLN) reduce nelfinavir (NFV)- or lopinavir/ritonavir (LPV/r)-related diarrhea. *J Int Assoc Phys AIDS Care (Chic Ill)* 2004;3(4):121–9.

71. Alak JI, Wolf BW, Mdurvwa EG, et al Supplementation with Lactobacillus reuteri or L. acidophilus reduced intestinal shedding of cryptosporidium parvum oocysts in immunodeficient C57BL/6 mice. *Cell Mol Biol (Noisy-le-grand)* 1999;45(6):855–63.

72. Reid G, Anand S, Bingham MO, et al. Probiotics for the developing world. *J Clin Gastroenterol* 2005;39(6):485–8.

73. Brink M, Todorov SD, Martin JH, Senekal M, Dicks LM. The effect of prebiotics on production of antimicrobial compounds, resistance to growth at low pH and in the presence of bile, and adhesion of probiotic cells to intestinal mucus. *J Appl Microbiol* 2006;100(4):813–20.

74. Simpore J, Zongo F, Kabore F, et al. Nutrition rehabilitation of HIV-infected and HIV-negative undernourished children utilizing spirulina. *Ann Nutr Metab* 2005;49(6):373–80.

75. Liu JJ, Reid G, Jiang Y, Turner MS, Tsai CC. Activity of HIV entry and fusion inhibitors expressed by the human vaginal colonizing probiotic Lactobacillus reuteri RC-14. *Cell Microbiol* 2007;9(1):120–30.

76. Botic T, Klingberg TD, Weingartl H, Cencic A. A novel eukaryotic cell culture model to study antiviral activity of potential probiotic bacteria. *Int J Food Microbiol* 2007;115(2):227–34.

77. Rao S, Hu S, McHugh L, et al. Toward a live microbial microbicide for HIV: commensal bacteria secreting an HIV fusion inhibitor peptide. *Proc Natl Acad Sci U S A* 2005;102(34):11993–8.

78. Jijon H, Backer J, Diaz H, et al. DNA from probiotic bacteria modulates murine and human epithelial and immune function. *Gastroenterology* 2004;126(5):1358–73.

79. Rachmilewitz D, Karmeli F, Takabayashi K, et al. Immunostimulatory DNA ameliorates experimental and spontaneous murine colitis. *Gastroenterology* 2002;122(5):1428–41.

80. Huang JS, Bousvaros A, Lee JW, Diaz A, Davidson EJ. Efficacy of probiotic use in acute diarrhea in children: a meta-analysis. *Dig Dis Sci* 2002;47(11):2625–34.

81. Szajewska H, Mrukowicz JZ. Probiotics in the treatment and prevention of acute infectious diarrhea in infants and children: a systematic review of published randomized, double-blind, placebo-controlled trials. *J Pediatr Gastroenterol Nutr* 2001;33 (Suppl 2):S17–25.

17 Role of Probiotics in the Management of *Helicobacter pylori* Infection

Philip M. Sherman and Kathene C. Johnson-Henry

Key Points

- *Helicobacter pylori* is a gram-negative organism that colonizes the stomach of humans and causes chronic-active gastritis, peptic ulcer disease, and gastric cancers.
- Currently, probiotics do not appear to have a role as sole therapy for use in either the prevention or treatment of *H. pylori* infection.
- A variety of probiotic agents are useful as adjunctive therapy, which can both enhance the success of eradicating the pathogen while reducing the frequency and severity of adverse effects arising from treatment regimens.
- Future studies should assess the role of prebiotics and probiotics as additional options for use in the prevention and treatment of *H. pylori* infection in humans.

Key Words: Adjunctive therapy, children, *Helicobacter pylori,* probiotics.

INTRODUCTION

Helicobacter pylori is a gram-negative, spiral-shaped, microaerophilic organism that colonizes the stomach of humans and causes chronic-active gastritis, peptic ulcer disease, and gastric cancers, including adenocarcinoma of the stomach and MALT (mucosal-associated lymphoid tumor) lymphomas [1]. Although the organism is now known to have infected humans for millennia [2], it was first identified and successfully cultured in the early 1980s. For their seminal discovery of this gastric bacterial pathogen, in 2005, Dr. Barry J. Marshall and Dr. J. Robin Warren were awarded the Nobel Prize in Medicine or Physiology (http://nobelprize.org/medicine).

It is now known that *H. pylori* colonizes the stomach of over half of the world's human population, primarily those who reside in poor socioeconomic circumstances and in developing nations. Infection is generally first acquired in children, who may be entirely asymptomatic, and then persists for life, unless specific eradication therapy is

From: *Nutrition and Health: Probiotics in Pediatric Medicine*
Edited by: S. Michail and P.M. Sherman © Humana Press, Totowa, NJ

initiated. All infected individuals have mucosal inflammation in the stomach (i.e., gastritis) in response to the organism, but only a subset will develop disease complications, such as an ulcer in the stomach or proximal duodenum and cancer in either the body or the antrum of the stomach [3], later on in life.

It is estimated that the lifetime risk of developing peptic ulceration is roughly 15%. However, this is an exceedingly important disease, because it has serious morbidity (i.e., pain, hemorrhage, and perforation) and mortality. The natural history of *H. pylori*-associated peptic ulcers is for recurrences of the ulceration, with attendant complications such as hemorrhage, perforation, and death. These complications are completely prevented by successful eradication of the gastric pathogen [4].

H. pylori infection is also associated with an increased risk of gastric adenocarcinoma and MALT (mucosa-associated lymphoid tissue) lymphoma. Indeed, *H. pylori* is the first bacterium ever to be classified as a class 1 carcinogen by the World Health Organization. Although the final verdict is not yet in, there is increasing evidence indicating that eradication of the gastric infection early in the sequence of events leading to carcinogenesis can prevent the development of malignant transformation [5]. The role of *H. pylori* infection in a variety of extra-gastric symptoms, such as sideropenic iron-deficiency anemia and immune thrombocytopenic purpura, is the subject of current research efforts [6].

CURRENT TREATMENTS TO ERADICATE *H. PYLORI* INFECTION

Eradication of *H. pylori* infection, both in animal models and in human subjects, is not successful when using antibiotics as monotherapy or dual therapy using combinations of an acid-suppressing agent and an antibiotic or two antibiotics without acid blockage [7]. Trial-and-error studies, first undertaken in infected adults, showed that to achieve eradication success rates in the range of >80% of treated subjects required the use of potent acid suppression in combination with two antibiotics—the so-called triple therapy [8]. First-line treatment regimens generally employ a proton pump inhibitor and two antibiotics (such as amoxicillin, metronidazole, or tetracycline) twice a day for 7–14 days. However, such combination therapy regimens suffer from suboptimal patient compliance and the frequent development of adverse side effects such as antibiotic-associated diarrhea. Moreover, a recent critical review of the literature available regarding eradication of *H. pylori* infection in children with a variety of combination treatment regimens raised concerns about the efficacy of current approaches, particularly in the developing world where antibiotic resistance profiles (which influence greatly successful responses to therapy) and the burden-of-illness are high [9]. These concerns have been confirmed by the review of a registry of European centers, which showed that overall eradication rates for *H. pylori*-infected children is just 65% [10], when employing triple therapy regimens that are based on studies previously undertaken in adults where eradication rates of >80% are considered to be acceptable criteria for first-line options of therapy [7]. Taken together, these studies show that the current management strategies to eradicate *H. pylori* infection in children are inadequate. Clearly, additional, novel approaches to the prevention and treatment of this gastric infection are urgently required [11].

PROBIOTICS IN VITRO AND IN TISSUE CULTURE EPITHELIAL CELL MODEL SYSTEMS

Multiple studies have shown that a number of probiotic strains are able to inhibit the growth of *H. pylori* when the organisms are cultured together in vitro [12]. A number of mechanisms of action appear to mediate the observed effects of probiotics. For instance, culture supernatants of *Lactobacillus* species possess anti-*Helicobacter* activity that are reported as both dependent [13–15] and independent [16] of lactic acid production and local pH. In one study, the inhibitory effects of the *Bacillus subtilis* 3 against *H. pylori* was secreted into the culture supernatant and reported as independent of both pH and concentration of organic acids. Rather, the probiotic produced and secreted active antibacterial compounds, including amicoumacin A [17].

Some studies show that probiotics are able to prevent pathogen binding to host cell receptors. For instance, in vitro modeling of colonization resistance has shown, by using a thin-layer chromatography overlay-binding assay, that some *Lactobacillus reuteri* strains (including JCM 1081 and TM 105) bind to gangliosides and sulfatides expressed on the plasma membrane of host epithelia and, thereby, block binding of *H. pylori* to cell surface receptors [18].

Cell surface-associated heat shock proteins, such as GroEL, expressed by lactic acid-producing organisms can result in the aggregation of *H. pylori*, which prevents pathogen binding to epithelial cells grown in tissue culture [19]. Heat-resistant and protease-sensitive materials elaborated by some, but not all, Bifidobacteria strains also inhibit the growth of *H. pylori* in vitro, irrespective of their antimicrobial resistance status [20].

One study showed that *L. gasseri* OLL2716 blocks *H. pylori*-induced release of the chemokine interleukin-8, responsible for attracting polymorphonuclear leukocytes to sites of injury and inflammation, from infected gastric MKN45 epithelial cells grown in tissue culture [21]. The effect of the probiotic on blocking chemokine production and secretion from infected epithelia was dependent on live probiotics. Both heat-killed and ultraviolet light-irradiated *L. gasseri* did not block interleukin-8 transcription and translation by gastric cells infected with *H. pylori*. Another study that emphasized differences between probiotic strains *Bifidobacterium bifidum* YIT 4007, clone BF-1 demonstrated a concentration-dependent inhibition of interleukin-8 production and secretion by *H. pylori*-infected gastric GCIY cells, whereas *Streptococcus thermophilus* YIT 2021 had no inhibitory effect [22]. Taken together, these in vitro studies highlight the potential mechanisms of the action of various probiotics and emphasize the importance of considering differences in the effects of various species and strains tested as probiotic agents.

PROBIOTICS IN ANIMAL MODELS OF *H. PYLORI* INFECTION

Probiotics have been shown to both reduce the frequency of *H. pylori* colonization and to ameliorate the severity of mucosal inflammation in the stomach of infected mice [23]. Using the mouse-adapted *H. pylori* strain SS-1, a mixture of probiotics was placed in the drinking water of mice both before and during the course of infection. Compared to mice provided drinking water without probiotics, a mixture of *L. helveticus,* strain R0052 [24] and *L. rhamnosus,* strain R0011 reduced the severity of gastric injury and the frequency of detectable *H. pylori* colonization in infected mice, without evidence of any adverse consequences on animal well being [23]. Another study showed similar results: *L. casei, strain Shirota* provided in the drinking water of mice infected with *H. pylori*, strain SS-1 reduced bacterial colonization and ameliorated inflammation in the stomach, but did not eradicate the gastric infection [25]. Similar beneficial effects of *L. salivarius* in reducing bacterial colonization and gastric inflammation was observed when employing a gnotobiotic mouse model of *H. pylori* infection [26]. Kabir and colleagues [27] reported that *L. salivarius* prevents *H. pylori* colonization of gnotobiotic mice only if the probiotic is provided in the drinking water in advance of orogastric challenge with the gastric pathogen. That is, *L. saliviruis* does not eradicate established *H. pylori* colonization—at least, in this animal model of infection.

The Mongolian gerbil serves as another small animal model of *H. pylori* infection. The combination of *L. helveticus* and *L. rhamnosus* has been provided to gerbils by intragastric lavage once just before challenge with the gastric pathogen and then once daily thereafter. Using this experimental approach, mucosal injury and inflammation in the stomach was partially prevented by probiotics, but not to the same extent as using traditional triple therapy to eradicate the gastric pathogen [28].

The choice of probiotic is likely to be an important variable that impacts on efficacy. For instance, *L. johnsonii* La1 provided in drinking water does not prevent *H. pylori*, strain SS-1 colonization of mice, even though the probiotic does block chemokine (interleukin-8) production and secretion by human gastric epithelial AGS cells grown in tissue culture [29]

PROBIOTICS AS SOLE THERAPY USED TO ERADICATE *H. PYLORI* INFECTION IN HUMANS

Clinical trials in adults indicate that probiotics are not effective as single therapy in eradicating established *H. pylori* infection in human subjects [22, 30]. Culture supernatants derived from a probiotic strain are able to suppress the growth of *H. pylori* both in vitro and in vivo, but does not eradicate the infection in humans when used together with a proton pump inhibitor, but without concurrent administration of antibiotics [31]. An open-label, uncontrolled trial of a probiotic drink containing a mixture of four bacterial strains (10^9 in 250 mL once daily of an equal mixture of *L. rhamnosus* GG, *L. rhamnosus* LC705, *P. freudenreichii* ssp. *shermanii* JS, and *B. lactis* Bb12) demonstrated no impact on gastric inflammation in a limited case series of adults infected with *H. pylori* [32]. Two-thirds of *H. pylori*-infected children in Chile had the infection successfully eradicated with triple therapy (proton pump inhibitor and amoxicillin and clarithromycin for 8 days), compared with just 12% of children treated with the yeast probiotic *Saccharomyces boulardii* and 7% of those treated with *L. acidophilus* LB. Both probiotics were given once daily for 8 weeks [33].

There is discordance between *H. pylori* susceptibility to a wide variety of products, including antibiotics and proton pump inhibitors, in vitro assays and rates of successful eradication of the organism from the stomach of humans in vivo. These differences serve to emphasize the importance of undertaking rigorous clinical trials to provide level 1 evidence (i.e., randomized and controlled prospective studies) documenting the efficacy of novel therapeutics, including probiotics, in defining optimal management strategies to prevent or eradicate *H. pylori* infections.

The role of probiotics in preventing the acquisition of *H. pylori* infection in uninfected subjects has not been investigated formally. Evidence from animal studies suggests that this may well prove to be a worthwhile area to pursue in greater detail. The potential for using probiotics in the management of subjects who are treated to eradicate the gastric infection, but are at high risk for reinfection [34], should be tested in the setting of a randomized, prospective clinical trial. Another study group to consider is the use of probiotics to prevent initial acquisition of *H. pylori* in young children (infants and toddlers) who reside in regions of the world with a high prevalence of infection, before their first exposure to the pathogen.

PROBIOTICS AS ADJUNCTIVE THERAPY TO TREAT *H. PYLORI*-INDUCED INFLAMMATION AND ULCERATION

Efficacy Studies

A recent study indicates that the effectiveness of an eradication therapy regimen can be enhanced by using probiotics [35]. In a randomized, controlled trial of 138 subjects who had previously failed a course of triple therapy, the rate of successful *H. pylori* eradication was significantly higher (85%) in subjects treated with quadruple therapy (omeprazole, amoxicillin, metronidazole, and bismuth subcitrate) and a yogurt containing a mixture of *L. acidophilus*, *L. bulgaricus*, *S. thermophilus*, and *B. lactis* (>10^9 organisms/mL, with roughly equal amounts of the four strains), compared to patients receiving quadruple therapy without probiotics (71%, $p < 0.05$ on an intent-to-treat analysis). Another study undertaken in Crakow, Poland, confirmed these results [36]. Supplementation with the combination of *L. helveticus* and *L. rhamnosus* in 53 subjects increased the efficacy of eradication of *H. pylori* using triple therapy to 94%, compared to 86% of 192 patients treated with triple therapy alone (proton pump inhibitor, amoxicillin, and clarithromycin). A more recent open, prospective trial undertaken in Italy showed that a mixture of nine probiotics and bovine-derived lactoferrin and inulin, as a prebiotic, increased the success rate of eradication to 89% in 105 subjects, compared to just 72% in 101 subjects ($p = 0.005$) treated with triple therapy alone for 7 days [37].

It is not certain if probiotics need to be delivered in a viable state in order to enhance the eradication *H. pylori* when used together with standard triple therapy regimens. For instance, one study reported that an inactivated preparation of *L. acidophilus* increased the success of eradication of *H. pylori* from 70% of 60 subjects treated with triple therapy (proton pump inhibitor and amoxiclliin and clarithromycin for 7 days) alone to 87% of 59 patients treated with triple therapy and inactivated probiotic ($p = 0.02$) [38].

One trial evaluated 86 *H. pylori*-infected children living in the Czech Republic. This prospective, randomized, and controlled study assessed the success of triple therapy (proton pump inhibitor, amoxicillin, and clarithryomycin) given for 7 days together with unfermented pasteurized milk, compared with the same triple therapy regimen and 10^{10} colony-forming units of *L. casei* DN-114 001 given once daily, in 100 mL of fermented milk, for 14 days [39]. Success of eradication was measured some 4 weeks later by two well-established indirect, but noninvasive, assays of gastric colonization status: urea breath and stool *H. pylori* antigen testing. On the basis of an intent-to-treat analysis, triple therapy alone (57.5%) was less successful than triple therapy and probiotic (84.6%) in eradicating

H. pylori infection ($p < 0.01$). By contrast, another study evaluating 65 *H. pylori*-infected children living in Argentina reported no benefit of adding yoghurt, containing 10^7 bacteria (*B. animalis* and *L. casei*) in 250 mL once daily for 3 months, to standard eradication triple therapy given for 7 days [40]. However, eradication rates—monitored by ^{13}C urea breath testing—were low in both groups (46% and 38%, respectively; $p = NS$).

Studies on Altering the Frequency of Adverse Events

As recently reviewed by Gotteland et al. [41], in six trials including a total of 607 subjects, probiotics were shown to be effective when employed as adjunctive therapy in reducing the frequency of adverse side effects of standard medical therapies used to eradicate *H. pylori* infection. For instance, a study on adults undertaken in Finland compared a combination of four probiotics administered in a fruit drink once daily (*L. rhamnosus* GG, *L. rhamnosus* LC705, *B. breve* Bb99, and *Propionibacterium freudenreichii* ssp. *shermanii* JS) to placebo (fruit drink alone) given during and for the 3 weeks following a course of anti-*Helicobacter* eradication therapy (7 days of proton pump inhibitor, amoxicillin and clarithromycin). Eradication rates were higher in the probiotics-treated group (91%) versus the placebo (79%), but the differences did not reach statistical significance—perhaps related to a relatively small sample size and a type 2 statistical error. However, the probiotic group reported statistically significant fewer treatment-related side effects, compared with those subjects who received placebo. There was a reduction in epigastric pain and bloating, but not diarrhea [42]. The precise mechanism(s) of action underlying this apparent benefit is not known. However, preliminary evidence suggests that it may relate to reducing alterations in the normal, commensal microbiota of the colon induced by anti-*Helicobacter* triple therapy regimens [43].

A study of 20 *H. pylori*-infected children in Italy showed that *L. reuteri* (10^8 colony-forming units daily) is more effective than placebo, given to an equal number of study subjects, in reducing both the frequency and severity of antibiotic-associated side effects while on a 10-day course of sequential therapy using 5 days of a proton pump inhibitor and amoxicillin followed by another 5 days of the acid-suppressing agent and clarithromycin and tinidazole [44].

META-ANALYSES

There are a number of published systematic reviews and meta-analyses of the English language biomedical literature related to the role of probiotics in the management of *H. pylori* infection [45, 46, 47, 48, 49]. Gotteland et al. [41] summarized ten clinical trials (eight in adults, two in children) showing that a variety of probiotic agents when used alone have limited efficacy in eradicating the organism from the stomach. This is not too surprising since antibiotics and acid-suppressing agents as monotherapy are also not effective in eradicating the gastric pathogen. A subsequent meta-analysis identified 14 randomized clinical trials involving 1,671 subjects, which showed that adding probiotics to standard *H. pylori* treatment regimens enhances eradication rates (83.6% versus 74.8%, summary odds ratio = 1.84, 95% confidence intervals: 1.34–2.54) and reduces therapy-related adverse effects (24.7% versus 38.5%; OR = 0.44; 95% CI: 0.30–0.66), in particular, diarrhea (OR = 0.34; 95% CI: 0.22–0.52) [50]. Evaluation using Egger's regression test and a funnel plot did not show evidence of a publication bias, but it is noted that none of the 14 trials included in the meta-analysis included patients of North America.

CLINICAL PRACTICE GUIDELINES AND CONSENSUS STATEMENTS

A number of expert opinion statements and clinical practice guidelines, from various parts of the world, have been published that relate to the management of children with *H. pylori* infection [51–54]. However, none of these reports considers the role of probiotics in the management of this gastric infection [55]. Surprisingly, the role of probiotics in the management of *H. pylori* infection in patients over 18 years was also not considered in the most recent consensus conference update of the European *Helicobacter* Study Group [56]. As summarized in the present systematic review, there now appears to be sufficient evidence published in the peer reviewed biomedical literature—related to both models of infection and studies in humans of various age groups—to indicate that a critical appraisal of the role of probiotics as an adjunct to treatment of *H. pylori* infection in children by a panel of international experts in the field is now most timely and well justified.

SUMMARY AND CURRENT RECOMMENDATIONS

To date, probiotics do not appear to have a role as sole therapy for use in either the prevention or treatment of *H. pylori* infection. On the other hand, there is increasing evidence that a variety of probiotic agents are useful as adjunctive therapy, which can both enhance the success of eradicating the gastric pathogen while, at the same time, reduce the frequency and severity of adverse effects arising from the other agents that are employed in current combination treatment regimens. Experimental studies, both in vitro and in animal models, support the use of probiotics as adjuncts to *Helicobacter* eradication regimens. Future studies should assess the role of prebiotics and synbiotics (i.e., the combination of pre- and probiotics) and products derived from probiotics (such as DNA and surface-layer proteins) as additional options for use in the prevention and treatment of *H. pylori* infection in humans.

REFERENCES

1. Ernst P, Peura DA, Crowe SE. The translation of *Helicobacter pylori* basic research to patient care. Gastroenterology 2006;130:188–2006.
2. Linz B, Balloux F, Moodley Y, et al. An African origin for the intimate association between humans and *Helicobacter pylori*. Nature 2007;445:915–918.
3. Falkow S. Is persistent bacterial infection good for your health? Cell 2006;124:699–702.
4. Gold B, Colletti RB, Abbott M, et al. *Helicobacter pylori* infection in children: recommendations for diagnosis and treatment. J Pediatr Gastroenterol Nutr 2003;31:490–497.
5. Matysiak-Budnik T, Megraud F. *Helicobacter pylori* infection and gastric cancer. Eur J Cancer 2006;42:708–716.
6. Sherman PM, Lin FYH. Extradigestive manifestions of *Helicobacter pylori* infection in children and adolescents. Can J Gastroenterol 2005;19:421–424.
7. Hunt RH, Smaill FM, Fallone CA, Sherman PM, Van Zanten SJV, Thomson ABR . Implications of antibiotic resistance in the management of *Helicobacter pylori* infection: Canadian Helicobacter Study Group. Can J Gastroenterol 2000;14:862–868.

8. Ford AC, Delaney BC, Forman D, Moayyedi P. Eradication therapy for peptic ulcer disease in *Helicobacter pylori* positive patients. Cochrane Database Syst Rev 2006; Apr. 19;(2):CD003840

9. Khurana R, Fischback L, Chiba N, et al. Meta-analysis: *Helicobacter pylori* eradication treatment efficacy in children. Aliment Pharmacol Ther 2007;25:523–536.

10. Oderda G, Shcherbakov P, Bonterns P, et al. Results of the pediatric European register for treatment of *Helicobacter pylori* (PERTH). Helicobacter 2007;12:150–156.

11. Emancipator D, Nedrud JG, Czinn SJ. *Helicobacter pylori* vaccines: is DNA the answer? Helicobacter 2006;11:513–516.

12. Rokka S, Pihlanto A, Korhonen H, Joutsjoki V. *In vitro* growth inhibition of *Helicobacter pylori* by lactobacilli belonging to the *Lactobacillus plantarum* group. Lett Appl Microbiol 2006;43:508–513.

13. Bhatia SJ, Kochar N, Abraham P, Nair NG, Mehta AP. *Lactobacillus acidophilus* inhibits growth of *Campylobacter pylori in vitro*. J Clin Microbiol 1989;27:2328–2330.

14. Midolo PD, Lambert JR, Hull R, Luo F, Grayson ML. *In vitro* inhibition of *Helicobacter pylori* NCTC 11637 by organic acids and lactic acid bacteria. J Appl Bacteriol 1995;79:475–479.

15. Lorca GL, Wadstrom T, Font de Valdez G, Ljungh A. *Lactobacillus acidophilus* autolysins inhibit *Helicobacter pylori in vitro*. Curr Microbiol 2001;42:39–44.

16. Coconnier M-H, Lievin V, Hemery E, Servin AL. Antagonistic activity against *Helicobacter* infection *in vitro* and *in vivo* by the human *Lactobacillus acidophilus* strain LB. Appl Environ Microbiol 1998;64:4573–4580

17. Pinchuk IV, Bressollier P, Verneuil B, et al. *In vitro* anti-*Helicobacter pylori* activity of the probiotic strain *Bacillus subtilis* 3 is due to the secretion of antibiotics. Antimicrob Agents Chemother 2001;45:3156–3161.

18. Mukai T, Assaka T, Sato E, Mori K, Matsumoto M, Ohori H. Inhibition of binding of *Helicobacter pylori* to glycolipid receptors by the probiotic *Lactobacillus reuteri*. FEMS Immunol Med Microbiol 2002;32:105–110.

19. Bergonzelli GE, Granato D, Pridmore RD, et al. GroEL of *Lactobacillus johnsonii* La1 (NCC 533) is cell surface associated: potential role in interactions with the host and the gastric pathogen *Helicobacter pylori*. Infect Immun 2006;74:425–434.

20. Collado MC, Gonzalez A, Gonzalez R, Hernandez M, Ferrus MA, Sanz Y. Antimicrobial peptides are among the antagonistic metabolites produced by *Bifidiobacterium* against *Helicobacter pylori*. Int J Antimicrob Agents 2005;25:385–391.

21. Tamura A, Kumai H, Nakamichi N, et al. Suppression of *Helicobacter pylori*-induced interleukin-8 production *in vitro* and within the gastric mucosa by a live *Lactobacillus* strain. J Gastroenterol Hepatol 2006;21:1399–1406.

22. Miki K, Urita Y, Ishikawa F, et al. Effect of *Bifidobacterium bifidum* fermented milk on *Helicobacter pylori* and serum pepsinogen in humans. J Dairy Sci 2007;90:2630–2640.

23. Johnson-Henry KC, Mitchell DJ, Avitzur Y, Galindo-Mata E, Jones NL, Sherman PM. Probotics reduce bacterial colonization and gastric inflammation in *H. pylori*-infected mice. Dig Dis Sci 2004;49:1095–1102.

24. Johnson-Henry KC, Hagen KE, Gordonpour M, Tompkins TA, Sherman PM. Surface-layer protein extracts from *Lactobacillus helveticus* inhibit enterohaemorrhagic *Escherichia coli* O157:H7 adhesion to epithelial cells. Cell Microbiol 2007;9:356–367.

25. Sgouras D, Maragkoudakis P, Petraki K, et al. *In vitro* and *in vivo* inhibition of *Helicobacter pylori* by *Lactobacillus casei* strain Shirota. Appl Environ Microbiol 2004;70:518–526.

26. Aiba Y, Suzuki N, Kabir AMA, Takagi A, Koga Y. Lactic acid-mediated suppression of *Helicobacter pylori* by the oral administration of *Lactobacillus salivarius* as a probiotic in a gnotbiotic murine model. Am J Gastroenterol 1998;93:2097–2101.

27. Kabir AMA, Aiba Y, Takagi A, Kamiya S, Miwa T, Koga Y. Prevention of *Helicobacter pylori* infection by lactobacilli in a gnotobiotic murine model. Gut 1997;41:49–55.

28. Brzozowski T, Konturek PC, Mierzwa M, et al. Effect of probiotics and triple eradication therapy on the cyclooxygenase (COX)-2 expression, apoptosis, and functional gastric mucosal impairment in *Helicobacter pylori*-infected Mongolian gerbils. Helicobacter 2006;11:10–20.

29. Sgouras DN, Panayotopoulou EG, Martinez-Gonzalez B, Petraki K, Michopoulos S, Mentis A. *Lactobacillus johnsonii* La1 attenuates *Helicobacter pylori*-associated gastritis and reduces levels of proinflammatory chemokines in C57BL/6 mice. Clin Diag Lab Immunol 2005;12:1378–1386.

30. Sakamoto I Igarashi M, Kimura K, Takagi A, Miwa T, Koga Y. Suppressive effect of *Lactobacillus gasseri* OLL 2716 (LG21) on *Helicobacter pylori* infection in humans. J Antimicrob Chemother 2001;47:709–710.
31. Michetti P, Dorta G, Wiesel PH, et al. Effect of whey-based culture supernatant of *Lactobacillus acidophilus (johnsonii)* La1 on *Helicobacter pylori* infection in humans. Digestion 1999;60:203–209.
32. Myllyluoma E, Kajander K, Mikkola H, et al. Probiotic intervention decreases serum gastrin-17 in *Helicobacter pylori* infection. Dig Liver Sci 2007;39:516–523.
33. Gotteland M, Poliak L, Cruchet S, Brunser O. Effect of regular ingestion of *Saccharomyces boulardii* plus inulin or *Lactobacillus acidophilus* LB in children colonized by *Helicobacter pylori*. Acta Paediatr 2005;94:1747–1751.
34. Halitim F, Vincent P, Michaud L, et al. High rate of *Helicobacter pylori* reinfection in children and adolescents. Helicobacter 2006;11:168–172.
35. Sheu B-S, Cheng H-C, Kao A-W, Wang S-T, Yang Y-J, Yang H-B, Wu J-J. Pretreatment with *Lactobacillus*- and *Bifidobacterium*-containing yogurt can improve the efficacy of quadruple therapy in eradicating residual *Helicobacter pylori* infection after failed triple therapy. Am J Clin Nutr 2006;83:864–869.
36. Ziemniak W. Efficacy of *Helicobacter pylori* eradication taking into account its resistance to antibiotics. J Physiol Pharmacol 2006;57(Suppl 3):123–141.
37. De Bortoli N, Leonardi G, Ciancia E, et al. *Helicobacter pylori* eradication: a randomized prospective study of triple therapy versus triple therapy plus lactoferrin and probiotics. Am J Gastroenterol 2007;102:951–956.
38. Canducci F, Armuzzi A, Cremonini F, et al. A lyophilized and inactivated culture of *Lactobacillus acidophilus* increases *Helicobacter pylori* eradication rates. Aliment Pharmacol Ther 2000;14:1625–1629.
39. Sykora J, Valeckova K, Amlerova J. Effects of a specially designed fermented milk product containing *Lactobacillus casei* DN-114 001 and the eradication of *H. pylori* in children. A prospective randomized double-blind study. J Clin Gastroenterol 2005;39:692–698.
40. Goldman CG, Barrado DA, Balcarce N, et al. Effect of a probiotic food as an adjuvant to triple therapy for eradication of *Helicobacter pylori* infection in children. Nutrition 2006;22:984–988.
41. Gotteland M, Brunser, Cruchet S. Systematic review: are probiotics useful in controlling gastric colonization by *Helicobacter pylori*? Aliment Pharmacol Ther 2006;23:1077–1086.
42. Myllyluoma E, Veijola L, Ahlroos T, et al. Probiotic supplementation improves tolerance to *Helicobacter pylori* eradication therapy – a placebo-controlled, double-blind randomized pilot study. Aliment Pharmacol Ther 2005;21:1263–1272.
43. Myllyluoma E, Ahlroos T, Veijola L, Rautelin H, Tynkkynen S, Korpela R. Effects of anti-*Helicobacter pylori* treatment and probiotic supplementation on intestinal microbiota. Int J Antimicrob Agents 2007;29:66–72.
44. Lionetti E, Miniello VL, Castellaneta SP, et al. *Lactobacillus reuteri* therapy to reduce side-effects during anti-*Helicobacter pylori* treatment in children: a randomized placebo controlled trial. Aliment Pharmacol Ther 2006;24:1461–1468.
45. Hamilton-Miller JMT. The role of probiotics in the treatment and prevention of *Helicobacter pylori* infection. Int J Antimicrob Agents 2003;22:360–366.
46. Felley C, Michetti P. Probiotics and *Helicobacter pylori*. Best Pract Res Clin Gastroenterol 2003;17:785–791.
47. Bleich A, Mahler M. Environment as a critical factor for the pathogenesis and outcome of gastrointestinal disease: experimental and human inflammatory bowel disease and *Helicobacter*-induced gastritis. Pathobiology 2005;72:293–307.
48. Lesbros-Pantoflickova D, Corthesy-Theulaz I, Blum AL. *Helicobacter pylori* and probiotics. J Nutr 2007;137:S812–S818.
49. Lenoir-Wijnkoop I, Sanders ME, Van Loo J, Sherman PM, et al. Probiotic and prebiotic influence beyond the intestinal tract. Nutr Rev 2007;65:469–489.
50. Tong JL, Ran ZH, Shen J, Zhang CX, Xiao SD. Meta-analysis: the effect of supplementation with probiotics on eradication rates and adverse events during *Helicobacter pylori* eradication therapy. Aliment Pharmacol Therap 2007;25:155–168.

51. Kato S, Kobayashi A, Sugiyama T, et al. Proposal of guidelines on the management of *Helicobacter pylori* in children (in Japanese). Jpn J Pediatr Gastroenterol Nutr 1997;11:173–176.

52. Sherman P, Hassall E, Hunt RH, et al. Canadian Helicobacter study group consensus conference on the approach to *Helicobacter pylori* infection in children and adolescents. Can J Gastroenterol 1999;13:553–559.

53. Drumm B, Koletzko S, Oderda G. *Helicobacter pylori* infection in children: a consdensus state of the European task force on *Helicobacter pylori*. J Pediatr Gastroenterol Nutr 2000;30;207–213.

54. Jones NL, Sherman PM, Fallone CA, et al. Canadian Helicobacter study group consensus conference: update to the approach to *Helicobacter pylori* infection in children and adolescents – an evidence-based evaluation. Can J Gastroenterol 2005;19:399–408.

55. Jones NL. A review of current guidelines for the management of *Helicobacter pylori* infection in children and adolescents. Pediatr Child Health 2004;9:709–713.

56. Malfertheiner P, Megraud F, O'Morain C, et al. Current concepts in the management of *Helicobacter pylori* infection: the Maastricht III consensus report. Gut 2007;56:772–781.

Section D
Probiotics Outside the Gut

18 Probiotics in Treatment and/or Prevention of Allergies

R. Fölster-Holst, B. Offick, E. Proksch, and J. Schrezenmeir

Approximately 20% of the population worldwide suffers from some form of allergy and the prevalence of allergic diseases is still rising (Warner et al. 2006). Atopic diseases[1] are associated with an immediate reaction against an antigen through activation of Th2 cells. This leads to various immunological diseases due to evasion of host defense mechanisms (Romagnani, 1996).

Although the etiology of the diseases remains elusive, much attention was given to environmental changes as a major factor in the development of allergic diseases. This is supported by the fact that the rise is most apparent in industrialized countries. In 1989, D.P. Strachan formulated the hygiene hypothesis as an explanation for the variation in allergy over time. According to his hypothesis, reduced family size and a reduction in childhood infections have reduced the exposure to microbes, which plays a crucial role in the maturation of the host immune system during the first years of life (Strachan, 2000).

Besides the societal and lifestyle changes, it has been shown that alterations in the intestinal microbiota can influence mucosal immunity. The composition of the intestinal microflora is affected by many factors, such as age, gender, diet, hygiene and use of antibiotics (Tlaskalová-Hogenova et al., 2005).

At birth, the immune system is not fully developed and for the sake of preventing in utero rejection, it tends to be directed towards a Th2 cell activation, even after birth

---

[1] Atopic diseases = an allergic hypersensitive reaction concerning bodily parts with no direct contact to the allergen. It includes eczema (atopic dermatitis), allergic rhinitis and asthma. Eczema affects especially young children and is characterized by a red, flaky, and itchy skin commonly appearing in the inner sides of elbows and knees. Allergic rhinitis is caused by aeroallergens (like pollen, fungi and house dust mites and pet allergens) and usually appears during middle childhood or adolescence. Symptoms are characterized by nasal itching, serial sneezing, rhinorrhea, congestion and conjunctivitis. Asthma is a chronic disease of the respiratory tract, including symptoms such as wheezing, breathlessness, chest tightness, and coughing. The main cause of asthma in infants is sensitization against indoor allergens in particular like house dust mites.

From: *Nutrition and Health: Probiotics in Pediatric Medicine*
Edited by: S. Michail and P.M. Sherman © Humana Press, Totowa, NJ

(Ouwehand, 2007). Although this distortion may be associated with allergic diseases, not all infants develop allergy. Microbial stimulation in early life shifts the Th1/Th2 balance toward a Th1 cell activity. It has been suggested that the absence of the exposure to microbes pre-disposes a child to develop atopic diseases (Ouwehand, 2007; Ogden, Bielory, 2005).

Oral exposure to allergens and the permeability of the gut for orally administered allergens may be of crucial importance for the disease development. At birth, the colon is sterile and evolves its own bacterial flora rapidly in the first few weeks of life, which is mainly recruited from the mother (Hopkins et al., 2002). Several studies indicate that the composition of the intestinal microflora differs between allergic versus non-allergic individuals and in industrialized versus developing countries (Björkstén et al., 1999, 2001; Kalliomäki et al., 2001a; Kirjavainen et al., 2001; Kirjavainen et al., 2002).

A comparison of the intestinal flora in children from countries with a high (Sweden) and low (Estonia) prevalence of allergic diseases showed that Lactobacilli and Bifidobacteria are more commonly found in the intestinal microflora of the non-allergic children, whereas *Staphylococcus aureus* and Clostridium were more common in allergic children (Björkstén et al., 1999, 2001; Sepp et al., 1997). This result was confirmed by several other studies (Kirjavainen et al., 2001a; Kalliomäki et al., 2001a; Watanabe et al., 2003). Mah et al. (2006) showed that infants with eczema had lower counts of Bifidobacteria and Clostridium. Among the different bifidobacterial species, a distinct pattern was observed in allergic versus non-allergic infants. Allergic infants had predominantly *B. adolescentis* in their stools, whereas *B. bifidum* was more commonly found in healthy infants (Ouwehand et al., 2001; He et al., 2001). Some studies, however, could not confirm these observations. The comparison of the commensal bacteria composition of 324 European infants showed no association between food sensitization or atopic dermatitis, and the intestinal microflora composition (Adlerberth et al., 2007). Another study also showed no difference in bacterial profile between healthy and allergic infants except an increased occurrence of *E. coli* in infants with atopic dermatitis (Penders et al., 2006). Even if the data are conflicting, most of these studies suggest that microbiota composition might be involved in allergic disease.

While the microflora in adults appears to be quite stable for a given individual over time, the intestinal microbiota of infants is vulnerable. Therefore, it may be possible to change the profile of bacteria in early life which in turn may influence the development of allergic diseases. Eventually this regime may also be suitable for the treatment of allergic diseases. One attempt to modulate the intestinal microbiota in early life is the administration of probiotics in infancy.

In the 1900s, Metchnikoff first described the therapeutic potential of lactic acid bacteria. He assumed that Lactobacilli could reduce or prevent the effects of microbes that cause gastrointestinal disease (Parvez et al., 2006). The term 'probiotics', literally mean 'for life', evolved much later (Schrezenmeir and de Vrese, 2001), since many study groups have demonstrated effects of oral intake of bacteria on various diseases, including allergic diseases.

Most studies dedicated to probiotics' use in allergy examined the effect of probiotics on overt allergic reactions. Not only the alleviation in clinical symptoms overall, but also the blockade of specific allergic mechanisms is an important aspect of allergy treatment. Prevention of allergy development is another option for subjects with a high risk of allergy (e.g. due to a family history of allergy). Both, prevention and treatment of allergic diseases have been examined.

MECHANISMS OF ACTION OF PROBIOTICS IN ALLERGIC REACTIONS

The mechanisms of action of probiotics are only partly known, though several in vivo and in vitro studies have examined various immune parameters (Table 18.1). As mentioned above, allergic diseases are associated with a disruption of the Th1/Th2 cytokine balance towards an activation of Th2 cells, which leads to an increase of Th2 cytokines such as interleukin-4 (IL-4), IL-5, and IL-13. This is followed by the induction of IgE and IgA synthesis and the activation and recruitment of mast cells and eosinophils which mediate most of the allergic symptoms (Kruisselbrink et al., 2001; Winkler et al., 2007). Probiotic bacteria have been found to inhibit the Th2 response and stimulate the Th1 response and the production of Th1 cytokines such as interferon-γ (IFN-γ), IL-2, and IL-12 (Isolauri et al., 2001; Winkler et al., 2007). The anti-inflammatory Th2 cytokine IL-10 is involved in the maintenance of immune homeostasis and may mediate the effects of probiotics through a down-regulatory effect on cytokine production. Another cytokine with a regulatory effect on immune cells is tumor necrosis factor-α (TNF-α), which is involved in systemic inflammation.

After ingestion of probiotic bacteria, they may modulate immunity by the mediation of Toll-like receptors TLR2 and TLR3, NOD, proteoglycan recognition proteins of enterocytes, dendritic cells, and mucosal immunocytes. This results in the activation of dendritic cells and a shift to activation of Th1 cells. The release of Th1 cytokines suppresses the activation of Th2 cells and increases the activation of macrophages and B cells to produce antigen-specific IgG (Winkler et al., 2007). In vitro studies showed, that preincubation with lactic acid bacteria strains slightly increases IFN-γ and IL-12 secretion by Dermatophagoides pteronyssinus (Dpt)-stimulated peripheral blood mononuclear cells (PBMC) or monocyte-derived dendritic cells from patients with house dust allergy. Also, this inhibited IL-4 and IL-5 response to the allergen (Pochard et al., 2002, 2005; Ghadimi et al., 2007). Another group reported an increase of the IFN-γ and IL-10 production and a decrease of the IL-5 production in PBMCs of healthy blood donors after stimulation with phytohaemagglutin (PHA) (Niers et al., 2005).

Similar results have been shown in vivo. In children with atopic diseases or food allergy, the ingestion of probiotic bacteria led to an increase of the IFN-γ production and a suppression of the IgE and allergen-induced IL-5, IL-10, and TNF-α production of specific allergen-incubated blood cells (Prescott et al., 2005; Taylor et al., 2006a; Flinterman et al., 2007). In contrast, in healthy or allergic subjects the effect of ingestion of probiotics on the cytokine production of human blood cells, stimulated with unspecific antigens, such as Concanavalin A (ConA) or PHA, showed no consistent pattern (Wheeler et al., 1997, Pohjavuori et al., 2004; Brouwer et al., 2006; Aldinucci et al., 2002; Christensen et al., 2006; Rosenfeldt et al., 2003; Pessi et al., 2000). Nevertheless, several in vivo studies with ovalbumin (OVA)-sensitised mice which were fed with probiotics showed an increase in Th1 cytokine (IFN-γ, IL-12) production, a decrease of the IgE, and a suppression of the OVA-induced Th2 cytokine (IL-4, IL-5) production (Fujiwara et al., 2004; Shida et al., 2002; Matsuzaki et al., 1998; Takahashi et al., 2006; Torii et al., 2007).

Table 18.1
Mechanisms of action of probiotic treatment

Author (year)	Study type (in vivo)[a]	Subjects (health status, age, n)[b]	Study design (duration treatment, s train, uptake [log cfu/d], preparation)[c]	Results[d]
Aattouri et al. (2002)	An: Ct (M)	r (Wistar), 4 w, F	4 w: L. bulgericus, S. thermophilus (7.3/ml, Y)	↑ proliferation (pp, sp, bl), IFN-γ (pp: p < 0.001, sp: p < 0.05; ConA or probiotics), B-cells (pp) ↔ macrophages, T cells
Aldinucci et al. (2002)	Cl: cC, pC (SM)	Al (allergic rhinopathy), He, 19–44 y, 20 (7 Al-T/6 Al-Ct7 He-Ct	4 m: L. acidophilus + Bifidobacteria (each 6–7.3, Y)	↑ IFN-γ (bl) ↓ IL-4 and IFN-γ (bl, PHA) ↔ IgE (bl, also placebo)
Berman et al. (2006)	Ob	He, 24–54 y, 10 (5 F/5 M)	8 w: L. rhamnosus, L. plantarum, L. salivarius, B. bifidum (total: 9.8, C)	↑ monocytes (bl, p = 0.0005), neutrophils (bl, p = 0.0122) ↔ NK cell activity, IgA (bl)
Blümer et al. (2007)	An: Ct (PBS)	m (BALB/c), sens (OVA), 6–8 w, F	60 d (ig 5× every 2.d before mating (=prenatal) and ig 25× every 2.d after delivery (=perinatal)): L. rhamnosus GG ATCC 53103 (HK) (8, PBS)	↑ prenatal: TNF-α (OVA, ConA, pla p < 0.05) ↓ perinatal: TNF-α (ConA, sp p < 0.05), IFN-γ (sp, OVA p < 0.05, ConA p < 0.001), IL-10 (OVA, ConA, sp, p < 0.05), IL-5 (OVA, ConA, sp, p < 0.05) ↔ IL-13, IL-4, specific IgG1 (OVA, sp), IgG2a, IgE (OVA, sp)
Chapat et al. (2004)	An: pC (steril 0.9% NaCl)	m (C57BL/6), sens (DNFB), 5–6 w, F	~26 d (d: 14 T/sens/12 T): L. casei DN-114,001 (1.6, FM)	↓ contact hypersensitivity (allergen-induced), CD8+T cells (sp, allergen-specific)
Christensen et al. (2006)	Cl:Rd, pC (microcristalline cellulose), dB	He, 18–40 y (mean: 25.6 y), 75 (46 F/25 M)	3 w (w: 2 RI/3 T/2 WO): B. animalis ssp. lactis Bb12 + L. paracasei CRL431 (8,9,10 or 11)	↑ phagocytic activity (bl, also placebo) ↔ IgA, IgG, IgM, IFN-γ, IL-10 (bl, also placebo), IgA (bl, fc, also placebo)

Study	Design	Subjects	Duration/Treatment	Outcomes
Ciprandi et al. (2004)	Ob: sB	Al (asthma, rhinitis, HDM), children, 10 (4 F/6 M)	4 w: *Bacillus clausii* spores (4 billion spores, Product: Enterogermina)	↑ IFN-γ (no, p < 0.05), IL-12 (no, p < 0.001), TGF-β (no, p < 0.05), IL-10 (no, p < 0.05) ↓ IL-4 (no, p < 0.01)
Ciprandi et al. (2005a)	Ob	Al (allergic rhinitis), mean: 22.3 y, 10	4 w: *Bacillus clausii* spores (6 billion spores, Product: Enterogermina)	↔ IL-1, IL-3, IL-6, IL-8 (no) ↑ IFN-γ (no, p = 0.038), TGF-β (no, p = 0.039), IL-10 (no, p = 0.009) ↓ IL-4 (no, p = 0.004)
Cukrowska et al. (2002)	Cl: Rd, pC (no probiotics), dB	He, nb, 61 (34 T/27 Ct)	4 w (2 and 3 w Fup): *E. coli* Nissle 1917 (8, suspension)	↑ specific *E. coli* Nissle IgA (bl, p < 0.0001) and IgM (bl, p < 0.01, also placebo: p < 0.05), total IgA (bl, p < 0.01, also placebo) and IgM (bl, p < 0.0001, also placebo: p < 0.05)
Díaz-Ropero et al. (2007)	An: Ct (SM)	m (Balb/c), 6 w, 24 (F, 2 × 8 T/8 Ct)	4 w (every 2. d): *L. salivarius* CECT5713 + *L. fermentum* CECT5716 (8.6, SM)	↑ IgA (L.f, mu, p < 0.05), IgE (L.f, bl, p = 0.1), IL-2 (sp, p < 0.05), IL-10 (sp, p < 0.05), IL-12 (L.f, sp, p < 0.05)
Feleszko et al. (2006)	An: Ct (water)	m (Balb/c), sens (OVA), He, 8 w, (F, 6–9/group)	8 w: *L. rhamnosus* GG ATCC 53103 or *B. lactis* Bb12 (9)	↔ IL-4 (sp), IgG (bl), IgA (bl) ↓ airway reactivity (p < 0.05), total IgE (bl, Bb12: p < 0.03, LGG: p < 0.003), specific IgE (bl, OVA, p < 0.003), specific IgG2 (bl, OVA, Bb12: p < 0.001, LGG: p < 0.03), eosinophilia (p < 0.05), IL-4, IL-5, IL-10, IFN-γ (all cytokines: MLN, OVA, LGG: p < 0.05) ↔ TGF-β
Flinterman et al. (2007)	Ob: Ct	Al (food allergy), children, 13 (7 T/6 Ct)	3 m	↑ proliferation, IFN-γ, IL-10, TNF-α (bl, additional probiotic cell stimulation) ↓ IgE (bl, additional probiotic cell stimulation), IL-10, TNF-α, IL-6 (tend) (bl) ↔ sensitisation to food allergens

(continued)

Table 18.1
(continued)

Author (year)	Study type (in vivo)[a]	Subjects (health status, age, n)[b]	Study design (duration treatment, strain, uptake [log cfu/d], preparation)[c]	Results[d]
Fujiwara et al. (2004)	An	m, sens (OVA)	20 w: L. paracasei KW3110	↑ IL-12 (sp) ↓ IgE (bl, OVA), IL-4 (sp)
Fukushima et al. (1998)	Ob	He, 15–31 m, 7 (3 F/4 M)	21 d: B. bifidum Bb12 (9, F)	↑ IgA (fc, $p < 0.05$)
Gill et al. (2001)	Ob: Rd, dB	He, 60–84 y (median: 69.5 y), 27 (16 F/11 M, 13 L/14 B)	3 w (w: 3 RI/3 T/3 WO): L. rhamnosus HN001 or B. lactis HN019 k (L:10.1 B:9.7, P)	↑ CD56⁺ cells (bl, L: $p = 0.0016$; B: $p = 0.0003$), tumoricidal activity (bl, L: $p = 0.001$; B: $p = 0.003$)
Hirose et al. (2006)	Cl: Rd, pC (dextrin), dB, pl	He, 40–64 y (A) and > 64 y (E) (mean: 56.3 y), 60 (30 F/30 M, 30 T/30 Ct)	12 w: L. plantarum L-137 (HK) (10 mg, C: LP20)	↑ proliferation (bl, ConA, $p = 0.036$), Th1/Th2 ratio (bl, $p = 0.002$), QOL (week 8: $p = 0.049$; week 12 $p = 0.092$)
Inoue et al. (2007a)	An: Ct (PBS)	m (NC/Nga), sens (induction of skinlesion), 22 (9 T/8 Ct/5 NT)	3 d: L. johnsonii NCC533 (10, PBS)	↓ IL-8, IL-10, IL-12, IL-23, CD86, CTLA-4, CD80 (all : Antigen-applied skin, < 0.05) ↔ IFN-γ, TGF-β, IL-18, CD28 (all: antigen-applied skin, also placebo)
Inoue et al. (2007b)	An: Ct (PBS)	m (NC/Nga), sens (induction of skin lesion: Der f), 3 w, 33 (14 F/19 M, 17 T/16 Ct)	3 d: L. johnsonii NCC533 (11.2)	↑ IgA (fc) ↓ atopic dermatitis development, total IgE (bl)
Kato et al. (1999)	An: Ct (distilled water)	m (Balb/c), 7–10 w, M	7 d: L. casei strain shirota (L) (9, P)	↑ IFN-γ (sp, ConA, $p < 0.01$) ↔ IL-4 (sp, ConA), IL-5 (sp, ConA) ↑ bothT: IFN-γ (sp)
Kim et al. (2005a)	An	m (C3H/HeJ), sens (OVA, CT)	7 w (start probiotics: 2 w before sens or 2 w after sens): B. bifidum BGN4	↓ preT: OVA -specific IgE and IgG1, tail symptoms (bl) postT: OVA-specific IgE (bl); bothT: IL-6, IL-18 (sp)

Reference	Design	Subjects/model	Treatment	Results
Kim et al. (2005b)	An: cC, Ct (no probiotics)	m (C3 H/HeJ), sens (OVA, CT), He, 3 w, 30 (F, 6 He/6 sens/6 B/6 L/6 E)	7 w: *B. bifidum* BGN4, *L. casei* 911, gram-negative *E. coli* MC4100 (0.2% of diet, Pe)	↓ specific IgE (OVA), total IgE/IgG1, mc degranulation, tail scabs (bl: B, L, E, $p < 0.05$), specific IgA/IgG1 (OVA, bl: B, L, $p < 0.05$)
Kishi et al. (1996)	C: Rd, pC	He, 60	4 w: *L. brevis* ssp *coagulans* (L&HK) (300 or 600 million bacteria)	↔ total IgA (fc), IgG2a (bl); ↑ IFN-α (virus-induced, $p < 0.05$, both doses, L) ↔ TNF-α (HK)
Marcos et al. (2004)	Ep: Rd, Ct (SM), pl	He (stress), 18–23 y, 155 (96 F/40 M)	6 w: *L. casei* DN-114001(8/ml, FM)	↑ lypmphocytes (bl, $p < 0.05$); ↓ placebo: lypmphocytes, CD56+ cells (bl, $p < 0.05$); ↔ IL-2, IL-4, IL-5, IL-10, TNF-α, IFN-γ (bl)
Mastrandrea et al. (2004)	Ob	Al (asthma, conjunctivitis, rhinitis, food allergy, atopic dermatitis, IBS), 6–48 y, 14 (5 F/9 M)	30 d: *L. acidophilus*, *L. delbrueckii*, *S. thermophilus* (9 total)	↓ CD34+ cells (bl, $p < 0.001$)
Matsumoto et al. (2007)	Cl: Rd, pC (Y), dB, co	Al (atopic dermatitis), mean: 22.1 y, 10 (4 F/6 M)	4 w (w: 4 T/4 WO/4 T): *B. animalis* ssp *lactis* LKM512 (7.7, Y)	↑ IFN-γ (bl, $p < 0.005$; also placebo: $p < 0.05$); ↔ IL-4, IL-5, IL-10, IL-12 (bl)
Matsuzaki et al. (1998)	An: Ct (no probiotics)	m (Balb/c), r (Wistar), sens (OVA), He, 7 w, 36 (6 NT/6 Ct/4 × 6 T)	21 d: *L. casei* Shirota (various, Pe) (m: fed *L. casei*; r: bl of m intradermally injected on shaved dorsal skin and OVA-injection)	↑ IFN-γ, IL-2, IL-12 (sp, OVA, $p < 0.05$); ↓ total IgE (bl; sp: OVA, $p < 0.05$), specific IgE (OVA, bl; sp, $p < 0.05$), IL-4, IL-5, IL-6, IL-10 (sp, OVA, $p < 0.05$)
Moreira et al. (2007)	Cl: Rd, pC	Al (allergic rhinitis, food allergy, atopic dermatitis, asthma, sensitized to birch pollen), 141	3 m: *L. rhamnosus* GG	↑ eosinophils (bl, also placebo); ↔ ECP, IgE (bl, also placebo)
Morita et al. (2006)	Ob	Al (perennial allergic rhinitis, allergic symptoms, high IgE), 17–56 y, 15 (8 F/7 M)	4 w: *L. gasseri* TMC0356 k (11, FM)	↑ Th1 cells (bl, $p < 0.05$); ↓ total IgE (bl, $p < 0.05$), specific IgE (bl, Acari, Japanese cedar, $p < 0.05$)

(continued)

Table 18.1
(continued)

Author (year)	Study type (in vivo)[a]	Subjects (health status, age, n)[b]	Study design (duration treatment, strain, uptake [log cfu/d], preparation)[c]	Results[d]
Nagao et al. (2000)	Ob: pC (M)	He, 20–40 y (mean: 32.7 y), 17 (10 F/7 M, 9 T/8 Ct)	3 m (Fup: 3 w, 2 m): L. casei strain shirota (10.6, FM)	↑ NK cell activity (bl, p = 0.005), ↔ NK cells, IFN-α, IFN-γ (bl)
Ogawa et al. (2006)	Cl: Rd, Ct (P) An: Ct (P)	He, 25–62 y, 14 (2 F/12 M, 7 T/7 Ct) m (NC/Nga), sens (Dpt- or picryl chloride- induced dermatitis), 6 w, 16 (M, 4 Ct/4 dextran/4 L.c/4 dextran + L.c)	4 w: L. casei ssp casei JCM1134 (9.7, P); 8 w: L. casei ssp casei JCM1134 (7, P)	↑ placebo: IgE (bl, p < 0.05), eosionophils (bl, p < 0.05) ↓ placebo: IFN-γ (bl) ↔ atopic dermatitis, IgE, TARC, IFN-γ, eosionophils (bl) ↓ atopic dermatitis (p < 0.05), IgE (bl, Dpt, p < 0.01)
Olivares et al. (2006)	Cl: Rd, pC (Y), dB	He, 23–43 y, 30 (15 F/15 M)	4 w (w: 2 RI/4 T/2 WO): L. gasseri CECT5714 + L. coryniformis CECT5711 (9.3 each, Y)	↑ phagocytic activity (bl, also placebo, p < 0.01), NK cells (bl, week 2: p < 0.05), IL-10 (bl, week 2: p < 0.05), IL-4 (bl, week 2: p < 0.05), IgA (fc, p < 0.05) ↓ IgE (bl, week 2: p < 0.01) ↔ IL-12, TNF-α, IgG (bl, also placebo), IgA (bl)
Parra et al. (2004a)	Cl: Rd, pC (M), dB	He, 51–58 y, 45 (24 F/21 M, 23 T/22 Ct)	8 w: L. casei DN114001 (10.5–12.5, FM)	↑ oxidative burst capacity of monocytes (bl, p = 0.029) ↔ immune cell proportion (bl)
Parra et al. (2004b)	Cl: Rd, pC (M), dB	He, 51–58 y, 45 (24 F/21 M, 23 T/22 Ct)	8 w: L. casei DN114001 (10.5–12.5, FM)	↑ oxidative burst capacity of monocytes (bl, p = 0.029), NK cell tumoricidal activity (bl, p = 0.023) ↔ immune cell proportion (bl)

Author	Design	Population	Probiotic	Results
Pelto et al. (1998)	Cl: Rd, Ct (M, dB, co	Al (milk hypersensitivity), He, 22–50 y (mean: 28 y), 17 (13 F/4 M, 9 He/8 Al)	1 w: L. rhamnosus GG ATCC 53103 (8.4, M)	$\downarrow$ expression of CR1, FcγRI, FcaR (bl, in neutrophils), CR1, CR3, FcaR (bl, in monocytes) (all milk-induced)
Pessi et al. (2000)	Ob	Al (atopic dermatitis, food allergy, CMA), 4–42 m (mean: 21 m), 9	4 w (w: 4 T/8 Fup): L. rhamnosus GG ATCC 53103 (10.3)	$\uparrow$ IL-10 (bl, $p < 0.001$)
Pohjavuori et al. (2004)	Cl: Rd, pC (microcristalline cellulose), dB	Al (atopic dermatitis), 1.4–11.5 m (mean: 6.5 m), 119 (46 F/73 M, 42 LGG/41 Mix/36 Ct)	4 w (w: 4 T/4 Fup): L. rhamnosus GG ATCC 53103 or MIX = L. rhamnosus GG, L. rhamnosus LC705, B. breve Bbi99, P. freudenreichii ssp. Shermanii JS (L:9.7 B:8.3 P:9.3, C)	$\uparrow$ IFN-γ (bl, LGG: CMA $p = 0.006$, IgE-ass. Atopic dermatitis $p = 0.017$), IL-4 (bl, Mix: CMA $p = 0.034$)
Prescott et al. (2005)	Cl: Rd, pC (maltodextran)	Al (atopic dermatitis), 6–18 m, 56 (24 F/29 M, 26 T/27 Ct)	8 w (w: 8 T/8 Fup): L. fermentum PCC (9.3, P)	$\uparrow$ IFN-γ (bl, PHA, SEB, $p < 0.05$, also placebo; probiotics: also after Fup) (bl, HDM, $p < 0.01$), TNF-α (bl, HKSa, $p = 0.011$) $\downarrow$ IL-13 (bl, HKSa)
Rinne et al. (2005)	Cl: Rd, pC	nb, 96	(probiotics pre- and postnatally): L. rhamnosus GG	$\uparrow$ IgM, IgA, IgG secreting cells ($p = 0.005$, $p = 0.03$, $p = 0.005$)
Sawada et al. (2006)	An: Ct (Pe)	m (Nc/Nga), sens (atopic skin lesion), 33 (16 T/17 Ct)	>12 w (from 14.d pregnancy + 4 w breastfed + 8 w Pe): L. rhamnosus GG ATCC 53103 (HK) (0.1–0.2, Pe)	$\uparrow$ IL-10 (bl, $p < 0.05$) $\downarrow$ atopic dermatitis, mast cells ($p < 0.001$), eosinophils ($p < 0.001$) $\leftrightarrow$ IgE, Treg cells, FOXP3, IL-1, IL-2, IL-4, IFN-γ, IL-6, IL-12, GM-CSF, TNF-α
Sheih et al. (2001)	Ob: Rd, sB	He, 44–80 y (median: 63.5 y), 52 (35 F/17 M, 25 LFM-L/27 LFM-LH-L)	3 w (w: 3 Rl/3 T/3 WO): L. rhamnosus HN001 (9/g, LFM or LFM-LH)	$\uparrow$ phagocytosis of PMN (bl, $p < 0.01$), NK cell activity (bl, $p < 0.01$)

(continued)

Table 18.1
(continued)

Author (year)	Study type (in vivo)[a]	Subjects (health status, age, n)[b]	Study design (duration treatment, strain, uptake [log cfu/d], preparation)[c]	Results[d]
Shida et al. (2002)	An: Ct (saline or *L. johnsonii*)	m (OVA23–3), sens (OVA), 8–10 w, 21 (6 NT/6 Ct/3 L.j)	4 w (OVA-diet, 3× probiotic-injection): *L. casei* strain shirota (HK) (200 µg/injection)	↑ IL-12, IFN-γ (both: sp, OVA, $p < 0.05$) ↓ IgE, IgG1 (both: sp, OVA, $p < 0.05$), specific and total IgE (bl, OVA, $p < 0.05$, 2.w), specific IgG1 (bl, OVA, $p < 0.01$), IL-4, IL-5 (both: sp, OVA, $p < 0.05$), anaphylaxis score ($p < 0.05$) ↔ IgG2a
Spanhaak et al. (1998)	Cl: Rd, pC (M), dB	He, 40–65 y (mean: 55.8 y), 20 (M, 10 T/10 Ct)	4 w (w: 2 RI/4 T/2 Fup): *L. casei* strain shirota (11.5, FM)	↑ Bb (fc, $p < 0.05$) ↓ Clostridium (fc, also placebo) ↔ NK cell activity, phagocytosis, cytokine production (bl)
Takahashi et al. (2006)	An: Ct (PBS)	m (Balb/c), sens (OVA), He, 7 w, 21 (F, 7 NT/7 T/Ct)	(probiotic on d 0–2 and 7–9 by gastric gavage): ODN BL07 S from *B. longum* (1 mg/ gavage)	↑ total and specific IgG2a (bl, OVA, $p < 0.05$), IL-12 (sp, OVA, $p = 0.09$), IFN-γ (sp, OVA, $p < 0.01$) ↓ specific IgE (bl, OVA, $p < 0.05$), total IgE (bl, $p = 0.09$), IL-4 (sp, OVA, $p = 0.10$), IL-5 (sp, OVA, $p = 0.06$) ↔ IL-10, TGF-β
Takeda et al. (2007)	Cl: Ct (M)	He (low NK-cell activity), 30–45 y (A) and 55–75 y (E), 19 (9 A/10 E)	3 w: *L. casei* strain shirota (10.6, FM)	↑ NK activity ($p < 0.01$) ↔ IFN-α/-γ (also placebo)
Taylor et al. (2006a)	Cl: Rd, pC (maltodextrin), dB	hR, nb, 231 (89 T/89 Ct)	6 m: *L. acidophilus* LAVRI-A1 (9.5, P)	↓ IL-5 (bl, SEB, $p = 0.044$), TGF-β (bl, SEB, $p = 0.015$), IL-10 (bl, TT, $p = 0.03$; HDM, $p = 0.014$), TNF-α (bl, HDM, $p = 0.046$) ↔ IL-6,IL-13, IFN-γ,TGF-β (bl)

Reference	Design	Population	Probiotic	Results
Taylor et al. (2006b)	Cl: Rd, pC (maltodextrin), dB An: Ct (saline)	m (Balb/c), sens (OVA), 6 w, 30 (6 NT/6 Ct/3 × 6 T)	6 m: *L. acidophilus* LAVRI-A1 (9.5, P)	↔ IL-5, IL-6, IL-10, IL-12, IL-13, TNF-α, IFN-γ, HLA-DR (bl) ↑ TGF-β (pp, OVA, $p < 0.05$), total IgA (pp, OVA, $p < 0.05$) ↓ specific IgE (bl, sp, OVA, $p < 0.05$), total IgE (sp, OVA, $p < 0.05$), IFN-γ (sp, OVA, $p < 0.05$), IL-4 (sp, OVA, $p < 0.05$), IL-10 (sp, OVA, $p < 0.05$)
Torii et al. (2007)	T/60 Ct, 60 F/58 M		8 w (w: 8 T/2 Fup): *L. acidophilus* strain L-92 (HK) (0.2, 1, 5 mg)	
Van de Water et al. (1999)	Cl: Rd, pC (no yoghurt), dB	Al, 20–40 y (A) and 50–70 y (E), 60 (20 Ct/20 HK/20 L)	1 y: (HK, L) (200 g, Y)	↓ allergic symptoms (A:E: $p < 0.05$), total IgE (E)
Viljanen et al. (2005a)	Cl: Rd, pC (microcristalline cellulose), dB	Al (atopic dermatitis, suspected CMA), 1.4–11.9 m (mean: 6.4 m), 230 (80 LGG/76 MIX/74 Ct)	4 w (w:4 T/4 Fup): *L. rhamnosus* GG ATCC 53103 or MIX = *L. rhamnosus* GG + *L. rhamnosus* LC705 + *B. breve* Bbi99 + *P. freudenreichii* ssp shermanii JS (L:9.7 B:8.3 P:9.3, C)	↔ specific IgE (bl, PHA, also placebo) ↑ IL-6 (bl, LGG, $p = 0.023$), IL-10 (bl, MIX, $p = 0.016$)
Viljanen et al. (2005b)	Cl: Rd, pC (microcristalline cellulose), dB	Al (atopic dermatitis, suspected CMA), 1.4–11.9 m (mean: 6.4 m), 230 (80 LGG/76 MIX/74 Ct)	4 w (w:4 T/4 Fup): *L. rhamnosus* GG ATCC 53103 or MIX = *L. rhamnosus* GG + *L. rhamnosus* LC705 + *B. breve* Bbi99 + *P. freudenreichii* ssp shermanii JS (L:9.7 B:8.3 P:9.3, C)	↑ IgA (fc, LGG, MIX $p = 0.064$, LGG: IgE-mediated CMA: $p = 0.014$) ↓ α1-antitrypsin (fc, $p = 0.033$), TNF-α (fc, LGG: IgE-mediated CMA: $p = 0.111$)

PREVENTION OF SENSITIZATION AND ALLERGIC DISEASES

The most important step in the prevention of allergic diseases is the prevention of sensitization (Table 18.2). In an epidemiologic study, Enomoto et al. investigated the relationship between allergy development and habitual ingestion of fermented milk products of 134 Japanese students. He reported a significant lower rate of allergy development among students eating fermented milk products compared with students not eating these products (Enomoto et al., 2006). Several intervention trials examined the effect of probiotics on sensitisation in high risk infants. The probiotic product was administered orally to the pregnant mother and/or their infants. In a randomized double-blinded placebo-controlled study, L. rhamnosus GG or placebo was given prenatally to mothers and postnatally to their infants at high risk of atopic disease. There was a 50% reduction in chronic relapsing atopic dermatitis at 2 year follow-up (Kalliomäki et al., 2001b). 4- and 7-year follow-up studies demonstrated that protection against allergic diseases by probiotics extended beyond infancy (Kalliomäki et al., 2003; Kalliomäki et al., 2007). Similarly, it was shown that repeated oral application of a probiotic E. coli strain in the early postnatal period prevented the incidence of allergies at 10 and 20 years of age (Lodinová-Zadnikova et al., 2003; Lodinová-Zadnikova et al., 2004). In other studies the incidence of IgE-associated dermatitis was reduced after the ingestion of probiotics only (Abrahamsson et al., 2007; Kukkonen et al., 2007). However, in a randomized double-blind placebo-controlled study Taylor could not confirm such effects. Administration of L. acidophilus could not reduce the risk of developing allergy in 231 infants (Taylor et al., 2007a, b). It should be noted that Taylor examined the effect of postnatal probiotic-supplementation, while other study groups (e.g. Kalliomäki et al., 2001b, 2003, 2007) combined pre- and postnatal probiotic-supplementation. Thus, the prenatal supplementation may be crucial for the preventive effect of probiotic bacteria.

TREATMENT OF ALLERGIES

Once allergic diseases have been developed the treatment focuses first on the blockage of allergic reactions and second on the alleviation of clinical symptoms. It was shown that probiotic supplementation decreased both the onset and severity of allergic diseases, such as atopic dermatitis and symptoms of food allergy compared to the control groups (Table 18.3). Most studies were performed with infants or children.

Majamaa and Isolauri investigated atopic dermatitis in infants who were fed an extensively hydrolysed formula containing L. rhamnosus GG for 1 month. Probiotic supplementation significantly improved the SCORAD (atopic dermatitis severity score) compared to control. However, 1 month after the cessation of the probiotic supplementation, both groups had similar median SCORAD scores that were significantly improved from initial scores (Majamaa, Isolauri, 1997).

The same study group examined the influence of probiotics in infants who developed atopic dermatitis during exclusive breast feeding. After 2 months of treatment, the SCORAD values of infants receiving the probiotic supplemented formulas (either B. lactis Bb-12 or L. rhamnosus GG) were significantly lower compared to those of infants who received unsupplemented formula. According to the first study of this

Table 18.2
Prevention of sensitization and allergic diseases

Author (year)	Study type (in vivo)[a]	Subjects[b] (health status, age, n)	Study design[c] (duration treatment, strain, uptake [log cfu/d], preparation)	Results[d]
Abrahamsson et al. (2007)	Cl: Rd, Ct, dB	hR, nb, 232	1 y (2 w prenatally/1 y postnatally/1 y Fup): L. reuteri ATCC55730 (8)	↓ IgE-associated eczema (1 y Fup, p = 0.02) ↔ eczema incidence, wheeze
Kalliomäki et al. (2001b)	Cl: Rd, pC (microcristalline cellulose), dB	hR, nb, 159	6.5–7 m (2–4 w prenatally/ 6 m postnatally/2 y Fup): L. rhamnosus GG ATCC 53103 (10, C)	↑ total IgE (bl, also placebo) ↓ atopic eczema (p = 0.008) ↔ SPT (also placebo)
Kalliomäki et al. (2003)	Cl: Rd, pC (microcristalline cellulose), dB	hR, nb, 159	6.5–7 m (2–4 w prenatally/ 6 m postnatally/4 y Fup): L. rhamnosus GG ATCC 53103 (10, C)	↓ atopic eczema
Kalliomäki et al. (2007)	Cl: Rd, pC (microcristalline cellulose), dB	hR, nb, 159	6.5–7 m (2–4 w prenatally/ 6 m postnatally/7 y Fup): L. rhamnosus GG ATCC 53103 (10, C)	↓ atopic eczema (p = 0.027)
Kukkonen et al. (2007)	Cl: Rd, pC (microcristalline cellulose/sugar syrup), dB	hR, nb, 1223 (610 T/613 Ct)	6.5–7 m (m: 0.5–1 prenatally/6 postnatally /2 y Fup): L. rhamnosus GG ATCC53103, L. rhamnosus LC705 DSM 7061, B. breve Bb99 DSM 13692, P. freudenreichii ssp shermanii JS DSM 7076 (L:9.7, B:8.3, P:9.3, C)	↓ IgE-associated diseases (p = 0.052), eczema (p = 0.035), atopic eczema (p = 0.025) ↔ cumulative incidence of allergic diseases
Lodinová-Zadnikova et al. (2004)	Cl: Ct	hR, nb	(10 y, 20 y Fup) probiotic E. coli	↓ infections (also after 10 y Fup), allergy (also after 10 y and 20 y Fup)

(continued)

Table 18.2
(continued)

Author (year)	Study type (in vivo)[a]	Subjects[b] (health status, age, n)	Study design[c] (duration treatment, strain, uptake [log cfu/d], preparation)	Results[d]
Lodinová-Zadnikova (2003)	Cl: Ct	hR, nb, 227 (150 = 20 y/ 77 = 10 y)	(10 y, 20 y Fup) probiotic *E. coli*	↓ allergy development (p < 0.01), infections (10 y Fup: p < 0.01) ↔ infections (20 y Fup)
Rautava et al. (2002)	Cl: Rd, pC (microcristalline cellulose), dB	hR, He, nb, 62 (30 T/32 Ct)	4 m (probiotics 1 m pre- and 3 m postnatally/ 2 y Fup): *L. rhamnosus* GG ATCC 53103 (10.3, C)	↑ TGF-$\beta2$ (bm, p = 0.018) ↓ atopic dermatitis development (2 y Fup: p = 0.0098)
Taylor et al. (2007a)	Cl: Rd, pC (maltodextrin), dB	hR, nb, 231 (58 T/60 Ct, 60 F/58 M)	6 m (m: 6 T/6 Fup): *L. acidophilus* LAVRI-A1 (9.5, P)	↑ sensitisation (SPT) (p = 0.03, also after 6 m Fup) ↔ atopic dermatitis rates, SCORAD
Taylor et al. (2007b)	Cl: Rd, pC (maltodextrin), dB	hR, nb, 231 (58 T/60 Ct, 60 F/58 M)	6 m (m: 6 T/6 Fup): *L. acidophilus* LAVRI-A1 (9.5, P)	↔ atopic dermatitis, FOXP3 expression (bl, unstimulated, HDM, OVA)

Table 18.3
Probiotics in treatment of allergies

Author (year)	Study type (in vivo)[a]	Subjects (health status, age, n)[b]	Study design (duration treatment, strain, uptake [log cfu/d], preparation)[c]	Results[d]
Brouwer et al. (2006)	CI: Rd, pC (F), dB	AI (atopic dermatitis, suspected CMA), <5 m, 50 (17 Lrh/16 LGG/17 Ct)	3 m (m: ~1 RI/3 TvCt): L. rhamnosus/ L. rhamnosus GG (9.7/ 100 ml, F)	↓ SCORAD (also placebo; p = 0.008), α1-antitrypsin (bl, also placebo), IL-4 (bl, also placebo, ConA, p = 0.039), IL-5 (bl, also placebo, ConA, p = 0.022) ↔ total IgE (bl, also placebo), specific IgE (CM, egg white, soy, peanut, cod, wheat, bl, also placebo), eosinophils (bl, also placebo), EPX (bl, also placebo), IFN-γ (bl, also placebo, ConA)
Ciprandi et al. (2005b)	CI: Ct (without probiotic)	AI (allergic rhinitis), 12–15 y (mean: 13.4 y), 20 (7 F/13 M; 10 T/19 Ct)	3 w: Bacillus clausii spores (6 billion spores, Product: Enterogermina)	↓ nasal symptoms (p = 0.049), eosinophils (no, p = 0.048)
Fölster-Holst et al. (2006)	CI: Rd, pC (microcristalline cellulose), dB	AI (atopic dermatitis), 1–55 m (median: 19 m), 54 (26 T/27 Ct, 20 F/34 M)	8 w (w: 8 T/4 Fup): L. rhamnosus GG (10, C)	↓ SCORAD (also placebo, p < 0.001), ECP (also placebo, fc, p = 0.04) ↔ total and specific IgE, CD30, α1-antitrypsin, calprotectin
Giovannini et al. (2007)	CI: Rd, pC (M), dB	AI (allergic asthma or allergic rhinitis), 2–5 y, 187 (67 F/120 M, 92 T/95 Ct, 119 asthma/131 rhinitis)	12 m: L. casei DN-114001 (10, FM)	↑ time free from asthma/rhinitis episodes (also placebo) ↓ nr of rhinitis episodes (p < 0.05) ↔ nr of asthma episodes, mean duration of asthma/rhinitis episodes
Hattori et al. (2003)	CI: Ct	AI (atopic dermatitis, B-deficient microflora), children, 15 (8 T/7 Ct)	1 m: B. breve M-16V	↓ cutaneous symptoms (p = 0.0176), total allergic symptoms (p = 0.0117)

(continued)

Table 18.3
(continued)

Author (year)	Study type (in vivo)[a]	Subjects (health status, age, n)[b]	Study design (duration treatment, strain, uptake [log cfu/d], preparation)[c]	Results[d]
Helin et al. (2002)	Cl: Rd, pC (microcristalline cellulose), dB	Al (birch pollen, apple), 14–36 y (mean: ~27 y), 38 (27 F/9 M, 18 T/18 Ct)	5.5 m (2 w RI/5.5 m T): L. rhamnosus GG ATCC 53103 (9.7, C)	↔ symptoms and medication
Ishida et al. (2005)	Cl: Rd, pC (M), dB	Al (perennial allergic rhinitis, high HD- or HDM-specific IgE), mean: 35.5 y, 52 (23 F/26 M, 25 T/24 Ct)	8 w (w: 1 RI/8 T/2 Fup): L. acidophilus L-92 (10.5, FM)	↓ nasal/ocular symptom-medication ($p < 0.01/p < 0.1$), swelling/colour nasal mucosa ($p < 0.05/p < 0.01$), HDM-specific IgE (bl, $p < 0.01$, also placebo: $p < 0.05$) ↔ HD-specific and total IgE (bl, both also placebo), Th1/Th2 ratio
Isolauri et al. (2000)	Cl: Rd, pC (EHF), dB	Al (atopic eczema-begun during exclusively breast-feeding), mean: 4.6 m, 27	2 m (m: 2 T/6 Fup): B. lactis (Bb-12) or L. rhamnosus GG ATCC 53103 (B:9/g L:8.5/g, EHF)	↓ SCORAD ($p = 0.002$), sCD4 (bl, $p = 0.005$), sCD8 (bl, $p > 0.05$, also placebo), IL-2sRa (bl, B: $p < 0.05$, L: $p > 0.05$, also placebo), TGF-β1 (bl, B: $p = 0.04$, L: $p = 0.07$) ↔ IL-1ra, TNF-α, GM-CSF, sICAM-1, RANTES, MCP-1 (bl)
Kirjavainen et al. (2003)	Cl: Rd, pC (EHF), dB	Al (CMA, atopic eczema), mean: 5.5 m, 35 (17 L/16 HK/10 Ct)	7.5 w: L. rhamnosus GG ATCC 53103 (L, HK) (9/g, EFH)	↓ SCORAD (L, $p = 0.02$)
Majamaa and Isolauri (1997)	Cl: Rd, pC (EHF), dB	Al (atopic eczema, CMA), postnatally: 2.5–15.7 m/perinatally: 0.6–8.5 m (mean: 4.4 m), 38 (27 postnatally/11 perinatally, postnatally: 13 T/14 Ct)	1 m (m: 1 T/2 Fup): L. rhamnosus GG ATCC 53103 (postnatally: 8.7/gm, perinatally: 10.6, EHF)	↓ postnatally: SCORAD ($p = 0.008$), α1-antitrypsin ($p = 0.03$), TNF-α (fc, $p = 0.003$), perin. SCORAD ($p = 0.007$) ↔ postnatally (CM, ConA): IL-4, IFN-γ, TNF-α, ECP (all: bl, also placebo)
Passeron et al. (2006)	Ep: Rd, pC (prebiotic), dB	Al (atopic dermatitis), 2–12 y (mean: 5.8 y), 48 (24 T/24 Ct)	3 m: L. rhamnosus Lcr35 + prebiotic (9.5)	↓ SCORAD (also placebo, $p < 0.0001$)

Peng and Hsu (2005)	Cl: Rd, pC (MP), dB	AI (perennial allergic rhinitis, HDM), mean: 15.7 y, 90 (36 F/54 M, 30 LGG/30 HK/30 Ct)	30 d: LP33 (L, HK) (10, C)	↓ frequency ($p < 0.0001$) and level of bother ($p < 0.004$)
Rosenfeldt et al. (2003)	Cl: Rd, pC (SM-P), dB, co	AI (atopic dermatitis), He, 1–13 y (median: 5.2 y), 43 (16 He/27 AI)	6 w (w: 2 RI/6 T/6 WO/6 T): L. rhamnosus 190702 + L. reuteri DSM 12246 (10.3 each, P)	↓ subjective eczema, extend of eczema ($p = 0.02$), ECP ($p = 0.03$), SCORAD (IgE-mediated allergy) ($p = 0.02$) ↔ SCORAD, IL-2, IL-4, IL-10, IFN-γ (bl, cytokines: also placebo)
Rosenfeldt et al. (2004)	Cl: Rd, pC (SM-P), dB, co	AI (atopic dermatitis), 1–13 y (median: 4 y), 41	6 w (w: 2 RI/6 T/6 WO/6 T): L. rhamnosus 190702 + L. reuteri DSM 12246 (10.3 each, P)	↓ frequency of gastrointestinal symptoms ($p = 0.002$), lactulose:mannitaol ratio ($p = 0.001$) ↔ SCORAD, IL-2, IL-4, IL-10, IFN-γ (bl)
Sistek et al. (2006)	Cl: Rd, pC (microcristalline cellulose), dB	AI (atopic dermatitis, food-sens), 1–10 y, 59 (29 T/30 Ct, 27 F/32 M, 43 sens/16 non-sens)	12 w (w: 2 RI/12 T/4 WO): L. rhamnosus, B. lactis (10.3/g, P)	↓ SCORAD (total: T:$p < 0.001$, WO: $p = 0.02$) (food-sensitized: T:$p < 0.0001$, WO:$p = 0.03$)
Tamura et al. (2007)	Cl: Rd, pC, dB	AI (allergic rhinitis, JCP)	8 w: L. casei strain shirota (FM)	↔ symptoms (also placebo)
Viljanen et al. (2005c)	Cl: Rd, pC (microcristalline cellulose), dB	AI (atopic dermatitis, suspected CMA), 1.4–11.9 m (mean: 6.4 m), 230 (80 L/76 MIX/74 Ct)	4 w (w:4 T/4 Fup): L. rhamnosus GG ATCC 53103 or MIX = L. rhamnosus GG + L. rhamnosus LC705, B. breve Bbi99 + P. freudenreichii ssp. shermanii JS (L:9.7 B:8.3 P:9.3, C)	↓ SCORAD (also placebo), SCORAD (IgE-sensitized, LGG: $p = 0.036$)
Wang et al. (2004)	Cl: Rd, pC (FM), dB	AI (perennial allergic rhinitis, HDM), 12.1–17.4 y, 80 (39 F/41 M, 60 T/20 Ct)	30 d: L. paracasei 33 (9.3, FM)	↓ frequency ($p = 0.037$), level of bother ($p = 0.022$)

(continued)

Table 18.3
(continued)

Author (year)	Study type (in vivo)[a]	Subjects (health status, age, n)[b]	Study design (duration treatment, strain, uptake [log cfu/d], preparation)[c]	Results[d]
Weston et al. (2005)	Cl: Rd, pC (maltodextran), dB	A1 (atopic dermatitis), 6–18 m, 53 (26 T/27 Ct)	8 w (w: 8 T/8 Fup): *L. fermentum* VRI-033 PCC (9.3)	↓ SCORAD (p = 0.03, also placebo)
Wheeler et al. (1997)	Cl: Rd, pC (Y), dB, co	A1 (allergic asthma), adult, 15	1 m (w: 4 T/4 WO/4 T): *L. acidophilus* (11.5, Y)	↑ IFN-γ (bl, ConA, p = 0.054) ↓ eosinophilia (bl) ↔ peripheral cell counts, IgE, IL-2, IL-4 (bl), QOL
Xiao et al. (2006a)	Cl: Rd, Ct (Y), dB	A1 (JCP), 23–61 y (mean : 36 y), 40 (23 F/17 M, 20 T/20 Ct)	14 w (w: 2 RI/14 T): *B. longum* BBS36 (7.3, Y)	↑ IL-10 (bl, also placebo, p < 0.001) ↓ eye symptoms (p = 0.044), IFN-γ (bl, also placebo, p < 0.05)
Xiao et al. (2006b)	Cl: Rd, pC (dextrin), dB	A1 (JCP), 28.4–44.6 y (mean : 36 y), 44 (18 F/26 M, 22 T/22 Ct)	13 w (w: 2 RI/13 T): *B. longum* BBS36 (10.7/2 g, P)	↑ total IgE, eosinophils (bl, p < 0.05) ↓ nr of persons with medication (p = 0.0056), rhinorrhea (p = 0.016), nasal blockage (p = 0.011), composite score (p = 0.033), total IgE (bl, p < 0.05, also placebo), JCP- specific IgE (bl, p < 0.01, also placebo), IFN-γ (bl, also placebo, p < 0.01), IL-10 (bl, p < 0.01) ↔ basophils, neutrophils, monocytes, lymphocytes (bl)
Xiao et al. (2007)	Cl: Rd, pC (dextrin), dB, co	A1 (JCP), 25–56 y, 24 (14 F/10 M)	4 w (w: 1 RI/4 T/2 WO/4 T): *B. longum* BBS36 (11, P)	↓ ocular symptoms (p = 0.033), disruption of normal activities (p = 0.011), prevalence of medication (p = 0.041) ↔ IgE (bl, also placebo)

group, the infants had similar improvement in SCORAD scores after 6 months (Isolauri et al., 2000). However, it is noticeable that infants of these Finnish studies had a very low SCORAD.

Other studies have confirmed a decrease of the SCORAD after probiotic consumption (Kirjavainen et al., 2003; Sistek et al., 2006). Some studies reported a probiotic-associated decrease of the SCORAD only in subjects with an IgE-mediated allergy (Viljanen et al., 2005c; Rosenfeldt et al., 2003). Some studies showed an improvement of the SCORAD value after the probiotic ingestion as well as after the placebo ingestion, which indicate that this effect was not due to the probiotic bacteria itself (Viljanen et al., 2005c; Fölster-Holst et al., 2006; Brouwer et al., 2006; Passeron et al., 2006; Weston et al., 2005). Taken together, these studies show a trend to a beneficial effect of probiotics on atopic dermatitis. Even if the decrease in the SCORAD score occurred in placebo-treated subjects as well, the probiotic-supplementation led to an accelerated improvement. However, all studies were performed in infants or children and some focusing on certain subgroups.

Helin et al. treated atopic patients who were allergic to birch pollen and apple food with *L. rhamnosus* GG during the birch-pollen season. Neither a reduction of the symptom score, nor of the sensitisation to birch pollen and apple occurred after probiotic intake (Helin et al., 2002). The consumption of *L. casei* strain Shirota in Japanese cedar pollen allergy had also no effect on the allergic symptoms (Tamura et al., 2007). Others reported that the ingestion of *B. longum* reduced ocular and nasal symptoms as well as the need for medication (Xiao et al., 2006a, b, 2007). Furthermore, in both, children and adult subjects with allergic rhinitis with or without house dust mite allergy, the intake of probiotic bacteria led to a reduction of the frequency and symptoms of the disease (Ishida et al., 2005; Peng et al., 2005; Wang et al., 2004). In a recent well-designed study *L. casei* DN-114,001 reduced the number of rhinitis episodes in 64 pre-school children with allergic rhinitis (Giovannini et al., 2007).

Thus far, there are few studies examining the treatment of allergic asthma with probiotics. The results of two studies concerning children or adults with allergic asthma showed no improvement after consumption of probiotic bacteria (Wheeler et al., 1997; Giovannini et al., 2007).

Others examined the effect of probiotic consumption on the sensitisation to several allergens (e.g. peanut, hen's egg, soy, wheat, milk, cat, dog), as determined by specific IgE production or skin prick test reaction (SPT). The authors could not find a difference before and after the treatment (Flinterman et al., 2007; Brouwer et al., 2006; Kalliomäki et al., 2001b).

SUMMARY AND FUTURE DIRECTIONS

Several human trials, as well as, numerous animal and in vitro studies indicate postitive effects of probiotics on allergic diseases thus giving a rationale for their application. However, positive effects of probiotics have not always been found, which may be due to differing study designs and to strain specifities. To clarify the effects of probiotics on allergic diseases, standardized multi-centre studies with uniform parameters regarding age of patients, severity of the allergic manifestations, strain and dosage of the probiotics, and the duration of application in a representative number of patients, should be performed.

References

Aattouri, N., Bouras, M., Tome, D., Marcos, A. and Lemonnier, D., Oral ingestion of lactic acid bacteria by rats increases lymphocyte proliferation and interferon-gamma production. *Br. J. Nutr.* 2002. 87: 367–373

Abrahamsson, T.R., Jakobsson, T., Böttcher, M.F., Fredrikson, M., Jenmalm, M.C., Björkstén, B. and Oldaeus, G., Probiotics in prevention of IgE-associated eczema: A double-blind, randomized, placebo-controlled trial. *J. Allergy Clin. Immunol.* 2007. 119: 1174–1180

Adlerberth, I., Strachan, D.P., Matricardi, P.M., Ahrné, S., Orfei, L., Aberg, N., Perkin, M.R., Tripodi, S., Hesselmar, B., Saalman, R., Coates, A.R., Bonanno, C.L., Panetta, V. and Wold, A.E., Gut microbiota and development of atopic eczema in 3 European birth cohorts. *J. Allergy Clin. Immunol.* 2007. 120: 343–350

Aldinucci, C., Bellussi, L., Monciatti, G., Passàli, G.C., Salerni, L., Passali, D. and Bocci, V., Effects of dietary yoghurt on immunological and clinical parameters of rhinopathic patients. *Eur. J. Clin. Nutr.* 2002. 56: 1155–1161

Berman, S.H., Eichelsdoerfera, P., Yima, D., Elmerb, G.W. and Wennera, C.A., Daily ingestion of a nutri-tional probiotic supplement enhances innate immune function in healthy adults. *Nutr. Res.* 2006. 26: 454–459

Björkstén, B., Naaber, P., Sepp, E. and Mikelsaar, M., The intestinal microflora in allergic Estonian and Swedish 2-year-old children. *Clin. Exp. Allergy.* 1999. 29: 342–346

Björkstén, B., Sepp, E., Julge, K., Voor, T. and Mikelsaar, M., Allergy development and the intestinal microflora during the first year of life. *J. Allergy Clin. Immunol.* 2001. 108: 516–520

Blümer, N., Sel, S., Virna, S., Patrascan, C.C., Zimmermann, S., Herz, U., Renz, H. and Garn, H., Perinatal maternal application of Lactobacillus rhamnosus GG suppresses allergic airway inflammation in mouse offspring. *Clin. Exp. Allergy.* 2007. 37: 348–357

Brouwer, M.L., Wolt-Plompen, S.A.A., Dubois, A.E.J., van der Heide, S., Jansen, D.F., Hoijer, M.A., Kauffman, H.F. and Duiverman, E.J., No effects of probiotics on atopic dermatitis in infancy: A rand-omized placebo-controlled trial. *Clin. Exp. Allergy.* 2006. 36: 899–906

Chapat, L., Chemin, K., Dubois, B., Bourdet-Sicard, R. and Kaiserlian, D., Lactobacillus casei reduces CD8+T cell-mediated skin inflammation. *Eur. J. Immunol.* 2004. 34: 2520–2528

Christensen, H.R., Nexmann Larsen, C., Kæstel, P., Rosholm, L.B., Sternberg, C., Fleischer Michaelsen, K. and Frøkiær, H., Immunomodulating potential of supplementation with probiotics: A dose-response study in healthy young adults. *FEMS Immunol. Med. Microbiol.* 2006. 47: 380–390

Ciprandi, G., Tosca, M.A., Milanese, M., Caligo, G. and Ricca, V., Cytokines evaluation in nasal lavage of allergic children after Bacillus clausii administration: A pilot study. *Pediatr. Allergy Immunol.* 2004. 15: 148–151

Ciprandi, G., Vizzaccaro, A., Cirillo, I. and Tosca, M.A., Bacillus clausii exerts immuno-modulatory activity in allergic subjects: a pilot study. *Allerg. Immunol. (Paris).* 2005a. 37: 129–134

Ciprandi, G., Vizzaccaro, A., Cirillo, I. and Tosca, M.A., Bacillus clausii effects in children with allergic rhinitis. *Allergy.* 2005b. 60: 702–710

Cukrowska, B., Lodinová-Zádniková, R., Enders, C., Sonnenborn, U., Schulze, J. and Tlaskalová-Hogenová, H., Specific proliferative and antibody repsponses of premature infants to intestinal coloni-zation with nonpathogenic probiotic E.coli strain Nissle 1917. *Scand. J. Immunol.* 2002. 55: 204–209

Díaz-Ropero, M.P., Martín, R., Sierra, S., Lara-Villoslada, F., Rodríguez, J.M., Xaus, J. and Olivares, M., Two Lactobacillus strains, isolated from breast milk, differently modulate the immune response. *J. Appl. Microbiol.* 2007. 102: 337–343

Enomoto, T., Shimizu, K. and Shimazu, S., Suppression of allergy development by habitual intake of fer-mented milk foods, evidence from an epidemiological study. *Arerugi* 2006. 55: 1394–1399

Feleszko, W., Jaworska, J., Rha, R.D., Steinhausen, S., Avagyan, A., Jaudszus, A., Ahrens, B., Groneberg, D.A., Wahn, U. and Hamelmann, E., Probiotic-induced suppression of allergic sensitization and airway inflammation is associated with an increase of T regulatory-dependent mechanisms in a murine model of asthma. *Clin. Exp. Allergy* 2006. 37: 498–505

Flinterman, A.E., Knol, E.F., van Ieperen-van Dijk, A.G., Timmerman, H.M., Knulst, A.C., Bruijnzeel-Koomen, C.A., Pasmans, S.G. and van Hoffen, E., Probiotics have a different immunomodulatory potential in vitro versus ex vivo upon oral administration in children with food allergy. *Int. Arch. Allergy Immunol.* 2007, 143: 237–244

Fölster-Holst, R., Müller, F., Schnopp, N., Abeck, D., Kreiselmaier, I., Lenz, T., von Rüden, U., Schrezenmeir, J., Christophers, E., and Weichenthal, M., Prospective, randomized controlled trial on Lactobacillus rhamnosus in infants with moderate to severe atopic dermatitis. *Br. J. Dermatol.* 2006. 155: 1256–1261

Fujiwara, D., Inoue, S., Wakabayashi, H. and Fujii, T., The anti-allergic effects of lactic acid bacteria are strain dependent and mediated by effects of both Th1/Th2 cytokine expression and balance. *Int. Arch. Allergy Immunol.* 2004. 135: 205–215

Fukushima, Y., Kawata, Y., Hara, H., Terada, A. and Mitsuoka, T., Effect of a probiotic formula on intestinal immunoglobulin A production in healthy children. *Int. J. Food Microbiol.* 1998. 42: 39–44

Ghadimi, D., Offick, B., Fölster-Holst, R., de Vrese, M., Winkler, P., Helwig, U., Heller, K. and Schrezenmeir, J., Probiotika und ihr Einfluss auf die Th1/Th2 Antwort. *Akt. Ernähr. Med.* 2007. 32

Gill, H.S., Rutherfurd, K.J. and Cross, M.L., Dietary probiotic supplementation enhances natural killer cell activity in the elderly: an investigation of age-related immunological changes. *J. Clin. Immunol.* 2001. 21: 264–271

Giovannini, M., Agostoni, C., Riva, E., Salvini, F., Ruscitto, A., Zuccotti, G.V. and Radaelli, G., A randomized prospective double blind controlled trial on effects of long-term consumption of fermented milk containing Lactobacillus casei in pro-school children with allergic asthma and/or rhinitis. *Pediatr. Res.* 2007. 62: 1–6

Hattori, K., Yamamoto, A., Sasai, M., Taniuchi, S., Kojima, T., Kobayashi, Y., Iwamoto, H., Namba, K. and Yaeshima, T., Effects of administration of bifidobacteria on fecal microflora and clinical symptoms in infants with atopic dermatitis. *Arerugi* 2003. 52: 20–30

He, F., Ouwehand, A.C., Isolauri, E., Hashimoto, H., Benno, Y., and Salminen S., Comparison of mucosal adhesion and species identification of bifidobacteria isolated from healthy and allergic infants. *FEMS Immunol. Med. Microbiol.* 2001. 30: 43–47

Helin, T., Haahtela, S. and Haahtela, T., No effect of oral treatment with an intestinal bacterial strain, Lactobacillus rhamnosus (ATCC 53103), on birch pollen allergy: A placebo-controlled double-blind study. *Allergy.* 2002. 57: 243–246

Hirose, Y., Murosaki, S., Yamamoto, Y., Yoshikai, Y. and Tsuru, T., Daily intake of heat-killed L. plantarum L-137 (HK-LP) augments acquired immunity in healthy adults. *J. Nutr.* 2006. 136: 3069–3073

Hopkins, M.J., Sharp, R. and Macfarlane G.T., Variation in human intestinal microbiota with age. *Dig. Liver Dis.* 2002. 34 (Suppl 2): S12–S18

Inoue, R., Otsuka, M., Nishio, A. and Ushida, K., Primary administration of *Lactobacillus johnsonii* NCC533 in waening period suppresses the elevation of proinflammatory cytokines and CD86 gene expression in skin lesions in NC/Nga mice. *FEMS Immunol. Med. Microbiol.* 2007a. 50: 67–76

Inoue, R., Nishio, A., Fukushima, Y. and Ushida, K., Oral treatment with probiotic *Lactobacillus johnsonii* NCC533 (La1) for a specific part of the weaning period prevents the development of atopic dermatitis induced after maturation in model mice, NC/Nga. *Br. J. Dermatol.* 2007b. 156: 499–509

Ishida, Y., Nakamura, F., Kanzato, H., Sawada, D., Hirata, H., Nishimura, A., Kajimoto, A., Kajimoto, O. and Fujiwara, S., Clinical effects of Lactobacillus acidophilus stain L-92 on perennial allergic rhinitis: a double-blind, placebo-controlled study. *J. Dairy Sci.* 2005. 88: 527–533

Isolauri, E., Arvola, T., Sütas, Y., Moilanen, E. and Salminen, S., Probiotics in the management of atopic eczema. *Clin. Exp. Allergy.* 2000. 30: 1604–1610

Isolauri, E., Sütas, Y., Kankaanpää, P., Arvilommi, H. and Salminen, S., Probiotics: effects on immunity. *Am. J. Clin. Nutr.* 2001. 73(Suppl): 444S–450S

Kalliomäki, M., Kirjavainen, P., Eerola, E., Kero, P., Salminen, S. and Isolauri, E., Distinct patterns of neonatal gut microflora in infants in whom atopy was and was not developing. *J. Allergy Clin. Immunol.* 2001a. 107: 129–134

Kalliomäki, M., Salminen, S., Arvilommi, H., Kero, P., Koskinen, P. and Isolauri, E., Probiotics in primary prevention of atopic disease: A randomized placebo-controlled trial. *Lancet* 2001b. 357: 1076–1079

Kalliomäki, M., Salminen, S., Poussa, T., Arvilommi, H. and Isolauri, E., Probiotics and prevention of atopic disease: A 4-year follow-up of a randomized placebo-controlled trial. *Lancet* 2003. 361: 1869–1971

Kalliomäki, M., Salminen, S., Poussa, T. and Isolauri, E., Probiotics during the first 7 years of life: A cumulative risk reduction of eczema in a randomized, placebo-controlled trial. *J. Allergy Clin. Immunol.* 2007. 119: 1019–1021

Kato, I., Tanaka, K. and Yokokura, T., Lactic acid bacterium potently induces the production of interleukin-12 and interferon-gamma by mouse splenocytes. *Int. J. Immunopharmacol.* 1999. 21: 121–131

Kim, H., Lee, S.Y. and Ji, G.E., Timing of bifidobacterium administration influences the development of allergy to ovalbumin in mice. *Biotechnol. Lett.* 2005a. 27: 1361–1367

Kim, H., Kwack, K., Kim, D.Y. and Ji, G.E., Oral probiotic bacterial administration suppressed allergic responses in an ovalbumin-induced allergy mouse model. *FEMS Immunol. Med. Microbiol.* 2005b. 45: 259–267

Kirjavainen, P.V., Apostolou, E., Arvola, T., Salminen, S.J., Gibson, G.R. and Isolauri, E., Characterizing the composition of intestinal microflora as a prospective treatment target in infant allergic disease. *FEMS Immunol. Med. Microbiol.* 2001. 32: 1–7

Kirjavainen, P.V., Arvola, T., Salminen, S.J. and Isolauri, E., Aberrant composition of gut microbiota of allergic infants : A target of bifidobacterial therapy at weaning? *Gut* 2002. 51: 51–55

Kirjavainen, P.V., Salminen, S.J. and Isolauri, E., Probiotic bacteria in the management of atopic disease: Underscoring the importance of viability. *J. Pediatr. Gastroenterol. Nutr.* 2003. 36: 223–227

Kishi, A., Uno, K., Matsubara, Y., Okuda, C. and Kishida, T., Effect of the oral administration of Lactobacillus brevis ssp coagulans on interferon-a producing capacity in humans. *J. Am. Coll. Nutr.* 1996. 15: 408–412

Kruisselbrink, A., Heijne den Bak-Glashouwer, M.-J., Havenith, C. E. G.; Thole, J. E. R. and Janssen, R., Recombinant Lactobacillus plantarum inhibits house dust mite-specific T-cell responses. *Clin. Exp. Immunol.* 2001. 126: 2–8

Kukkonen, K., Savilahti, E., Haahtela, T., Juntunen-Backman, K., Korpela, R., Poussa, T., Tuure, T. and Kuitunen, M., Probiotics and prebiotic galacto-oligosaccharides in the prevention of allergic diseases: A randomized, double-blind, placebo-controlled trial. *J. Allergy Clin. Immunol.* 2007. 119: 192–198

Lodinová-Zádniková, R., Cukrowska, B. and Tlaskalova-Hogenova, H., Oral administration of probiotic Escherichia coli after birth reduces frequency of allergies and repeated infections later in life (after 10 and 20 years). *Int. Arch. Allergy Immunol.* 2003. 131: 209–211

Lodinová-Zádniková, R., Prokesová, L., Tlaskalová, H., Kocourková, I., Zizka, J. and Stranák, Z., Influence of oral colonization with probiotic E. coli strain after birth on frequency of recurrent infections, allergy and development of some immunologic parameters. Long-term studies. *Ceska. Gynekol.* 2004. 69 (Suppl 1): 91–97

Mah, K.W., Björkstén, B., Lee, B.W., van Bever, H.P., Shek, L.P., Tan, T.N., Lee, Y.K. and Chua, Y.K., Distinct pattern of commensal gut microbiota in toddlers with eczema. *Int. Arch. Allergy Immunol.* 2006. 140: 157–163

Majamaa, H. and Isolauri, E., Probiotics: a novel approach in the management of food allergy. *J. Allergy Clin. Immunol.* 1997. 99: 179–185

Marcos, A., Wärnberg, J., Nova, E., Gómez, S., Alvarez, A., Alvarez, R., Mateos, J.A. and Cobo, J.M., The effect of milk fermented by yoghurt cultures plus Lactobacillus casei DN-114001 on the immune response of subjects under academis examination stress. *Eur. J. Nutr.* 2004. 43: 381–389

Mastrandrea, F., Coradduzza, G., Serio, G., Minardi, A., Manelli, M., Ardito, S. and Muratore, L., Probiotics reduce the CD34 + hemopoietic precursor cell increased traffic in allergic subjects. *Allerg. Immunol. (Paris)* 2004. 36: 118–122

Matsumoto, M., Aranami, A., Ishige, A., Watanabe, K. and Benno, Y., LKM512 yoghurt consumption improves the intestinal environment and induces the T-helper type 1 cytokine in adult patients with intractable atopic dermatitis. *Clin. Exp. Allergy* 2007. 37: 358–370

Matsuzaki, T., Yamazaki, R., Hashimoto, S. and Yokokura, T., The effect of oral feeding of Lactobacillus casei strain shirota on immunoglobulin E production in mice. *J. Dairy Sci.* 1998. 81: 48–53

Moreira, A., Kekkonen, R., Korpela, R., Delgado, L. and Haahtela, T., Allergy in marathon runners and effect of Lactobacillus GG supplementation on allergic inflammatory markers. *Respir. Med.* 2007. 101: 1123–1131

Morita, H., He, F., Kawase, M., Kubota, A., Hiramatsu, M., Kurisaki, J.I. and Salminen, S., Preliminary human study for possible alteration of serum immunoglobulin E production in perennial allergic rhinitis with fermented milk prepared with Lactobacillus gasseri TMC0356. *Microbiol. Immunol.* 2006. 50: 701–706

Nagao, F., Nakayama, M., Muto, T. and Okumura, K., Effects of a fermented milk drink containing Lactobacillus casei strain shirota on the immune system in healthy human subjects. *Biosci. Biotechnol. Biochem.* 2000. 64: 2706–2708

Niers, L.E.M., Timmerman, H.M., Rijkers, G.T., van Bleek, G.M., van Uden, N.O.P., Knol, E.F., Kapsenberg, M.L., Kimpen, J.L.L. and Hoekstra, M.O., Identification of strong interleukin-10 inducing lactic acid bacteria which down-regulate T helper type 2 cytokines. *Clin. Exp. Allergy* 2005. 35: 1481–1489

Ogawa, T., Hashikawa, S., Asai, Y., Sakamoto, H., Yasuda, K. and Makimura, Y., A new synbiotic, Lactobacillus casei subsp. Casei together with dextran, reduces murine and human allergic reaction. *FEMS Immunol. Med. Microbiol.* 2006. 46: 400–409

Ogden, N.S. and Bielory L., Probiotics: a complementary approach in the treatment and prevention of pediatric atopic disease. *Curr. Opin. Allergy Clin. Immunol.* 2005. 5: 179–184

Olivares, M., Díaz-Ropero, P., Gómez, N., Lara-Villoslada, F., Sierra, S., Maldonado, J.A., Martín, R., Rodríguez, J.M. and Xaus, J., The consumption of two new probiotic strains, Lactobacillus gasseri CECT5714 and Lactobacillus coryniformis CECT5711, boost the immune system of healthy humans. *Int. Microbiol.* 2006. 9: 47–52

Ouwehand, A.C., Antiallergic effects of probiotics. *J. Nutr.* 2007. 137: 794S–797S

Ouwehand, A.C., Isolauri, E., He, F., Hashimoto, H., Benno, Y. and Salminen S., Differences in bifidobacterium flora composition in allergic and healthy infants. *J. Allergy Clin. Immunol.* 2001. 108: 144–145

Parra, D., De Morentin, B.M., Cobo, J.M., Mateos, A. and Martinez, J.A., Monocyte function in healthy middle-aged people receiving fermented milk containing Lactobacillus casei. *J. Nutr. Health Aging.* 2004a. 8: 208–211

Parra, D., De Morentin, B.M., Cobo, J.M., Mateos, A. and Martinez, J.A., Daily intake of fermented milk containing Lactobacillus casei DN114001 improves innate-defense capacity in healthy middle-aged people. *J. Physiol. Biochem.* 2004b. 60: 85–91

Parvez, S., Malik, K,A., Ah Kang, S. and Kim, H.-Y., Probiotics and their fermented food products are beneficial for health. *J. Appl. Microbiol.* 2006. 100: 1171–1185

Passeron, T., Lacour, J.P., Fontas, E. and Ortonne, J.P., Prebiotics and synbiotics: two promising approaches for the treatment of atopic dermatitis in children above 2 years. *Allergy* 2006. 61: 431–437

Pelto, L., Isolauri, E., Lilius, E.M., Nuutila, J. and Salminen, S., Probiotic bacteria down-regulate the milk-induced inflammatory response in milk-hypersensitive subjects but have an immunostimulatory effect in healthy subjects. *Clin. Exp. Allergy* 1998. 28: 1474–1479

Penders, J., Stobberingh, E.E., Thijs, C., Adams, H., Vink, C., van Ree, R. and van den Brandt, P.A., Molecular fingerprinting of the intestinal microbiota of infants in whom atopic eczema was or was not developing. *Clin. Exp. Allergy.* 2006. 36: 1602–1608

Peng, G.C. and Hsu, C.H., The efficacy and safety of heat-killed Lactobacillus paracasei for treatment of perennial allergic rhinitis induced by house-dust mite. *Pediatr. Allergy Immunol.* 2005. 16: 433–438

Pessi, T., Sütas, Y., Hurme, M. and Isolauri, E., Interleukin-10 generation in atopic children following oral Lactobacillus rhamnosus GG. *Clin. Exp. Allergy.* 2000. 30: 1804–1808

Pochard, P., Gosset, P., Grangette, C., Andre, C., Tonnel, A.B., Pestel, J. and Mercenier, A., Lactic acid bacteria inhibit Th2 cytokine production by mononuclear cells from allergic patients. *J. Allergy Clin. Immunol.* 2002. 110: 617–623

Pochard, P., Hammad, H., Ratajczak, C., Charbonnier-Hatzfeld, A.S., Just, N., Tonnel, A.B. and Pestel, J., Direct regulatory immune activity of lactic acid bacteria on Der p 1-pulsed dendritic cells from allergic patients. *J. Allergy Clin. Immunol.* 2005. 116: 198–204

Pohjavuori, E., Viljanen, M., Korpela, R., Kuitunen, M., Tiittanen, M., Vaarala, O. and Saviiahti, E., Lactobacillus GG effect in increasing IFN-γ production in infants with cow's milk allergy. *J. Allergy Clin. Immunol.* 2004. 114: 131–136

Prescott, S.L., Dunstan, J.A., Hale, J., Breckler, L., Lehmann, H., Weston, S. and Richmond, P., Clinical effects of probiotics are associated with increased interferon-y responses in very young children with atopic dermatitis. *Clin. Exp. Allergy* 2005. 35: 1557–1564

Rautava, S., Kalliomäki, M. and Isolauri, E., Probiotics during pregnancy and breast-feeding might confer immunomodulatory protection against atopic disease in the infant. *J. Allergy Clin. Immunol.* 2002. 109: 119–121

Rinne, M., Kalliomäki, M., Arvilommi, H., Salminen, S. and Isolauri, E., Effect of probiotics and breast-feeding on the bifidobacterium and lactobacillus/enterococcus microbiota and humoral immune responses. *J. Pediatr.* 2005. 147: 186–191

Romagnani, S., TH1 and TH2 in human diseases. *Clin. Immunol. Immunopathol.* 1996. 80: 225–235

Rosenfeldt, V., Benfeldt, E., Dam Nielsen, S., Fleischer Michaelsen, K., Jeppesen, D.L., Valerius, N.H. and Paerregaard, A., Effect of probiotic Lactobacillus strains in children with atopic dermatitis. *J. Allergy Clin. Immunol.* 2003. 111: 389–395

Rosenfeldt, V., Benfeldt, E., Valerius, N.H., Paerregaard, A. and Fleischer Michaelsen, K., Effect of probiotics on gastrointestinal symptoms and small intestinal permeability in children with atopic dermatitis. *J. Pediatr.* 2004. 145: 612–616

Sawada, J., Morita, H., Tanaka, A., Salminen, S., He, F. and Matsuda, H., Ingestion of heat-treated Lactobacillus rhamnosus GG prevents development of atopic dermatitis in NC/Nga mice. *Clin. Exp. Allergy.* 2006. 37: 296–303

Schrezenmeir, J. and de Vrese, M., Probiotics, prebiotics, and synbiotics-approaching a definition. *Am. J. Clin. Nutr.* 2001. 73: 361S-364S

Sepp, E., Julge, K., Vasar, M., Naaber, P., Björkstén, B. and Mikelsaar, M., Intestinal microflora of Estonian and Swedish infants. *Acta. Paediatr.* 1997. 89: 956–961

Sheih, Y.H., Chiang, B.L., Wang, L.H., Liao, C.K. and Gill, H.S., Systemic immunity-enhancing effects in healthy subjects following dietary consumption of the lactic acid bacterium Lactobacillus rhamnosus HN001. *J. Am. Coll. Nutr.* 2001. 20: 149–156

Shida, K., Takahashi, R., Iwadate, E., Takamizawa, K., Yasui, H., Sato, T., Habu, S., Hachimura, S. and Kaminogawa, S., Lactobacillus casei strain Shirota suppresses serum immunoglobulin E and immunoglobulin G1 responses and systemic anaphylaxis in a food allergy model. *Clin. Exp. Allergy.* 2002. 32: 563–570

Sistek, D., Kelly, R., Wickens, K., Stanley, T., Fitzharris, P. and Crane, J., Is the effect of probiotics on atopic dermatitis confined to food sensitized children? *Clin. Exp. Allergy.* 2006. 36: 629–633

Spanhaak, S., Havebaar, R. and Schaafsma, G., The effect of consumption of milk fermented by Lactobacillus casei strain shirota on the intestinal microflora and immune parameters in humans. *Eur. J. Clin. Nutr.* 1998. 52 : 899–907

Strachan, D.P., Family size, infection and atopy: The first decade of the "hygiene hypothesis". *Thorax* 2000. 55 (Suppl 1): S2–S10

Takahashi, N., Kitazawa, H., Iwabuchi, N., Xiao, J.Z., Miyaji, K., Iwatsuki, K. and Saito, T., Oral administration of an immunostimulatory DNA sequence from Bifidobacterium longum improves Th1/Th2 balance in a murine model. *Biosci. Biotechnol. Biochem.* 2006. 70: 2013–2017

Takeda, K. and Okumura, K., Effects of a fermented milk drink containing Lactobacillus casei strain shirota on the human NK-cell activity. *J. Nutr.* 2007. 137: 791S–793S

Tamura, M., Shikina, T., Morihana, T., Hayama, M., Kajimoto, O., Sakamoto, A., Kajimoto, Y., Watanabe, O., Nonaka, C., Shida, K. and Nanno, M., Effects of probiotics on allergic rhinitis induced by Japanese cedar pollen: randomized double-blind, placebo-controlled clinical trial. *Int. Arch. Allergy. Immunol.* 2007. 143: 75–82

Taylor, A.L., Hale, J., Wiltschut, J., Lehmann, H., Dunstan, J.A. and Prescott, S.L., Effects of probiotic supplementation for the first 6 months of life on allergen- and vaccine-specific immune response. *Clin. Exp. Allergy.* 2006a. 36: 1227–1235

Taylor, A.L., Hale, J., Wiltschut, J., Lehmann, H., Dunstan, J.A. and Prescott, S.L., Evaluation of the effects of probiotic supplementation from the neonatal period on innate immune development in infancy. *Clin. Exp. Allergy.* 2006b. 36: 1218–1226

Taylor, A.L., Dunstan, J.A. and Prescott, S.L., Probiotic supplementation for the first 6 months of life fails to reduce the risk of atopic dermatitis and increases the risk of allergen sensitization in high-risk children: a randomized controlled trial. *J. Allergy Clin. Immunol.* 2007a. 119: 184–191

Taylor, A.L., Hale, J., Hales, B.J., Dunstan, J.A., Thomas, W.R. and Prescott, S.L., FOXP3 mRNA expression at 6 months of age is higher in infants who develop atopic dermatitis, but is not affected by giving probiotics from birth. *Pediatr. Allergy Immunol.* 2007b. 18: 10–19

Tlaskalová-Hogenová, H., Tuckova, L., Mestecky, J., Kolinska, J., Rossmann, P., Stepankova, R., Kozakova, Hudcovic, T., Hrncir, T., Frolova, L. and Kverka, M., Interaction of mucosal microbiota with the innate immune system. *Scand. J. Immunol.* 2005. 62 (Suppl 1): 106-113

Torii, A., Torii, S., Fujiwara, S., Tanaka, H., Inagaki, N. and Nagai, H., Lactobacillus acidophilus strain L-92 regulates the production of Th1 cytokine as well as Th2 cytokines. *Allergol. Int.* 2007. 56: 1–9

Van de Water, J., Keen, C.L. and Gershwin, M.E., The influence of chronic yoghurt consumption on immunity. *J. Nutr.* 1999. 129: 1492S-1495S

Viljanen, M., Pohjavuori, E., Haahtela, T., Korpela, R., Kuitunen, M., Sarnesto, A., Vaarala, O. and Savilahti, E., Induction of inflammation as a possible mechanism of probiotic effect in atopic-eczema-dermatitis syndrome. *J. Allergy Clin. Immunol.* 2005a. 115: 1254–1259

Viljanen, M., Kuitunen, M., Haahtela, T., Juntunen-Backman, K., Korpela, R. and Savilahti, E., Probiotic effects on faecal inflammatory markers and on faecal IgA in food allergic atopic eczema/dermatitis syndrome infants. *Pediatr. Allergy Immunol.* 2005b. 16: 65–71

Viljanen, M., Savilahti, E., Haahtela, T., Juntunen-Backman, K., Korpela, R., Poussa, T., Tuure, T. and Kuitunen, M., Probiotics in the treatment of atopic eczema/dermatitis syndrome in infants: A double-blind placebo-controlled trial. *Allergy* 2005c. 60: 494–500

Wang, M.F., Lin, H.C., Wang, Y.Y. and Hsu, C.H., Treatment of perennial allergic rhinitis with lactic acid bacteria. *Pediatr. Allergy Immunol.* 2004. 15: 152–158

Warner, J.O., Kaliner, M.A., Crisci, C.D., Del Giacco, S.D., Frew, A.J., Liu, G.H., Maspero, J., Moon, H.B., Nakagawa, T., Potter, P.C., Rosenwasser, L.J., Singh, A.B., Valovirta, E. and van Cauwenberge, P., Allergy Practice Worldwide: A Report by the World Allergy Organization Specialty and Training Council. *Int. Arch. Allergy Immunol.* 2006. 139: 166–174

Watanabe, S., Narisawa, Y., Arase, S., Okamatsu, H., Ikenaga, T., Tajiri, Y. and Kumemura, M., Differences in fecal microflora between patients with atopic dermatitis and healthy control subjects. *J. Allergy Clin. Immunol.* 2003. 111: 587–591

Weston, S., Halbert, A., Richmond, P. and Prescott, S.L., Effects of probiotics on atopic dermatitis: A randomised controlled trial. *Arch. Dis. Child.* 2005. 90: 892–897

Wheeler, J.G., Shema, S.J., Bogle, M.L., Shirrell, M.A., Burks, A.W., Pittler, A. and Helm, R.M., Immune and clinical impact of Lactobacillus acidophilus on asthma. *Ann. Allergy Asthma Immunol.* 1997. 79: 229–233

Winkler, P., Ghadimi, D., Schrezenmeir, J. and Kraehenbuhl, J.P., Molecular and cellular basis of microflora-host interactions. *J. Nutr.* 2007. 137: 755S–771S

Xiao, J.Z., Kondo, S., Yanagisawa, N., Takahishi, N., Odamaki, T., Iwabuchi, N., Iwatsuki, K., Kokubo, S., Togashi, H., Enomoto, K. and Enomoto, T., Effect of probiotic Bifidobacterium longum BBS36 in relieving clinical symptoms and modulating plasma cytokine levels of japanese cedar pollinosis during the pollen season. A randomized double-blind, placebo-controlled trial. *J. Investig. Allergol. Clin. Immunol.* 2006a. 16: 86–93

Xiao, J.Z., Kondo, S., Yanagisawa, N., Takahishi, N., Odamaki, T., Iwabuchi, N., Miyaji, K., Iwatsuki, K., Togashi, H., Enomoto, K. and Enomoto, T., Probiotics in the treatment of Japanese cedar pollinosis: A double-blind placebo-controlled trial. *Clin. Exp. Allergy* 2006b. 36: 1425–1435

Xiao, J.Z., Kondo, S., Yanagisawa, N., Miyaji, K., Enomoto, K., Sakoda, T., Iwatsuki, K. and Enomoto, T., Clinical efficacy of probiotic Bifidobacterium longum for the treatment of symptoms of Japanese cedar pollen allergy in subjects evaluated in an environmental exposure unit. *Allergol. Int.* 2007. 56: 67–75

19 The Role of Probiotics in the Treatment and Prevention of Asthma

Michael D. Cabana

Key Points

- Asthma is one of the most common chronic diseases.
- The number of studies focusing on the treatment of asthma have been small and shown little, if any, effect.
- To date there is insufficient data to support the use of probiotics for the prevention of asthma.

Key Words: Asthama, eczema, hygiene hypothesis.

INTRODUCTION

Asthma is one of the most common chronic diseases. In the USA alone, 32.6 million persons are affected by asthma during their lifetime.[1] Asthma is a chronic, obstructive respiratory disease characterized by intermittent exacerbations, due to pulmonary bronchoconstriction and mucus production in the small airways of the lungs. Symptoms include wheezing, cough, and shortness of breath and/or chest pain. Between exacerbations or asthma "attacks," pulmonary function is relatively normal. These exacerbations can be triggered by any number of exposures, including upper respiratory infections, allergies, exercise, or exposure to environmental irritants such as tobacco smoke.

Given the burden of disease, there is great interest in the development of preventive therapies for asthma. As asthma has an episodic nature, with intermittent exacerbations, it is important to define the different levels of prevention. Primary prevention refers to attempts to avert the initial development of asthma. Once the disease has been diagnosed, efforts to prevent further exacerbations are referred to as tertiary prevention,[2] which includes treatment to prevent or mitigate an asthma exacerbation.

Although there has been much work on the effects of probiotics on gastrointestinal disorders and infectious diseases, there are few trials on the effects of probiotics in the prevention or the treatment of asthma. In recent years, there has been growing interest in this area. It is hypothesized that probiotic bacteria may have an immunomodulatory effect,

From: *Nutrition and Health: Probiotics in Pediatric Medicine*
Edited by: S. Michail and P.M. Sherman © Humana Press, Totowa, NJ

and as a result, the effectiveness of probiotics have been examined in the context of treatment or tertiary prevention of asthma. In addition, several studies have explored the use of probiotics for primary prevention of atopic disease, and specific studies are underway to examine the use of probiotics in the context of primary prevention of asthma.

This chapter summarizes current work in probiotic effects on the primary and tertiary prevention of asthma.

GUT FLORA AND ATOPIC DISEASE

Asthma is one of several atopic diseases, which include eczema and rhinitis. As a patient with one atopic disease has increased likelihood of having additional atopic disorders, insight regarding atopic disease in general may be applicable to asthma.

Broad ecologic studies have noted differences in the intestinal microflora among infants from different countries and among those persons that have different dietary lifestyles.[3] These differences in microflora may correspond to the differences in the prevalence of different allergic diseases in children from such groups.

For example, lower levels of *Clostridium difficile* and higher levels of lactobacilli have been noted in stool samples from Estonian children, compared to stool samples from Swedish children. Estonian children have decreased consumption of processed foods and higher levels of fermented food products, which may help account for the differences noted. The differences in intestinal microflora have been noted to correspond not only with dietary differences, but also with lower levels of asthma and allergy in these countries.[4]

Observational studies have taken advantage of examining the effects of an anthroposophic diet, which includes vegetables spontaneously fermented by lactobacilli, as well as a restrictive use of antibiotics on gut microflora and allergic disease. Fecal samples from anthroposophic children, compared to controls, have been noted to have higher numbers of enterococci and lactic acid bacteria.[5] These differences in gut microflora are associated with the decreased likelihood of atopic sensitization and atopic disease, such as rhinitis, that have been noted in children from anthroposophic families.[6] It is difficult to attribute which specific facets of an anthroposophic lifestyle are associated with decreased allergic disease. A cross-sectional multicenter study including 4,606 children with anthroposophic lifestyles and 2,024 controls noted a decreased likelihood of rhino-conjunctivitis, atopic eczema, and atopic sensitization. In this cohort, decreased use of antibiotics, antipyretics, and immunizations were associated with a reduced risk of allergic disease.[7]

Several studies have examined specific associations between gastrointestinal microflora populations and atopic diseases; however, the majority of these studies have focused on atopic dermatitis or atopic sensitization, as opposed to asthma (Table 19.1). As a result, the link between gastrointestinal colonization and asthma still needs further clarification.

A case-control study of 98 children with and without atopic dermatitis in Japan noted that children with atopic dermatitis had lower colony counts of bifidobacteria. Fecal samples were not prospectively obtained and as a result, represent colonization with current disease, not necessarily colonization before disease development. However, the severity of eczema was inversely related to fecal levels of bifidobacteria.[8]

Table 19.1

Studies that link associations between stool colonization and development of atopic disease

Author	Study design	Determination of stool colonization	Determination of atopic disease	Association noted
Penders et al. (2007)	KOALA prospective birth cohort ($n = 957$) (Excluded pre-term infants and those infants with antibiotic exposure in first month)	At 1 month of age, stool sample obtained and analyzed using quantitative real-time PCR	At 2 years of age, eczema and history of recurrent wheezing determined by parental questionnaires. Sensitization determined by IgE level > 0.3 IU against one or more of tested food or inhalant allergens	• *Clostridium difficile* colonization associated with increased likelihood of eczema (OR: 1.40; 95% CI: 1.02, 1.91), recurrent wheeze (OR: 1.75; 95% CI: 1.09, 2.80), atopic dermatitis (OR: 1.73; 95% CI: 1.08, 2.78), or sensitization (OR: 1.54; 95% CI: 1.02, 2.31). • *Escherichia coli* colonization associated with increased likelihood of eczema (OR: 1.87; 95% CI: 1.15, 3.04), but not recurrent wheeze, atopic dermatitis or sensitization. • No association found between level of bifidobacteria colonization, presence of *Bacteroides fragilis* or presence of lactobacilli colonization.
Watanabe et al. (2003)	Case-control study of 30 children with atopic dermatitis and 68 sex-matched control subjects.	Fecal samples collected within 1 week of survey	Atopic dermatitis based on Japanese Dermatological Association criteria.	Bifidobacteria colony counts lower in patients with atopic dermatitis
Kalliomaki et al. (2001)	Prospective cohort ($n = 76$) of infants with a family history of atopic disease	Fecal samples at 3 weeks of age and 3 months of age. Bacterial culture, gas-liquid chromatography (GLC) of bacterial fatty acids and quantitative fluorescent in-situ hybridization (FISH) of bacterial cells.	Atopic sensitization evaluated by skin prick testing at 12 months.	At 3 weeks of age, using FISH, atopic children had more clostridia ($p = 0.04$); and a reduced ratio of bifidobacteria to clostridia ($p = 0.03$)

(continued)

Table 19.1
(continued)

Author	Study design	Determination of stool colonization	Determination of atopic disease	Association noted
Bjorksten et al. (2001)	Description of 18 allergic infants and 26 nonallergic infants. "The two groups were selected from participants in a prospective study of the development of immune responses to allergens and the development of allergy in relation to environmental factors."	Fecal samples at 5–6 days, 1, 3, 6, and 12 months.	"Allergic children had atopic dermatitis and/or at least 1 positive skin prick test result."	Allergic infants less likely to be colonized with bifidobacteria in the first year of life. Allergic infants less likely to be colonized with enterococci in the first year of life. Allergic infants more likely to be colonized with clostridia at 3 months of life.
Bottcher et al. (2000)	Convenience sample of 25 allergic and 47 nonallergic children participating in a prospective study.	Stool culture at 13 months of age. Microflora characteristics assessed based on concentrations of eight different short-chain fatty acids, conversion of cholesterol to coprostanol, and fecal tryptic activity.	At 11–13 months of age, allergy determined by at least one positive skin prick test to one of five allergens and allergic symptoms	Allergic infants had higher levels of i-caproic acid (which has been associated with *C. difficile*)
Bjorkstein et al. (1999)	Description of 29 Estonian and 33 Swedish 2-year-old children who were participating in, "a prospective study of allergic disease in relation to environmental factors starting at birth. The children were selected from a larger cohort based on a convincing history of either the presence or absence of allergic disease up to 2 years of age."	Fecal samples collected at 2 years of age	Allergic defined as atopic dermatitis and positive skin prick test.	Allergic children less frequently colonized with lactobacilli. Allergic children less frequently colonized with bifidobacteria

PCR, polymerase chain reaction; OR, odds ratio; CI, confidence interval.

A similar cross-sectional study of a convenience sample of 62 Estonian and Swedish children with and without allergic disease (defined as atopic dermatitis and a positive skin prick test), noted that allergic children were less frequently colonized with bifidio-bacteria and *Lactobacillus*.[9]

Stronger study designs that include prospective collection of stool samples have noted similar observations. One prospective study included children from Estonia and Sweden who were selected from a sample of children already participating in a prospective study of the development of allergy. Allergy was defined as atopic dermatitis or at least one positive skin prick test result. A prospective comparison of these children without allergy noted that allergic infants were less likely to be colonized with Bifidobacetria and Enterococci in the first year of life. Allergic infants were more likely to be colonized with clostridia at 3 months of life.[10]

Large sample sizes may be needed to detect significant clinical differences in stool colonization. In addition, traditional bacterial stool culture may not be sensitive in detecting subtle changes in gut microflora for these studies. Other techniques have been employed to help characterize stool colonization in these populations.

A study of a convenience sample of 25 allergic and 47 nonallergic children participating in a prospective study included an analysis of microflora-associated characteristics such as formation of short-chain fatty acids. Stool culture was obtained at 13 months of age and analyzed for concentrations of different short-chain fatty acids. Allergic infants had significantly higher levels of i-caproic acid, which has been associated with *C. difficile*.[11]

In Finland, a cohort of 76 infants compared fecal samples at 3 weeks of age to later development of atopic sensitization at 12 months of age. At 3 weeks of age, although there was no difference in cultured fecal microflora, further assessment using fluorescent in situ hybridization (FISH) of bacterial cells revealed that atopic children had greater bacterial counts of clostridia ($p = 0.04$); and a reduced ratio of bifidobacteria to clostridia ($p = 0.03$).[12]

The strongest link between fecal microflora early in life to the later development of recurrent wheezing is the large-scale prospective study of the KOALA cohort, which examined gut microbial composition of 957 infants in the Netherlands.[13] Infants were recruited during the prenatal period at 34 weeks gestation. The final study cohort excluded infants who were premature, who received antibiotics during the first year of life, or those for whom insufficient stool samples were obtained.

Stool samples were obtained at 1 month of age and analyzed using quantitative real-time polymerase chain reaction. At 2 years of age, a history of recurrent wheezing, which was defined as at least four episodes of wheezing, was determined using parent interviews.

C. difficile colonization at 1 month was associated with increased likelihood of eczema (OR: 1.40; 95% CI: 1.02, 1.91), recurrent wheeze (OR: 1.75; 95% CI: 1.09, 2.80), atopic dermatitis (OR: 1.73; 95% CI: 1.08, 2.78), or sensitization (OR: 1.54; 95% CI: 1.02, 2.31). Escherichia *coli* colonization at 1 month was associated with increased likelihood of eczema (OR: 1.87; 95% CI: 1.15, 3.04), but not recurrent wheeze, atopic dermatitis or sensitization. No association was found between higher levels of bifidobacteria colonization (compared to low levels), or with *Bacteroides fragilis* or lactobacilli colonization.

It is difficult to establish the diagnosis of asthma at a young age, since a significant proportion of children who wheeze have transient symptoms and never wheeze again.[14] In addition, there are many different causes for wheezing in young children, such as bronchiolitis. However, the use of recurrent wheezing is a reasonable but limited marker for the later development of asthma. Castro-Rodriguez et al. used frequent wheezing as part of a clinical index based on data collected from parents of children at 3 years of age. The index, which included frequent wheezing, had a positive predictive value of 0.48 (and a negative predictive value of 0.92) for predicting the later development of asthma at 6 years of age.[15]

PROBIOTICS FOR THE TREATMENT OF ASTHMA

Collectively, the studies demonstrate the importance of gut microbial community to "extraintestinal" manifestations of disease. Certain patterns are noteworthy. In many studies, early colonization with bifidobacteria and decreased colonization with clostridia seem to have a protective effect from the development of atopic disease, such as eczema. Shifts in the microbial community composition and abundance of specific bacterial species correlate with development of atopy. However, the link to asthma is not as well defined due to limited studies in this area.

Further characterization of how the infant intestinal microflora is linked to atopic disease is ongoing. As described in previous chapters, there are many hypothesized mechanisms by which probiotics produce a healthy effect for gastrointestinal disorders. These include competitive inhibition with pathogenic bacteria, as probiotic organisms may compete for receptor sites in the intestinal lumen or compete with pathogens for nutrients. Other proposed mechanisms include enhancement of host immune defenses via intensification of tight junctions between enterocytes, stimulation of cytokines, increasing immunoglobulin A production, and production of substances thought to secondarily act as protective nutrients, such as arginine, glutamine, and short-chain fatty acids.[16]

Probiotic supplementation may attenuate the inflammatory response. Studies using animal models have showed that treatment with *Lactobacillus reuteri* leads to attenuation of an allergic airway response, as defined by hyperresponsiveness, influx of eosinophils into the airway lumen and parenchyma, cytokine responses, such as reduced levels of TNF, IL-5, and IL-13. Further work is needed to detail more specific mechanism of how changes in gut microflora affect regulators of allergic airways disease.[17]

LIMITED EVIDENCE AND SUCCESS FOR PROBIOTIC TREATMENT OF ASTHMA

Use of probiotics for the treatment of asthma has not been as successful as their use for the treatment of atopic dermatitis. Although results have been mixed,[18] some studies using rigorous, double-blind, placebo-controlled designs have been successful for certain subsets of patients. For atopic dermatitis, probiotic treatment is more likely to be successful when patients are younger, with more severe disease and when subjective outcomes are measured.[19,20,21]

There is limited data on the effectiveness of probiotics for the treatment of asthma and the few studies are reviewed below, as well as in Table 19.2.

Table 19.2
Probiotic trials for the prevention or treatment of asthma

Author	Treatment (T) or Prevention (P)	Study design/ Location/ Date	Subjects Inclusion criteria Exclusion criteria	Intervention description	Association noted
Giovannini et al. (2007)	T	Randomized Double-blind placebo-controlled trial Northern Italy April 2003–March 2004	$N = 176$ children 2–5 years Allergy based on skin prick test Allergic asthma and/or rhinitis (Excluded children with cow's milk allergy, lactose intolerance, severe food allergy and other severe chronic disease, perinatal respiratory problems, antibiotic use in the preceding 4 weeks)	12 months of daily oral supplementation of fermented milk containing two yogurt cultures of *Lactobacillus bulgaricus* 10^7 cfu/mL and *Streptococcus thermophilus* 10^8 cfu/ mL and *L. casei* CN-114 10^8 cfu/mL versus non-fermented milk control	• No difference in the duration of asthma episodes. • No difference in the time free from episodes of asthma. • No difference in the mean of the cumulative number of episodes of asthma
Stockert et al. (2007)	T	Randomized Double-blind placebo-controlled trial Vienna, Austria Recruitment date not stated	$N = 17$ children 6–12 years 1-year history of intermittent or mild persistent asthma FEV1 $\leq 85\%$ of predicted, $\geq 12\%$ reversibility of FEV1 and $\geq 15\%$ diurnal variation in peak expiratory flow. (Excluded children received systemic or inhaled corticosteroids or laser acupuncture treatment in last 6 months or any severe concomitant disease.	10 treatments of laser acupuncture once a week plus 6×10^7 non-pathogenic *Enterococcus faecalis* three times a day for 7 weeks versus control of laser acupuncture (without laser light) and placebo.	• No difference in quality of life scores • No difference in use of beta-agonists, inhaled corticosteroids, or cromolyn sodium

(continued)

Table 19.2
(continued)

Author	Treatment (T) or Prevention (P)	Study design/ Location/ Date	Subjects Inclusion criteria Exclusion criteria	Intervention description	Association nnoted
Kukkonen et al. (2007)	P	Double-blind placebo-controlled trial Helsinki, Finland November 2000–March 2003	$N = 1,223$ newborn infants	2–4 weeks prenatally twice daily and postnatally for 6 months of 5×10^9 cfu $L.$ $rhamnosus$ GG (ATCC 53103); 2×10^8 $Bifidobacterium$ $breve$ Bb99(CSM13692(; 2×10^9 $Propionbacterium$ $freudenreichii$ ssp. $shermanii$ JS (DSM 7076). Post-natal intervention also included 0.8 g of galacto-oligosaccharides once daily.	• No differences in the cumulative effect on any allergic disease—combined for food allergy, ecze,ma, asthma, and allergic rhinitis. (OR: 0.85; 95% CI: 0.64. 1.12). • When adjusted for confounding factors, there were differences in IgE-associated disease, eczema and atopic eczema, but not for asthma.
Wheeler et al. (1997)	T	Double-blind placebo-controlled cross-over trial Arkansas, USA Study dates not stated	$N = 15$ asthmatics with moderate asthma	1 month treatment phase of $L.$ $acidophilus$ ($8 \times 108/g$ yogurt, 450 g yogurt/d) + $S.$ $thermophilus$ ($3 \times 10^8/g$) and $L.$ $bulgaricus$ ($3 \times 108/g$) strain designations not provided	• No differences in pulmonary function tests • No differences in quality of life index • No differences in IL-2, IL-4, IgE or peripheral cell counts.

A small cross-over double-blinded trial examined the effects of probiotics on the treatment of asthma. The subjects included 15 patients with a history of asthma, who required daily asthma medications but were clinically stable. Subjects were assigned to 1 month of 250 g of yogurt with *L. acidophilus* (average concentration 7.6×10^8 bacteria/g), *L. bulgaricus* (average concentration 3.0 to 3.4×10^8 bacteria/g), and *Streptococcus thermophilus* (average concentration 3.1 to 3.7×10^8 bacteria/g), or 1 month of the same yogurt without *L. acidophilus*. Outcomes were based on pulmonary function tests, such as average peak flows, and quality of life assessment, peripheral cell counts, immunoglobulin E (IgE) or IL-2 and IL-4 levels. For all outcomes, there were no differences in the two groups.[22]

A randomized double-blind study assessed the effect of probiotic *Enterococcus faecalis* and acupuncture on pulmonary lung function tests for children with asthma. The combination of probiotic therapy and acupuncture was thought to be more consistent with the principles of traditional Chinese medicine practices, which would include a multimodal approach to lung disease. As a result, those in the intervention group ($n = 7$) received 6×10^7 non-pathogenic *E. faecalis* three times per day combined with 10 weeks of laser acupuncture, compared to placebo ($n = 9$). In the final analysis, there was no effect on forced expiratory volume (FEV1) or quality of life scores.[23]

A larger study with a longer intervention duration examined the effect of fermented milk containing *L. casei* (10^8 cfu/mL) on the number of episodes of asthma and allergic rhinitis.24 Subjects included 187 children, between 2 and 5 years of age. The groups received either 12 months of daily supply of a control non-fermented milk product or the intervention fermented milk containing yogurt cultures of *L. bulgaricus* 10^7 cfu/mL and *S. thermophilus* 10^8 cfu/mL and *L. casei* CN-114 10^8 cfu/mL. After 12 months, there was no statistical difference in the time free from episodes of asthma or the mean number of episodes of asthma.

There is limited data on the effectiveness of probiotics for the treatment of asthma, once the disease has been diagnosed and established (Table 19.2). Current studies have been limited by small sample sizes, which limit the ability to detect significant clinical effects from the intervention.

PROBIOTICS FOR THE PREVENTION OF ASTHMA

The potential role of probiotics for asthma may lie in primary prevention. Environmental factors during early infancy affect immune system development and as a result, may also affect the subsequent risk for allergic disease.[25] Within the mature immune system, T-helper (Th) cells help recognize foreign antigens and secrete cytokines to help activate other components of the immune system. The two subtypes of Th cells, Th-1 cells and Th-2 cells, are defined for the most part by the specific cytokines they produce. The hygiene hypothesis suggests that the absence of infectious exposure at a critical point in immune system development leads to an unfavorable Th1/Th2 balance and subsequently, a greater risk for the later development of atopic disease and asthma.[26] There are considerable arguments in favor and against this hypothesis.[27,28]

If the hygiene hypothesis is accurate, it may be possible to devise strategies that can establish a Th1/Th2 balance that blocks the onset of asthma or slows the progression of disease. The mucosal immune system of the gastrointestinal tract plays a role in early priming and the development of tolerance to antigens.[29] In addition, the importance of bacterial polysaccharide in developing a Th-1 response has also been documented.[30] With shared anatomy in the pharynx, as well as the mucocilliary clearance of the nasal cavity and sinuses, upper respiratory exposures may overlap as gastrointestinal exposures, triggering a subsequent effect.[31] As a result, probiotics may be a promising and practical exposure that may lead to a Th phenotype that is not associated with atopic conditions.

There are many attractive aspects of the use of probiotics for primary prevention of asthma or allergic disease. First, the exposure is feasible and practical. Probiotics can be introduced into the diet as early as infancy, as some infant formulas contain probiotic supplements.[32] Even prenatal exposure has been associated with a potential benefit in both clinical trials[33] and also animal models.[34] Probiotics have a relatively long safety record and present a justifiable risk to the patient.[35] Although the potential risks of probiotic supplementation are low, care should be taken when probiotics are used with infants that are immunosuppressed or have complicated medical histories. Finally, probiotic supplementation could potentially be a passive method to prevent asthma with large-scale public benefits, similar to folic acid fortification of grains[36] or universal salt iodization.[37] Given the prevalence of asthma, the impact of such an intervention could potentially be tremendous.

EFFECT OF PROBIOTICS FOR PRIMARY PREVENTION OF ATOPIC DISEASE AND ASTHMA

Attempts to utilize probiotics in allergic disease have mostly focused on atopic dermatitis, as opposed to asthma. Atopic dermatitis is another common childhood condition that is strongly associated with pediatric asthma.[38] Some studies also suggest a potential benefit of probiotics for the primary prevention of atopic dermatitis, which is associated with the later development of asthma.

A double-blind, randomized controlled trial of 62 mother–infant pairs to evaluate the effect of probiotic supplementation to the pregnant and lactating mothers suggested that probiotic supplementation decreased the infant's risk of developing atopic eczema during the first 2 years of life.[39]

For example, randomized controlled trials of a probiotic exposure, *Lactobacillus*, suggest benefit in decreasing the risk of eczema. A randomized, controlled, double-blind study of 159 newborns, found that early *Lactobacillus* exposure as a probiotic supplement leads to decreased risk of atopic disease. In addition, a follow-up study found that such effects are sustained past infancy.[33] Although the benefits of *Lactobacillus* exposure are only associated with the prevention of atopic dermatitis, early development of eczema is associated with later development of asthma.

Other studies that have utilized other *Lactobacillus* strains have not yielded similar results. The results from a randomized controlled trial of a 6 month exposure of *L. acidophilus* to 231 infants showed that early probiotic supplementation did not reduce the risk of atopic dermatitis.[40]

Only one published study thus far, has examined the effect on asthma. A randomized controlled, double-blind study of 1,223 mother-child pairs examined the effectiveness of probiotics and prebiotic supplementation in preventing allergic disease, including asthma.

Those randomized to the intervention received a twice daily dose of a combination of probiotics (*L. rhamnosus, Bifidobacterium breve*, and *Propionibacterium freudenreichii*) for 2 to 4 weeks before delivery. The infant received a similar probiotic supplement as well as galacto-oligosaccharides daily for the first 6 months of life. Outcome measures were the presence of food allergy, eczema, asthma, or allergic rhinitis at 2 years of age. Although supplementation reduced eczema (OR: 0.74; 95% CI: 0.55, 0.98) and atopic eczema (OR: 0.66; 95% CI: 0.46, 0.95), there was no reported effect on the prevalence of asthma. However, at 2 years of age, the prevalence in the study population was only 3.2%. Differences may be more notable at later ages.[41]

Additional studies are needed to replicate these findings with different populations in different settings. The Trial of Infant Probiotic Supplementation (TIPS) is an ongoing study in the USA to test the effectiveness of a daily infant probiotic supplement taken during the first 6 months of life in preventing the development of early markers of asthma. Unlike other studies, the intervention is post-natal. In addition, patients are being recruited from a community with limited infant exposure to probiotics. As a result, it may be possible that the effect of probiotic supplementation may be more pronounced in this community.[42]

SUMMARY

There are few studies that have rigorously examined the effect of probiotic supplementation in the treatment or prevention of asthma. The few studies that have focused on the treatment of asthma have been small and shown little, if any, effect. Although there is evidence for the effect of probiotics for the primary prevention of eczema, to date there is no data to support the use of probiotics for the prevention of asthma. Further studies are needed to examine the potential effects of probiotics in different settings for different aspects of asthma. This work funded in part by the National Institutes of Health (HL080074) and the Clinical and Translational Science Institute (UL1RR024131) at the University of California, San Francisco.

REFERENCES

1. Akinbami L. Asthma prevalence, health care use and mortality: United States, 2003–5. http://www.cdc.gov/nchs/products/pubs/pubd/hestats/ashtma03–05/asthma03–05.htm. Accessed July 1, 2007.
2. Last JM. Scope and Methods of Prevention. In: Last JM, Wallace RB, (eds) *Public Health and Preventive Medicine*. 13th ed;1992.
3. Simhon A, Douglas JR, Drasar BS, Soothill JF. Effect of feeding on infants' faecal flora. *Arch Dis Child.* 1982;57:54–8
4. Sepp E. Julge K, Vasar M, Naaber P, Bjorksten B, Mikelsaar M. Intestinal microflora of Estonia and Swedish infants. *Acta Paediatr.* 1997;86:956–1061.
5. Alm JS, Swartz J, Björkstén B, Engstrand L, Engström J, Kühn I, et al. An anthroposophic lifestyle and intestinal microflora in infancy. *Ped All Immun.* 2002;13:402–11.
6. Alfvén T, Braun-Fahrländer C, Brunekreef B, von Mutius E, Riedler J, Scheynius A, et al. Allergic diseases and atopic sensitization in children related to farming and anthroposophic lifestyle--the PARSIFAL study. *Allergy* 2006;61:414–20.
7. Flöistrup H, Swartz J, Bergström A, Alm JS, Scheynius A, van Hage M, et al. Allergic disease and sensitization in Steiner school children. *J Allergy Clin Immunol.* 2006;117:59–66.

8. Watanabe, S., et al., Differences in fecal microflora between patients with atopic dermatitis and healthy control subjects. *J Allergy Clin Immunol.* 2003;111(3):587–91.

9. Bjorksten B, Naaber P, Sepp E, Mikelsaar M. The intestinal microflora in allergic Estonian and Swedish 2-year-old children. *Clin Exp Allergy* 1999; 29:342–6.

10. Bjorksten B, Sepp E, Julge K, Voor T, Mikelsaar M. Allergy development and the intestinal microflora during the first year of life. *J Allergy Clin Immunol.* 2001;108:516–20.

11. Bottcher M, Sandin A, Norin E, Midtvedt T, Bjorksten B. Morcoflora associated characteristics in faeces from allergic and non-allergic children. *Clin Exp Allergy* 2000;30:590–96.

12. Kalliomaki M, Kirjavainen P, Eerola E, Kero P, Salminen S Isolauri E. Distinct patterns of neonatal gut microflora in infants in whom atopy was and was not developing. *J Allergy Clin Immunol.* 2001;107(1):129–34.

13. Penders J, Thijs C vandenBrandt P, Kummeling I, Snijders B, Stelma F, et al. Gut microbiota composition and development of atopic manifestations in infancy: the KOALA birth cohort study. *Gut* 2007;56:661–7.

14. Martinez FD, Wright AL, Taussig LM, Holberg CJ, Halonen M, Morgan WJ. Asthma and wheezing in the first six years of life. *New Engl J Med.* 1995;332:133–8.

15. Castro-Rodriguez JA, Holberg CJ, Wright AL, Martinez FD. A clinical index to define risk of asthma in young children with recurrent wheezing. *Am J Respir Crit Care Med.* 2000;162:1403–06.

16. Duggan C, Gannon J, Waker WA. Protective nutrients and functional foods for the gastrointestinal tract. *Am J Clin Nutr.* 2002;75:789–808.

17. Forsythe P. Inman MD, Bienenstock J. Oral treatment with live *Lactobacillus reuteri* inhibits the allergic airway response in mice. *Am J Respir Crit Care Med.* 2007;175:561–69.

18. Brouwer ML, Wolt-Plompen SAA, Dubois AEJ, et al. No effects of probiotics on atopic dermatitis in infancy: a randomized placebo-controlled trial. *Clin Exp Allergy* 2006;36:899–906.

19. Isolauri E, Arvola T, Sutas Y, Moilanen E, Salminen S. Probiotics in the management of atopic eczema. *Clin Exp Allergy* 2000;30:1604–10.

20. Viljanen M, Savilahti E, Haahtela T, et al. Probiotics in the treatment of atopic eczema/dermatitis syndrome in infants: a double-blind placebo-controlled trial. *Allergy* 2005; 60:494–500.

21. Rosenfeldt V, Benfeldt E, Nielsen SD, et al. Effect of probiotic Lactobacillus strains in children with atopic dermatitis. *JACI* 2003;111:389–95.

22. Wheeler JG, Shema SJ, Bogle ML, et al. Immune and clinical impact of Lactobacillus acidophilus on asthma. *Ann All Asthma Immunol.* 1997;79:229–33.

23. Stockert K, Schneider B, Porenta G, Rath R, Nissel H, Eichler I. Laser acupuncture and probiotics in school-aged children with asthma. *Pedriatr Allergy Immunol.* 2007;18:160–66.

24. Giovannini M, Agosoni C, Riva E, Salvini F, Ruscitto A, Zuccotti GV. et al. A randomized prospective double blind controlled trial on effects of long-term consumption of fermented milk containing Lactobacillus casei in pre-school children with allergic asthma and/or rhinitis. *Pediatr Res.* 2007;62:215–20.

25. Prescott SL, Macaubas C, Smallacombe T, Holt BJ, Sly PD, Holt PG. Development of allergen-specific T-cell memory in atopic and normal children. *Lancet.* 1999;353:196–200.

26. Martinez FD, Holt PG. Role of microbial burden in aetiology of allergy and asthma. *Lancet.* 1999;354 s12–15.

27. Von Mutius E. The increase in asthma can be ascribed to cleanliness. *Am J Respir Crit Care Med.* 2001;164:1106–69.

28. Platts-Mills TA, Woodfolk JA, Sporik RB. The increase in asthma cannot be ascribed to cleanliness. *Am J Respir Crit Care Med.* 2001;164:1106.

29. Backhed F, Ley RE, Sonnenburg JL, Peterson DA, Gordon JI. Host-bacterial mutualism in the human intestine. *Science.* 2005;307:1915–20.

30. Mazmanian SK, Liu CH, Tzianabos AO, Kasper DL. An immunomoduatory molecule of symbiotic bacteria directs maturation of the host immune system. *Cell.* 2005;122:107–18.

31. Noverr MC, Huffnagle GB. Does the microbiota regulate immune responses outside the gut? *Trends Mirco.* 2004;12:562–66.

32. Ghisolfi J, Roberfroid M, Rigo J, Moro G, Polanco I. Infant formula supplemented with probiotics or prebiotics. *J Ped Gastro Nutr.* 2002;35:467–69.

33. Kalliomaki M, Salminen S, Poussa T, Arvilommi H, Isolauri E. Probiotics and prevention of atopic disease: 4- year follow-up of a randomized placebo-controlled trial. *Lancet.* 2003;361:1869–71.
34. Blumer N, Sel S, Virna S, Patrascan CC, Zimmerman S, Herz U, et al. Perinatal maternal application of *Lactobacillus rhamnosus GG* suppresses allergic airway inflammation in mouse offspring. *Clin Exp Allergy.* 2007;37:348–57.
35. Borriello SP, Hammes WP, Holzapfel W, et al. Safety of probiotics that contain *Lactobacilli* or *Bifidobacteria. Clin Inf Dis.* 2003;36:775–80.
36. Castilla EE, Orioli IM, Lopez-Camelo JS, Dutra Md Mda G, Nazer-Herrera J. Preliminary data on changes in neural tube defect prevalence rates after folic acid fortification in South America. *Am J Med Genet.* 2003;123:123–8.
37. Delange F, de Benoist B, Pretell E, Dunn JT. Iodine deficiency in the world: where do we stand at the turn of the century? *Thyroid.* 2001;11:437–47.
38. Gustafsson D, Sjoberg O, Foucard T. Development of allergies and asthma in infants and yound children with atopic dermatitis: a prospective follow-up to 7 years of age. *Allergy.* 2000;55:240–45.
39. Rautava S, Kalliomaki M, Isolauri E. Probiotics during pregnancy and breast-feeding might confer immunomodulatory protection against atopic disease in the infant. *J Allergy Clin Immunol.* 2002;109:119–20.
40. Taylor AL, Dunstan JA, Prescott SL. Probiotic supplementation for the first 6 months of life fails to reduce the risk of atopic dermatitis and increases the risk of allergen sensitization in high-risk children: a randomized controlled trial. *J Allergy Clin Immunol.* 2007;119:184–91.
41. Kukkonen K, Savilahti E, Haahtela T, Juntunen-Backman K, Korpela R, Poussa T et al. Probiotics and prebiotic galactooliosaccharides in the prevention of allergic diseases: a randomized, double-blind, placebo-controlled trial. *J Allergy Clin Immunol.* 2007; 119:192–98.
42. Cabana MD. McKean M, Wong AR, Chao C, Caughey AB. Examining the hygiene hypothesis: the trial of infant probiotic supplementation. *Pediatr Perinat Epidemiol.* (in press).

20 The Impact of Probiotics on Maternal and Child Health: Clinical Evidence

Kingsley C. Anukam and Gregor Reid

Key Points

- Alleviating the problems of maternal and child health in countries with large malnourished and/or HIV-infected populations, will require multidimensional approaches including holistic and pharmaceutical interventions.
- Urogenital infections have a major role in preterm labor and the well-being of newborns.
- Probiotics show potential in reducing the risk of recurrence of urinary tract infection (UTI).
- There is some evidence to suggest that probiotics can have a role to play in bacterial vaginosis (BV) and maternal health.
- The role of probiotics in a number of newborn, and childhood diseases is reviewed in this chapter.

Key Words: Diarrhea, maternal and child health, preterm birth, Probiotics.

INTRODUCTION

It has been 100 years since Nobel Laureate Dr. Elie Metchnikoff hypothesized that fermented food product consumption could prolong life [1]. While commercial-fermented milk products have been available for over 70 years, the "antibiotic era" has arguably stalled in-depth investigations into the benefits of lactic acid bacteria for prevention and treatment of illness and prolongation of life. It has taken advances in modern science, problems with pharmaceutical therapies and demands from consumers for natural products, to finally push forward research in this area. This progress has been particularly noticeable in the past 6 years.

In 2001, the Food and Agriculture Organization of the United Nations and the World Health Organization assembled an Expert Panel to determine if there was evidence of efficacy of probiotics, and to develop a modern and more appropriate definition from

From: *Nutrition and Health: Probiotics in Pediatric Medicine*
Edited by: S. Michail and P.M. Sherman © Humana Press, Totowa, NJ

those that had, up to that point, focused on gut benefits and some in vitro bacterial properties. From this meeting came several important outcomes, the first of which was a new definition: "Live microorganisms which when administered in adequate amounts confer a health benefit on the host" [2]. The Expert Panel reviewed the literature and concluded that there was evidence that probiotics could provide health benefits, notably with strong evidence for diarrhea alleviation in children.

CREATING A CLIMATE FOR IMPLEMENTATION OF PROBIOTICS IN DEVELOPING COUNTRIES

The Expert Panel recommendations also stated that "Efforts should be made to make probiotic products more widely available, especially for relief work and populations at high risk of morbidity and mortality" [2]. This type of commitment has also been echoed in the United Nations' Millennium Development Goals (MDG) 4, 5, and 6, which are concerned with child mortality, maternal mortality, HIV/AIDS, and malaria [3]. Unfortunately, the recommendations of both these documents has shown little evidence of being brought to fruition, for example by using beneficial microbes (probiotics) to reduce maternal and child mortality associated with infection.

Although, poverty, mismanagement of resources and lack of political will influence access to good health care, it is the strength of an economy and the political health priorities that determine expenditure on health for rural and urban populations. A study on the level of political priority given to maternal mortality reduction in Guatemala, Honduras, India, Indonesia, and Nigeria showed that factors which shape political priority are international agency efforts to establish a global norm and the generation of clear policy alternatives to demonstrate that a given problem is surmountable [4]. Alleviating the problems of maternal and child health in countries with large malnourished and/or HIV-infected populations, will require multidimensional approaches including holistic and pharmaceutical interventions. Such approaches are all the more challenging given that governmental systems (regulatory, trade, health, agriculture), nongovernmental agencies and educational programs (teaching physicians and health care professionals) have not been set up to understand, utilize, regulate, or implement natural therapeutics, like probiotics. Indeed, there is an inherent lack of knowledge about what probiotics are and how they can benefit people [5], reflecting, in part, a failure of member nations to implement the FAO/WHO Expert Panel Report. In addition, there has been a shift in food production and intake, in part due to global warming causing droughts, for example in sub-Saharan Africa, as well as in the introduction of Western/Northern foods designed with long shelf life rather than meeting nutritional needs, and by older customs of producing fermented foods not being passed to successive generations.

The net effect is that in many populations, lactic acid bacterial intake has decreased significantly over the past 50 years, maternal and childhood deaths still remain unacceptably high in developing countries, and the pharmaceutical or high tech approaches have not adequately addressed the problems. In this chapter, we will explore the potential applications of probiotics for maternal and child health in developed and developing countries.

IMPORTANT MATERNAL HEALTH PROBLEMS

There are many factors, which influence maternal and fetal health, but urogenital infections have a major role in preterm labor and the well-being of newborns. Bacterial vaginosis (BV) is a condition with an etiology that is still evolving, but which basically consists of a depletion or loss of lactobacilli in the vagina, colonization by Gram-negative (*Prevotella, Mobiluncus, Gardnerella*) and Gram-positive (*Atopobium*) anaerobes or, in some cases, aerobes such as enterococci and *Escherichia coli* [7]. Although often without symptoms [8], BV is common in women of all age groups, and it can be associated with odor, discharge, and an alkaline pH. The treatment consists of metronidazole or clindamycin orally or vaginally, but neither is optimally effective and recurrences are common [9,10]. All too often, the diagnosis of BV is missed, and in many instances patients self-treat with antifungal therapies believing the problem is caused by yeast [11]. Unfortunately, the use of antifungals can increase the resultant incidence of BV [12].

A recent study evaluated the risk of urinary tract infection (UTI) in pregnant women with BV diagnosed by Amsel's criteria. A total of 76 women had BV and 246 women did not; and 18 women (23.6%) with BV had UTI, compared with 24 (9.8%) of those without. The study showed that BV was associated with an increased risk of UTI (odds ratio (OR) 3.05; 95% CI: 1.47 - 6.33), thereby confirming a previous study [13] and emphasizing the need to better manage this condition. Many women do not realize their increased risk of acquiring sexually transmitted infections (STIs) when BV is present [14–17].

The results of a meta-analysis involving women screened for BV, diagnosed either by clinical criteria or Gram-stain findings confirmed that BV is a risk factor for preterm delivery and maternal infectious morbidity, and a strong risk factor for late miscarriage [18]. A study examined the role of first trimester BV and the level of BV-associated microorganisms, and the risk of second trimester pregnancy loss among urban women. The report indicated that there was a twofold increased risk of second trimester pregnancy loss, and low amounts or the absence of *Lactobacillus* spp. in the first trimester also significantly increased the risk of second trimester pregnancy loss [19].

Preterm labor/birth has a high impact on the quality of life of the women [20] and is a leading cause of infant mortality and morbidity in the USA [21, 22] and Canada, but more so in developing countries [23]. Low-birth-weight infants, born after a preterm birth (PTB) or secondary to intrauterine growth restriction, account for much of the increased morbidity, mortality, and high cost. Wide disparities exist in both preterm birth and growth restriction among different population groups. Poor and black women, for example, have twice the preterm birth rate and higher rates of growth restriction than do most other women. Studies have linked low birth weight with a greater risk of adult chronic medical conditions, such as diabetes, hypertension, and heart disease [22].

Of interest, maternal thinness is a strong predictor of both preterm birth and fetal growth restriction. Yet, in the USA, several nutritional interventions, including high-protein diets, caloric supplementation, calcium and iron supplementation, and various other vitamin and mineral supplementations, have not generally reduced preterm birth (PTB) or growth restriction. Bacterial intrauterine infections play an important role in the etiology of the earliest preterm births, but, at least to date, antibiotic treatment either before labor for risk factors such as BV or during preterm labor have not consistently reduced the preterm birth rate [24]. Although, macrolides and clindamycin given during the second trimester may reduce the rate of preterm delivery [25]. Pharmaceutical interventions, such as antibiotics, have been suboptimally effective and have failed to reduce the incidence of PTB. The absence of lactobacilli in the vagina, a specific feature of BV, raises the question as to whether restoration of lactobacilli, by probiotic therapy, can restore the normal flora and improve the chances of having a healthy term pregnancy.

CLINICAL EVIDENCE FOR PROBIOTICS AGAINST UTI AND BV

In the late 1980s, human studies were carried out in which *L. rhamnosus* GR-1 in a douche suspension was instilled into the vagina to show that the organism could colonize for a period of time [26]. This was followed by studies using a gelatin capsule containing freeze-dried lactobacilli inserted into the vagina [27]. In both cases, the process did not result in any adverse events but did show a potential to reduce the risk of recurrence of UTI. The use of orally administered lactobacilli was more recently tested, on the basis that if pathogens infect the host from the anal skin, why couldn't lactobacilli also ascend from the anus to the vagina and repopulate the area? This concept was verified in several labs [28–33], and *Lactobacillus* strains GR-1 and RC-14 were shown to reduce UTI, BV, and yeast pathogens as well as infections [29]. The mechanism of action is likely multifactorial and could include the ingested lactobacilli ascending from the rectal skin to the vagina, or causing a reduced pathogen ascension, or influencing the immune or host system in a way that reduces infectivity.

As this approach to restoration and maintenance of women's health has become more recognized, other groups have undertaken studies using different strains. A prospective clinical pilot study was performed to confirm the safety and effectiveness of *Lactobacillus* vaginal suppositories against the recurrence of UTI. The patients enrolled in the study were instructed to administer vaginal suppositories containing the strain *L. crispatus* GAI 98322. A significant reduction in the number of recurrences was noted, without any adverse complication ($P = 0.0007$). The administration of vaginal suppositories containing *L. crispatus* GAI 98332 seemed to be a safe and promising treatment for the prevention of recurrent UTI [34]. Delai et al. [35] demonstrated the effectiveness of the contemporary oral administration of *L. paracasei* ssp. *paracasei* F19 in association with vaginal suppositories containing an unnamed *L. acidophilus* in the treatment of BV. The study had a potentially fatal flaw in that not all the 60 subjects had confirmed diagnosis of BV. The subjects were randomized in two groups: Group A treated with vaginal suppositories containing *L. acidophilus*; Group B treated with the same vaginal suppositories + *L. paracasei* ssp. *paracasei* F 19 for oral administration. There was a significant reduction of vaginal pH, an improvement in the amine sniff test and in subjective symptomatology after 3 months of treatment and follow-up (3 months). This study needs to be repeated with larger sample size, but nevertheless, reviews of the evidence from microbiological and clinical studies have indicated that probiotics can be beneficial for preventing recurrent UTI in women in a safe manner [36–38].

The usefulness of orally administered lactobacilli for urogenital health has been demonstrated in several other important studies. In a randomized, double-blind, placebo controlled trial, 106 women with BV were given a single oral dose of metronidazole

(500 mg) twice daily from 1 to 7 days, plus oral *L. rhamnosus* GR-1 and *L. reuteri* RC-14 or placebo twice daily from 1 to 30 days [39]. The cure rate in the antibiotic/probiotic group was 88% compared to 40% in the antibiotic/placebo group ($p < 0.001$). High counts of *Lactobacillus* sp. (>10^5 CFU/ml) were recovered from the vagina of 96% of probiotic treated subjects compared to 53% controls at day 30. In another study using the same probiotics, there was a 88% cure of BV following intravaginal administration of the probiotic alone, compared to 50% cure with intravaginal metronidazole treatment [40]. In the case, 40 women diagnosed with BV were randomized to receive either two dried capsules containing *L. rhamnosus* GR-1 and *L. reuteri* RC-14 each night for 5 days, or 0.75% metronidazole gel, applied vaginally twice a day (in the morning and evening). Follow-up at day 6, 15, and 30 showed cure of BV in significantly more probiotic treated subjects (16, 17, and 18/20, respectively) compared to metronidazole treatment (9, 9, and 11/20: $P = 0.016$ at day 6, $P = 0.002$ at day 15, and $P = 0.056$ at day 30). This is the first proven cure of BV using probiotics and provides hope that alternative remedies to antibiotics can be found.

THE PATHWAY OF UROGENITAL INFECTIONS IN CAUSING PRETERM BIRTH

One of the most common pathways for urogenital pathogens to cause preterm labor is the natural movement of bacterial organisms from the rectal skin and subsequent ascension to the upper urogenital tract [41,42]. A number of BV organisms secrete sialidase, an enzyme which facilitates attachment and breakdown of mucin, and mucinases, which assist pathogen ascension into uterine tissues [43]. In addition some BV organisms release proteolytic enzymes that may act directly on cervical collagen and fetal membranes leading to premature cervical ripening and weakening of the fetal membranes with subsequent preterm premature rupture of the membranes [44]. The organisms associated with BV are invariably detected by the host as foreign, resulting in chemotactic influx of monocytes and macrophages, production of phospholipase A2 and other inflammatory mediators. Phospholipase A2 is an enzyme that liberates arachidonic acid from the phospholipids of the membranes, and this forms a cascade leading to the synthesis of prostaglandins E2 and F2a by the placental membranes [45]. Correspondingly, protease toxins may activate the decidua and fetal membranes to produce cytokines such as tumor necrosis factor, interleukins (IL-1a, IL-1b, IL-6, IL-8) and granulocyte-macrophage colony-stimulating factor. In response to the activation of local inflammatory reactions, prostaglandins synthesis and release are stimulated [46], causing premature contractions and preterm labor.

The rationale for probiotic use in pregnant women to prevent BV and preterm birth is quite strong [47,48]. *L. rhamnosus* GR-1 and *L. reuteri* RC-14 can safely populate the vagina after oral and vaginal administration, displace and kill pathogens including *Gardnerella vaginalis* and *E. coli*, and modulate the immune response to interfere with the inflammatory cascade that leads to PTB (Fig. 20.1). In addition, a recent study of 22 pregnant women in Poland showed that the elevated pH associated with BV could be normalized to pH 4.5 in over 70% cases by daily oral lactobacilli GR-1 and RC-14 treatment for 30 days (unpublished data). Thus, there is some evidence to suggest that probiotics can have a role to play in maternal health.

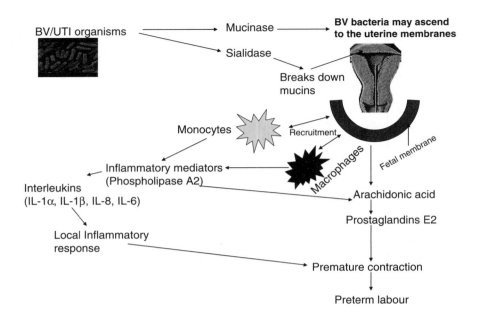

Fig. 20.1. Possible pathway of how urogenital pathogens might induce preterm birth

USE OF PROBIOTICS TO PREVENT PRETERM BIRTH

Although there have not yet been any studies to test whether probiotics can prevent PTB, some are currently being undertaken. One study has evaluated the safety of probiotics for preventing preterm labor and birth [30]. It was conducted in Japan, and it enrolled 24 women after 34 weeks of pregnancy. The probiotic *L. johnsonii* La1120 was used in fermented milk daily for 2 weeks, while the control group received placebo-fermented milk. The only outcome assessed was the presence of BV after completion of treatment.

As high rates of BV are observed with in vitro fertilization (IVF) patients [49–52], abnormal vaginal microbiota presumably explain, at least to some extent, reproductive failure as well as the increased risk of adverse pregnancy outcome seen in these patients. One mechanism could be the induction of an inflammatory response that prevents the sperm from fertilizing the egg. At present, a screen-and-treat procedure to restore the normal vaginal microbiota is not a routine part of the infertility work-up and treatment. While Gram staining of vaginal smears would offer an inexpensive and validated means for screening and diagnosing BV, probiotic therapy might provide a means to safely reconstitute the lactobacilli population prior to IVF treatment [53].

NEWBORN, AND CHILDHOOD USE OF PROBIOTICS

At birth, low weight newborns are at high risk of necrotizing enterocolitis (NEC), a severe and often fatal infection of the intestine. Several studies have been undertaken using lactobacilli to reduce the risk of NEC, and all have reported an element of success. The first was an open label study, which compared a previous year of NEC incidence with a treatment year using a strain of *L. acidophilus* [54]. This is not the ideal comparison as NEC can occur in clusters. Still, the incidence during the treatment year was halved as were the deaths compared to the previous year. Additional studies recently summarized by Deshpande et al. [55] have shown that NEC deaths can indeed be prevented by a variety of lactic acid bacteria, some of which are proven probiotics. Development of abnormal patterns of bowel colonization is a complication in preterm infants and a recent study has demonstrated that administration of probiotics colonized the gastrointestinal tract and improved feeding tolerance in 37% of the preterms [56].

In early childhood, UTI is one of the commonest bacterial infections, ranking second only to those of the respiratory tract [57] Vesicoureteral reflux (VUR) is a risk factor for recurrent UTI [58] and elevated urine interleukin 8 has been found to be a marker [59]. There is reason to believe that undetected and therefore untreated attacks of pyelonephritis can cause renal scarring and later life renal damage and the development of hypertension, which occurs in about 10% of children and accounts for around 20% of the children that enter into dialysis and transplant programs [60]. UTI is almost always an ascending infection caused by bacteria which originate in the person's own bowel. Since the bacterial composition of stools is influenced by the diet, the risk of UTI may be altered by dietary modifications, such as intake of cranberry products. Probiotics have not been adequately tested for prevention of UTI in children, and it remains to be seen if similar strains that have an effect in adults can also benefit children [61]. As UTI in childhood increases the risk of the condition recurring in adulthood [62], it could be argued that early probiotic intervention could decrease the risk of infection later in life. Such long-term follow-up studies are needed when probiotic strains have been successfully used as a prophylaxis in pediatric UTI [63]. So-called probiotics are marketed in several countries for use in all age groups, and pediatric health care providers appear to have had some clinical benefits in children [64]. One study has shown that orally administered *Saccharomyces boulardii* probiotics, known to alleviate diarrhea, can decrease *E. coli* numbers in the colon in children [65], but whether this reduces UTI episodes remains to be determined.

There is strong evidence that certain strains of lactobacilli and bifidobacteria have a major part in the maintenance and restoration of health in children especially for diarrhea [66,67] and some indications that they may prevent allergic conditions [68]. Probiotic intervention in the first months of life, as tested using *L. rhamnosus* GG, has been found to be well tolerated and did not significantly interfere with long-term composition or quantity of gut microbiota [69]. Indeed, intestinal colonization during and immediately following birth represents the first contact for the newborn with microbes, which in turn act to prime the maturation of the immune system. A study was designed to characterize both the mother-infant bifidobacteria transfer at birth and the development of bifidobacteria microbiota during the first weeks of life, in infants whose mothers received *L. rhamnosus* GG or placebo. Results indicated that specific changes in the transfer and initial establishment of bifidobacteria in neonates took place as consequence of the consumption of *L. rhamnosus* GG by the mothers [70].

In another study designed to assess the impact of probiotics and breast-feeding on gut microecology, mothers were randomized to receive placebo or *L. rhamnosus* GG before delivery, and the infants then received it for 6 months thereafter. Evaluation of gut microbiota, humoral immune responses, and soluble cluster of differentiation 14 (sCD14) in colostrum in 96 infants was performed [71]. Fecal *Bifidobacterium* and *Lactobacillus/Enterococcus* counts were higher in breast-fed than formula-fed infants at 6 months ($P < 0.0001$ and $P = 0.01$, respectively). At 3 months, the total number of immunoglobulin (Ig)G-secreting cells in breast-fed infants supplemented with probiotics exceeded those in breast-fed infants receiving placebo ($P = 0.05$), and their number correlated with the concentration of sCD14 in colostrum. Total numbers of IgM-, IgA-, and IgG-secreting cells at 12 months were higher in infants breast-fed exclusively for at least for 3 months and supplemented with probiotics, as compared to breast-fed infants receiving placebo ($P = 0.005$, $P = 0.03$, and $P = 0.04$, respectively). The study also found an interaction between probiotics and breast-feeding with respect to the number of Ig-secreting cells, suggesting that probiotics taken during breast-feeding can positively influence gut immunity.

SUMMARY AND TRANSLATION TO MOTHERS AND CHILDREN WORLDWIDE

It is noteworthy that almost all of the basic and clinical trials on probiotics have been carried out in the western hemisphere, where the disease burden is arguably less remarkable. The developing world bears the weight of most infectious diseases, and children are highly disadvantaged. The concept that probiotic bacteria, formulated into food or dietary supplements, could have a role to play in reducing preterm deliveries, morbidity, and mortality of newborns and infants suffering from gastroenteritis, is worthy of urgent action. Such efforts should not be at the expense of safety and long-term follow-up studies to ensure that no major adverse effects arise due to this early intervention. On the other hand, as probiotics become increasingly accepted by consumers and health care providers, too many products have failed to meet the standards required for use of the term probiotic, regardless of whether or not they are approved by regulatory agencies who themselves often do not understand the concepts or adhere to FAO/WHO Guidelines. Regulatory agencies should strive to ensure that probiotic products are identified to the species, strain level, and most importantly be shown to confer tangible, measurable benefits on the consumers. The international community, whether or not driven by documents from the United Nations, World Health Organization or nongovernmental organizations, should increase their efforts towards enshrining the probiotic concept into all levels of society in rural and urban areas. Scientists meanwhile, must continue to design studies to better understand the role of the indigenous and probiotic microbes in health, and translate this knowledge into products whose activities are properly and fairly communicated to the general public.

Acknowledgments Support from NSERC, ONF, AFMnet, OMAF, and CIHR is appreciated

Table 20.1
Probiotics for newborns and adults, including some for pregnant women

Product	Microbial strain	Clinical data	Producer/source
Culturelle	*Lactobacillus rhamnosus* GG (LGG)	Reduce antibiotic-associated diarrhea, atopy, and respiratory infection in day care centers	Valio, Finland
Florastor	*Saccharomyces cerevisiae boulardii*	Treat and prevent antibiotic-associated diarrhea	MFI Pharma, Biocodex France
VSL#3	8 strains	Remission of pouchitis and ulcerative colitis (IBD)	VSL Pharmaceuticals, Italy
Urex-cap-5 under various brand names	*L. rhamnosus* GR-1 and *L. reuteri* RC-14.	Anti-inflammatory effect in women Treatment of BV Prevention of urogenital infection	Urex Biotech Inc, Canada and Chr. Hansen Denmark
Align	*B. infantis* 35624	Relief from IBS	Procter & Gamble USA
Activia yogurt	*B. animalis* DN 117–001.	Improves transit time	Danone France
Yakult	*L. casei* Shirota	Reduce bladder cancer recurrences	Yakult, Japan
Reuteri	*L. reuteri* SD2112	Gut health, reduces colic in babies	Biogaia, Sweden
Howaru	*B. lactis* HN019 (DR10) *L. rhamnosus* HN001 (DR20)	Immune enhancement	Danisco, Denmark
Actimel DanActive	*L. casei* DN114001	Immune enhancement	Danone, France
Proviva	*L. plantarum* 299	Reduce infection and hospital stay in seriously ill patients	Probi AB, Sweden
	L. rhamnosus R0011 *L. acidophilus* R0052	Intestinal health	Institut Rosell

(continued)

Table 20.1
(continued)

Others	*L. rhamnosus* LB21		Essum AB, Sweden
	Lactococcus lactis L1A		
	L. salivarius UCC118		University College Cork, Ireland
	B. longum BB536		Morinaga Milk Industry Co., Ltd. Japan
	L. acidophilus NCFM®	In many US yogurts	Danisco, Denmark
	L. fermentum VRI003 (PCC)		Probiomics, Australia
	L. johnsonii Lj-1 (same as NCC533)	In yogurts	Nestlé, Switzerland
	Escherichia coli Nissle 1917	Treatment of colitis	Ardeypharm, Germany
	L. gasseri OLL 2716	Suppressed *H. pylori* and gastric mucosal inflammation	Lacteol Laboratory
			Meiji Milk products, Japan
Bio K Plus	*L. acidophilus CL-128 and L. casei*	Antibiotic associated diarrhea	Bio K Canada
Various product names	*L. acidophilus LA-1*	Gut health	Chr. Hansen, Denmark
	L. paracasei		
	CRL 431		
	B. lactis Bb-12		

REFERENCES

1. Metchnikoff E. The prolongation of life: Optimistic studies. New York: Putman's Sons, 1908, 161–183

2. FAO/WHO (2001) Evaluation of health and nutritional properties of probiotics in food including powdered milk and live lactic acid bacteria. Food and Agriculture Organization of the United Nations and World Health Organization Report. Available at: http://www.fao.org/es/ESN/probio/probio.htm. 2001; Accessed 28 April 2007.

3. World Health Organization. Health and the Millennium Development Goals. Available at: http://www.who.int.proxy1.lib.uwo.ca:2048/mdg. Accessed 5 May 2006.

4. Shiffman J. Generating political priority for maternal mortality reduction in 5 developing countries. *Am J Public Health.* 2007 May;97(5):796–803.

5. Anukam KC, Osazuwa EO, Reid G. Knowledge of probiotics by Nigerian clinicians. *Int J Probiotics Prebiotics* 2006; 1: 57–62.

6. Burton JP, Devillard E, Cadieux PA, Hammond J-A, Reid G. Detection of *Atopobium vaginae* in post menopausal women by cultivation-independent methods warrants further investigation. *J Clin Microbiol.* 2004;42:1829–31.

7. Donder GG, Vereecken A, Bosmans E, Dekeersmaecker A, Salembier G, Spitz B. Definition of a type of abnormal vaginal flora that is distinct from bacterial vaginosis: aerobic vaginitis. *BJOG.* 2002;109(1):34–43.

8. Klebanoff MA, Schwebke JR, Zhang J, Nansel TR, Yu KF, Andrews WW. Vulvovaginal symptoms in women with bacterial vaginosis. *Obstet Gynecol.* 2004;104(2):267–72.

9. Livengood CH 3rd, Thomason JL, Hill GB. Bacterial vaginosis: diagnostic and pathogenetic findings during topical clindamycin therapy. *Am J Obstet Gynecol.* 1990;163:515–20.

10. Schmitt C, Sobel JD, Meriwether C. Bacterial vaginosis: treatment with clindamycin cream versus oral metronidazole. *Obstet Gynecol.* 1992;79:1020–3.

11. Ferris DG, Nyirjesy P, Sobel JD, Soper D, Pavletic A, Litaker MS. Over-the-counter antifungal drug misuse associated with patient-diagnosed vulvovaginal candidiasis. *Obstet Gynecol.* 2002;99(3):419–25.

12. Pawlaczyk M, Friebe Z, Pawlaczyk MT, Sowinska-Przepiera E, Wlosinska J. The effect of treatment for vaginal yeast infection on the prevalence of bacterial vaginosis in early pregnancy. *Acta Dermatovenerol Croat.* 2006;14(1):26–9.

13. Sharami SH, Afrakhteh M, Shakiba M. Urinary tract infections in pregnant women with bacterial vaginosis. *J Obstet Gynaecol.* 2007 Apr;27(3):252–4.

14. Bhalla P, Chawla R, Garg S, Singh MM, Raina U, Bhalla R, Sodhanit P. Prevalence of bacterial vaginosis among women in Delhi, India. *Ind J Med Res.* 2007 Feb;125:167–72.

15. Cherpes, T.L., Meyn, L.A., Krohn, M.A., and Hillier, S.L. 2003. Risk factors for infection with herpes simplex virus type 2: role of smoking, douching, uncircumcised males, and vaginal flora. *Sex Transm Dis.* 30(5):405–10.

16. Sewankambo, N., R. H. Gray, M. J. Wawer, L. Paxton, D. McNaim, F. Wabwire-Mangen, D. Serwadda, C. Li, N. Kiwanuka, S. L. Hillier, L. Rabe, C. A. Gaydos, T. C. Quinn, and J. Konde-Lule. 1997. HIV-1 infection associated with abnormal vaginal flora morphology and bacterial vaginosis. *Lancet.* 350(9077):546–50.

17. Wiesenfeld HC, Hillier SL, Krohn MA, Landers DV, Sweet RL. Bacterial vaginosis is a strong predictor of *Neisseria gonorrhoeae* and *Chlamydia trachomatis* infection. *Clin Infect Dis.* 2003 Mar 1;36(5):663–8.

18. Leitich H, Kiss H. Asymptomatic bacterial vaginosis and intermediate flora as risk factors for adverse pregnancy outcome. *Best Pract Res Clin Obstet Gynaecol.* 2007;21(3):375–90.

19. Nelson DB, Bellamy S, Nachamkin I, Ness RB, Macones GA, Allen-Taylor L. First trimester bacterial vaginosis, individual microorganism levels, and risk of second trimester pregnancy loss among urban women. *Fertil Steril.* 2007;88:1396–1403.

20. Hill PD, Aldag JC. Maternal perceived quality of life following childbirth. *J Obstet Gynecol Neonatal Nurs.* 2007;36(4):328–34.

21. Callaghan WM, MacDorman MF, Rasmussen SA, Qin C, Lackritz EM. The contribution of preterm birth to infant mortality rates in the United States. *Pediatrics*. 2006;118(4):1566–73.

22. Goldenberg RL, Culhane JF. Low birth weight in the United States. *Am J Clin Nutr*. 2007 Feb;85(2):584S–90S.

23. Ngoc NT, Merialdi M, Abdel-Aleem H, Carroli G, Purwar M, Zavaleta N, Campodonico L, Ali MM, Hofmeyr GJ, Mathai M, Lincetto O, Villar J. Causes of stillbirths and early neonatal deaths: data from 7993 pregnancies in six developing countries. *Bull World Health Organ*. 2006 Sep;84(9):699–705.

24. McDonald HM, Brocklehurst P, Gordon A. Antibiotics for treating bacterial vaginosis in pregnancy. *Cochrane Database Syst Rev*. 2007 Jan 24;(1):CD000262.

25. Morency AM, Bujold E. The effect of second-trimester antibiotic therapy on the rate of preterm birth. *J Obstet Gynaecol Can*. 2007; 29(1):35–44.

26. Bruce AW, Reid G. Intravaginal instillation of lactobacilli for prevention of recurrent urinary tract infections. *Can J Microbiol*. 1988;34:339–43.

27. Reid G, Bruce AW, Taylor M. Installation of *Lactobacillus* and stimulation of indigenous organisms to prevent recurrence of urinary tract infections. *Microecol Ther*. 1995;23:32–45.

28. Reid G, Bruce AW, Fraser N, Heinemann C, Owen J, Henning B. Oral probiotics can resolve urogenital infections. *FEMS Microbiol Immunol*. 2001;30:49–52.

29. Reid G, Charbonneau D, Erb J, Kochanowski B, Beuerman D, Poehner R, and Bruce A.W. Oral use of *Lactobacillus rhamnosus* GR-1 and *L. fermentum* RC-14 significantly alters vaginal flora: randomized, placebo-controlled trial. *FEMS Immunol Med Microbiol*. 2003;35:131–4.

30. Nishijima K, Shukunami K, Kotsuji F. Probiotics affects vaginal flora in pregnant women, suggesting the possibility of preventing preterm labor. *J Clin Gastroenterol*. 2005;39(5):447–8.

31. Vasquez A, Ahrne S, Jeppsson B, Molin G. Oral administration of *Lactobacillus* and *Bifidobacterium* strains of intestinal and vaginal origin to healthy human females: re-isolation from feces and vagina. Microbial Ecol. *Health Dis*. 2005; 17: 15–20.

32. Antonio MA, Rabe LK, Hillier SL. Colonization of the rectum by Lactobacillus species and decreased risk of bacterial vaginosis. *J Infect Dis*. 2005;192(3):394–8.

33. Morelli L, Zonenenschain D, Del Piano M, Cognein P. Utilization of the intestinal tract as a delivery system for urogenital probiotics. *J Clin Gastroenterol*. 2004;38(6 Suppl):S107–10.

34. Uehara S, Monden K, Nomoto K, Seno Y, Kariyama R, Kumon H. A pilot study evaluating the safety and effectiveness of *Lactobacillus* vaginal suppositories in patients with recurrent urinary tract infection. *Int J Antimicrob Agents*. 2006;28(1 Suppl):S30–4.

35. Delia A, Morgante G, Rago G, Musacchio MC, Petraglia F, De Leo V. Effectiveness of oral administration of *Lactobacillus paracasei* subsp. paracasei F19 in association with vaginal suppositories of *Lactobacillus acidofilus* in the treatment of vaginosis and in the prevention of recurrent vaginitis. *Minerva Ginecol*. 2006 Jun;58(3):227–31.

36. Falagas ME, Betsi GI, Tokas T, Athanasiou S. Probiotics for prevention of recurrent urinary tract infections in women: a review of the evidence from microbiological and clinical studies. *Drugs*. 2006;66(9):1253–61.

37. Reid G, Bruce AW. Probiotics to prevent urinary tract infections: the rationale and evidence. *World J Urol*. 2006 Feb;24(1):28–32.

38. Hoesl CE, Altwein JE. The probiotic approach: an alternative treatment option in urology. *Eur Urol*. 2005 Mar;47(3):288–96.

39. Anukam KC, Osazuwa EO, Ahonkhai I, Ngwu M, Osemene G, Bruce AW and Reid G Augmentation of antimicrobial metronidazole therapy of bacterial vaginosis with oral probiotic *Lactobacillus rhamnosus* GR-1 and *Lactobacillus reuteri* RC-14: randomized, double-blind, placebo controlled trial. *Microbes Infect*. 2006;8(6):1450–54.

40. Anukam KC, Osazuwa E, Osemene GI, Ehigiagbe F, Bruce AW, Reid G. Clinical study comparing probiotic *Lactobacillus* GR-1 and RC-14 with metronidazole vaginal gel to treat symptomatic bacterial vaginosis. *Microbes Infect*. 2006;8 (12–13):2772–76.

41. Bruce AW, Chadwick P, Hassan A, VanCott GF. Recurrent urethritis in women. *Can Med Assoc J*. 1973; 108(8):973–6.

42. Fowler JE Jr, Stamey TA. Studies of introital colonization in women with recurrent urinary infections. VII. The role of bacterial adherence. *J Urol*. 1977;117(4):472–76.

43. Cauci S, McGregor J, Thorsen P, Grove J, Guaschino S. Combination of vaginal pH with vaginal siali-dase and prolidase activities for prediction of low birth weight and preterm birth. *Am J Obstet Gynecol.* 2005;192(2):489–96.

44. Lockwood CJ. Recent advances in elucidating the pathogenesis of preterm delivery, the detection of patients at risk, and preventative therapies. *Curr Opin Obstet Gynecol.* 1994;6:7–18.

45. Bejar R, Curbelo V, Davis C, Gluck L. Premature labor. II. Bacterial sources of phospholipase. *Obstet Gynecol.* 1981;57(4):479–82.

46. Park JS, Park CW, Lockwood CJ, Norwitz ER. Role of cytokines in preterm labor and birth. *Minerva Ginecol.* 2005;57(4):349–66.

47. Onderdonk AB. Probiotics for women's health. *J Clin Gastroenterol.* 2006 Mar;40(3):256–59.

48. Reid G, Bocking A. The potential for probiotics to prevent bacterial vaginosis and preterm labor. *Am J Obstet Gynecol.* 2003;189(4):1202–8.

49. Spandorfer SD, Neuer A, Giraldo PC, Rosenwaks Z, Witkin SS. Relationship of abnormal vaginal flora, proinflammatory cytokines and idiopathic infertility in women undergoing IVF. *J Reprod Med.* 2001;46(9):806–10

50. Wilson JD, Ralph SG, Rutherford AJ. Rates of bacterial vaginosis in women undergoing in vitro ferti-lisation for different types of infertility. *BJOG.* 2002;109(6):714–7.

51. Eckert LO, Moore DE, Patton DL, Agnew KJ, Eschenbach DA Relationship of vaginal bacteria and inflammation with conception and early pregnancy loss following in-vitro fertilization. *Infect Dis Obstet Gynecol.* 2003;11(1):11–7

52. Deb K, Chatturvedi MM, Jaiswal YK. Gram-negative bacterial endotoxin- induced infertility: a birds eye view. *Gynecol Obstet Invest.* 2004;57(4):224–32

53. Verstraelen H, Senok AC. Vaginal lactobacilli, probiotics, and IVF. *Reprod Biomed Online.* 2005;11(6):674–5

54. Hoyos AB. Reduced incidence of necrotizing enterocolitis associated with enteral administration of *Lactobacillus acidophilus* and *Bifidobacterium infantis* to neonates in an intensive care unit. *Int J Infect Dis.* 1999;3(4):197–202.

55. Deshpande G, Rao S, Patole S. Probiotics for prevention of necrotising enterocolitis in preterm neonates with very low birthweight: a systematic review of randomised controlled trials. *Lancet.* 2007;369(9573):1614–20

56. Lee SJ, Cho SJ, Park EA. Effects of probiotics on enteric flora and feeding tolerance in preterm infants. *Neonatology.* 2007;91(3):174–9.

57. Twaij M. Urinary tract infection in children: a review of its pathogenesis and risk factors. *J R Soc Health.* 2000;120(4):220–26.

58. Nuutinen M, Uhari M. Recurrence and follow-up after urinary tract infection under the age of 1 year. *Pediatr Nephrol.* 2001;16(1):69–72.

59. Galanakis E, Bitsori M, Dimitriou H, Giannakopoulou C, Karkavitsas NS, Kalmanti M. Urine inter-leukin-8 as a marker of vesicoureteral reflux in infants. *Pediatrics.* 2006;117:e863–7.

60. Jodal UThe natural history of bacteriuria in childhood. *Infect Dis Clin North Am.* 1987;1(4):713–29

61. Kontiokari T, Nuutinen M, Uhari M. *Dietary factors affecting susceptibility to urinary tract infection Pediatr Nephrol.* 2004;19(4):378–83.

62. Reid G. The potential role of probiotics in pediatric urology. *J Urol.* 2002;168(4 Pt 1):1512–7.

63. Gerasimov SV. Probiotic prophylaxis in pediatric recurrent urinary tract infections. *Clin Pediatr (Phila).* 2004 Jan–Feb;43(1):95–8.

64. NASPGHAN Nutrition Report Committee; Michail S, Sylvester F, Fuchs G, Issenman R. Clinical efficacy of probiotics: review of the evidence with focus on children. J Pediatr Gastroenterol Nutr. 2006 Oct;43(4):550–7.

65. Akil I, Yilmaz O, Kurutepe S, Degerli K, Kavukcu S. Influence of oral intake of *Saccharomyces boul-ardii* on *Escherichia coli* in enteric flora. *Pediatr Nephrol.* 2006 Jun;21(6):807–10.

66. Szajewska H, Ruszczynski M, Radzikowski A. Probiotics in the prevention of antibiotic-associated diarrhea in children: a meta-analysis of randomized controlled trials. *J Pediatr.* 2006;149(3):367–72.

67. Sazawal S, Hiremath G, Dhingra U, Malik P, Deb S, Black RE. Efficacy of probiotics in prevention of acute diarrhoea: a meta-analysis of masked, randomised, placebo-controlled trials. *Lancet Infect Dis.* 2006;6(6):374–82.

68. Kukkonen K, Savilahti E, Haahtela T, Juntunen-Backman K, Korpela R, Poussa T, Tuure T, Kuitunen M. Probiotics and prebiotic galacto-oligosaccharides in the prevention of allergic diseases: a randomized, double-blind, placebo-controlled trial. *J Allergy Clin Immunol.* 2007;119(1):192–8.

69. Rinne M, Kalliomaki M, Salminen S, Isolauri E. Probiotic intervention in the first months of life: short-term effects on gastrointestinal symptoms and long-term effects on gut microbiota. *J Pediatr Gastroenterol Nutr.* 2006;43(2):200–5.

70. Gueimonde M, Sakata S, Kalliomaki M, Isolauri E, Benno Y, Salminen S. Effect of maternal consumption of *Lactobacillus* GG on transfer and establishment of fecal bifidobacterial microbiota in neonates. *J Pediatr Gastroenterol Nutr.* 2006 Feb;42(2):166–70.

71. Rinne M, Kalliomaki M, Arvilommi H, Salminen S, Isolauri E. Effect of probiotics and breastfeeding on the *Bifidobacterium* and *Lactobacillus/Enterococcus* microbiota and humoral immune responses. *J Pediatr.* 2005;147(2):186–91.

Section E
Probiotics Products

21 Probiotics in Foods and Supplements

Steven J Czinn and Samra Sarigol Blanchard

Key Points

- The number of commercially marketed probiotic products in the USA has increased dramatically.
- There is a paucity of information regarding the dosage and viability of the different probiotic strains and products.
- This chapter will provide a practical overview of the different probiotic preparations available to clinicians.

Key Words: Probiotic foods (yogurt, kefir) and probiotic supplements available in USA,

INTRODUCTION

In the past 10 years, the number of commercially marketed probiotic products in the USA has tripled. Probiotics are available in foods and dietary supplements. In food products, the most common used species are *Lactobacillus*, *Bifidobacterium*, or *Streptococcus thermophilus*. In addition to yogurt and kefir, the types of foods delivering probiotics have expanded to granola, cereal, and juices.

The supplement market contains many products of single or multistrain probiotics in capsule, liquid, or powder form. The suitable description of a probiotic product as reflected on the label should include genus and species identification, with nomenclature consistent with currently recognized names, strain designation, viable count of each strain at the end of shelf life, recommended storage conditions, safety, recommended dose and an accurate description of the physiological effect, as allowed by law. Finally, physicians and consumers should wary that the probiotic strains listed on the label may not actually be contained in the product.

The term probiotic was defined by a group of experts convened by the Food and Agriculture Organization (FAO) of the United Nations and the World Health Organization (WHO) as "live microorganisms administered in adequate amounts which confer a beneficial health effect on the host".[1] In recent years, there has been an

From: *Nutrition and Health: Probiotics in Pediatric Medicine*
Edited by: S. Michail and P.M. Sherman © Humana Press, Totowa, NJ

upsurge in medical research assessing the therapeutic benefits of probiotics, as well as growing commercial interest in the probiotic food concept.

Probiotic food constitutes a sizeable part of the functional food market, and continues to grow with a potential for market growth estimated at a staggering $120 million per month. However, major concerns regarding the quality, labeling, and verification of claims attributed to some of these products still remain.[2]

Probiotics are available in the USA as conventional foods, dietary supplements, medical foods and drugs. Dietary supplements are subcategory of foods created in 1994 by the Dietary Supplement Health and Education Act.[3] These products are meant to be used as oral supplements to the diet. However, labels can stipulate a target population. Medical foods are used under medical supervision for patients needing special dietary supplementation for a medical condition. Despite the facts that sales of probiotics are skyrocketing, there are currently no probiotic drugs approved by FDA for human use in the USA.

In recent months, the diversity of food products containing probiotics has expanded considerably. "Guidelines for the Evaluation of Probiotics in Food" require the probiotic to be identified at the genus, species, and strain level, using appropriate molecular and physiological techniques. The strain should be deposited in an internationally recognized culture collection so that scientists are able to replicate published research on the strain. Properly controlled studies must be conducted to document the safety and health benefit in the target host. It is also necessary to keep the probiotic viable at a minimum required level in the final product through the end of shelf life.

When prescribing probiotics, we should consider the probiotic formulation, including live, dead, compounded preparations or their products, the effective dose necessary to achieve a benefit and the type of disease targeted. It is also important for the prescribing physician to realize that the US Food and Drug Administration does not currently regulate probiotic products.

There is no governing agency overseeing quality control, and the actual number of viable organisms in commercial products may be quite different from what is being advertised. Nutritional probiotics are microbial food supplements also known as functional foods that are added to foods but cannot claim a medical indication since they are not required to demonstrate clinical efficacy or the same degree of safety as required by pharmaceutical probiotics.

The main probiotic preparations currently on the market are the lactic acid-producing bacteria: *Bifidibacterium* and *Lactobacillus*. These genera initiated their role as probiotics through their association with healthy human intestinal tracts and, in the case of lactobacilli, their presence in fermented foods. However, studies are also investigating potential probiotic roles of other microbes such as yeast, *Saccharomyces boulardii*, *Escherichia*, *Enterococcus,* and *Bacillus*.

Food Products

Although fermented dairy products such as yogurt and kefir are typically associated with delivery of "beneficial cultures," the types of foods claiming to deliver probiotics have expanded to include granola and candy bars, frozen yogurt, cereal, and cookies. In food products, the probiotics used are primarily species of *Lactobacillus*, *Bifidobacterium*, or *S. thermophilus*. Yogurt is one of the common probiotic food source in the markets. In the USA, yogurt is required to be produced by the fermentation by *Lactobacillus bulgaricus* and *S. thermophilus*. As long as a yogurt is not heat treated after fermentation, the yogurt should contain high numbers of both of these bacteria. This is the situation with all yogurts that display the Live Active Culture Seal (a program administered by the National Yogurt Association). The National Yogurt Association's criteria for "live and active culture yogurt" require that product contain 100 million (10^8) organisms per gram that remain active throughout the stated shelf life.[2,4] However, post-fermentation heat treatment of yogurt, which kills all live cultures, is allowed. FDA regulations require that all yogurts be made with active cultures. Only those that are not heat treated, however, retain live and active cultures when they reach consumers. Other probiotic bacteria such as *Lactobacillus* can be added to yogurt to promote a probiotic effect.

In the dairy category, new products abound, including *Dannon's Activia* yogurt featuring *Bifidobacterium animalis* DN173010, *DanActive* fermented milk with *L. casei* DN114001, and *Danimals* yogurt drink with *L. rhamnosus* GG. All three products contain the yogurt starter cultures *L. bulgaricus* and *S. thermophilus*.[4] Yogurts produced by *Stonyfield Farms* are supplemented with six species of bacteria. The yogurt starter culture bacteria, *S. thermophilus* and *L. bulgaricus*, are present along with unspecified strains of *Bifidobacterium* species, *L. casei, L. acidophilus* and *L. reuteri. Stonyfield Farms* yogurts also contain inulin.

Adequate number of viable cells, namely the "therapeutic minimum" must be consumed regularly for the transfer of the probiotic effect to consumers. Therefore, consumption should be in excess of 100 g per day of bio-yogurt containing more than 10^6 colony forming units (cfu) ml.[5]

Some additional dairy products currently available with live cultures added for beneficial health effects are frozen yogurt (TCBY), cheese (Kraft LiveActive Cheddar Cheese) and kefir (Lifeway® Real Lowfat Kefir Plain; Lifeway Foods, Inc., Morton Grove, IL).

Kefir is a self-carbonated fermented milk made from kefir grains, a complex and specific mixture of bacteria and yeast held together by a polysaccharide matrix. This product contains active probiotic cultures of *S. lactis, S. cremoris, S. diacetylactis, L. plantarum, L. casei, Saccharomyces fragilis,* and *Leuconostoc cremoris*.

Cheeses with long ripening times have also been manufactured using probiotic strains, which multiply and survive throughout the ripening cycle without altering the quality of the product.[6]*Kraft LiveActive* cheese is the first cheddar cheese in Canada that contains the beneficial probiotics *B. lactis* and *L. rhamnosus*. New products such as *LiveActive Cottage Cheese, Kraft LiveActive Cheese Sticks* and *Cheese Cubes* with probiotics continue to become available. Horizon Organic Dairy includes *L. acidophilus* and *Bifidobacterium* in all its yogurt and cottage cheese products.

Historically dairy products have dominated the probiotic concept for foods. In the past year, a number of other foods containing live cultures have hit the market, including granola and candy bars (*Attune*), cereal (*Kashi*), and wafers (*Mrs. Freshley's*). Attune Foods recently introduced both chocolate bars and granola bars containing "over five times the live active cultures as found in yogurt." Three strains *L. acidophilus, L. casei* and *B. lactis* are included in these products at a concentration of 10^{10}cfu/bar good until the end of room temperature shelf life. This is a unique offering in USA market and provides a convenient format for a food containing live active cultures. Kashi has also launched a probiotic-containing cereal called "Vive" In addition to containing 10^9 cfu/serving of *L. acidophilus* LA14, it also contains several other functional food ingredients. Probiotic drinks are more widely used in Europe where probiotic fortified fruit juices are available.

Despite the documented technical challenges involved with the formulating nondairy probiotic foods[7], fruit juice could serve as a good medium for functional ingredients like probiotics[8].

Probiotic-coated drinking straws and bottle caps are also marketed. The straws designed for single use are coated on the inside with probiotic powder. As the beverage is sipped, the coating dissolves and probiotic is consumed along with the drink. The bottle caps hold a dose of probiotic powder. Before drinking the contents, the bottle is shaken and the powder blends with the liquid. In USA, *BioGaia* has two products: *BioGaia Probiotic straw* and *BioGaia LifeTop Cap*. The probiotic straws consist of a telescopic polypropene drinking straw, with a Reuteri oil droplet attached to its inner part. Drinking 100 ml will release the required dose. Each straw provides a minimum of 100 million active colonies of *L. reuteri*. This application is suitable for any drink that is either cold or at room temperature.

Nestlé has launched first FDA approved probiotic-supplemented infant formula, *Good Start Supreme with Natural Cultures*, containing *BIFIDUS BL* (*B. lactis* Bb 12) with data showing immune benefits. Fukushima et al. reported that the levels of total fecal IgA increased significantly during intake of the probiotic formula in healthy infants[9].

To continue to develop new functional foods, technologically suitable probiotic strains must be found since the manufacturing process poses a serious challenge to survival and viability. The product environment and storage condition also may adversely impact on viability of the probiotic. This is a particular concern, given that high levels (at least 10^7/g or ml) of live microorganisms are recommended for probiotic products. More than 100 companies in the USA market probiotic products in supplement form. Unfortunately, many of the products currently on the market are not clearly tied to research documenting beneficial effects.

Dietary Supplements

The dietary supplement market for probiotic cultures seems to be a more diverse and more active market than probiotics to supplement dairy products. The supplement market contains many different product formats and contents, including capsules, liquids, tablets, and even food-like formats. If properly prepared and stored, probiotic bacteria can remain viable in dried form and reach the intestine alive when consumed. A diverse array of bacterial genera and species are represented in these products, including many different Lactobacilli, Bifidobacteria and less commonly, *Enterococcus, Bacillus, Escherichia coli* and yeast. Dietary supplement products are purchased primarily in health food stores or natural foods grocery stores.

The two most popular forms of probiotic supplement are capsules and freeze-dried (lyophilized) powders. Probiotics may be sold as a single microorganism or a mixture of several types. As virtually all liquid probiotics lose their potency within 2 weeks after they are produced, they should be avoided. (Most liquids don't even make it to store shelves within that period of time.) Liquid acidophilus, for example, must be handled like a perishable dairy product, with distinct expiration dates and strict requirements for refrigeration at all times. Some companies resort to adding buffering agents to prevent the product from becoming sour or bitter. Such additives interfere with the bacteria's optimum performance. There are liquid preparations available in both Europe and the USA such as *BioGaia Probiotic* drops, which provide 100 million live *L. reuteri* in 5 drops (5 drops = 0.17 ml).

A probiotic preparation must contain a certain minimum number of colony forming units (cfu). Although no dose–effect relation study is currently available, the probiotic-induced changes are rarely seen at daily doses of less than 10^8 to 10^{-10} cfu[3]. Over-the-counter products may contain more than 50 billion cfu per dose. Doses used in therapeutic and preventive trials also vary greatly. A daily intake of minimum 10^9 to 10^{10} cfu is required to show a health effect.[10] The beneficial effects of probiotics seem to be strain-specific and dose-dependent. Because of this, accurate labeling is important. The suitable description of a probiotic product as reflected on the label should include: genus and species identification, with nomenclature consistent with currently recognized names, strain designation, viable count of each strain at the end of shelf life, recommended storage conditions, safety, recommended dose and accurate description of the physiological effect, as allowed by law.[11] Several studies have documented that the probiotic strains listed on the label may not actually even be contained in the product. Finally, products sold for medicinal purposes tend to be of higher quality than probiotics used in supplements.

Probiotics are considered dietary supplements and are subject to the "Dietary Supplement, Health, and Education Act." This act was passed by Congress in 1994 and provides a framework for the regulation of dietary supplements by the FDA. Probiotic dietary products require FDA approval or GRAS (Generally Recognized as Safe) status, which means nonpathogenic strains with no adverse health effects. It should be kept in mind, however, that "GRAS" status is only for a specified use of probiotic. The microorganisms themselves are not considered GRAS, but their traditional use in dairy foods is accepted as safe.[4]

Although there are numerous probiotic preparations in the market, most contain a small number of species such as *Lactobacillus*, *Bifidobacterium*, *Streptococcus*, and the nonpathogenic yeast, *Saccharomyces*. Probiotic combinations may increase the beneficial health effects as compared to individual strains. Combinations of probiotic strains may have synergistic adhesion effects, but such combinations also need to be assessed in clinical studies. The common commercial probiotics and their contents are reviewed in Table 21.1.

Probiotic lozenges and chewing gums are additional products marketed for oral health to prevent halitosis and gingival disease. Though their effectiveness has not been scientifically clear yet, probiotic lozenges and gums are already available in US markets. A small number of studies suggest that probiotic bacterial strains originally sourced from the indigenous oral flora of healthy humans may have potential application to reduce the severity of halitosis.[12,13]*L. rheuteri Prodentis* is the active agent in *BioGaia* lozenges and gum and *S. salivarius K 12* in the *Active K-12* product manufactured by *TheraBreath*.

Table 21.1
Common probiotics supplements

Product	Content	Labeled or recommended dose
Align (Proctor & Gamble)	*Bifidobacterium infantis* 4 mg/capsule	1 capsule daily
BifidoBiotics (Allergy Research Group)	*Lactobacillus sporogenes* *L. acidophilus* *B. breve* *B. longum* Prebiotic 4 billion organisms/capsule	1 capsule twice a day
Culturelle (Amerifit Nutrition, Inc)	*L. rhamnosus-* *strain GG* inulin 10 billion per capsule	1 capsule twice a day
Florastor (Biocodex)	*Saccharomyces boulardii* 250 mg (5 billion bacteria) per capsule or packet	1–2 capsule or packet twice a day
Nature's Biotics (Life Science Products)	*L. acidophilus* *B. bifidum* *Bacillus subtilis* *Bacillus licheniformis* *L. bulgaricus* *L. lactis*	Children's chewable tablets 1–2 capsule daily
Primal Defense Kids (Garden of Life)	*B. breve* *B. longum* *B. infantis* *Saccharomyces boulardii* Four billion cfu^{3}per ¼ tsp	Daily value is not established
Probiotica (McNeil Consumer Healthcare)	*L. reuteri* Hundred million cells per tablet	1 tablet daily
ABC Dophilus powder for * infants and children* (Solgar)	*B. infantis* *B. bifidum* *Streptococcus thermophilus* 1 billion organism per ½ tsp	½ tsp daily

VSL#3
(Nature's Pharmaceuticals,
Inc)
(Requires *refrigeration*)
	L. casei
	L. plantarum
	L. acidophilus
	L. bulgaricus
	B. longum
	B. breve
	B. infantis
	S. thermophilus
	450 billion bacteria per pack
		1 packet twice a day
		Higher doses for
		   pouchitis or
		   ulcerative colitis

(continued)

Table 21.1
(continued)

Product	Content	Labeled or recommended dose
Flora.Q (Bradley Pharmaceutical, Inc)	L. acidophilus Bifidobacterium L. paracasei S. thermophilus 8 billion CFU per capsule	1 capsule daily (Flora.Q2 is the double strength form with 16 billion cfu per capsule)

SUMMARY AND CONCLUSION

In spite of the paucity of information regarding the dosage and viability of probiotic strains, lack of standardization and potential safety issues, there are considerable potential benefits of probiotics over a wide range of clinical conditions, which were reviewed in previous chapters. Ongoing research will continue to identify and characterize existing strains of probiotics, identifying strain-specific outcomes, determine optimal doses and assess their stability through processing and digestion. While gene technology will play a role in developing new strains, food industry research will focus on prolonging the shelf life and survival of probiotics through the intestinal tract, optimizing adhesion capacity, developing proper production, handling, and packaging procedures to ensure that the desired benefits are delivered to the consumer.

REFERENCES

1. FAO/WHO. Evaluation of health and nutritional properties of powder milk and lactic acid bacteria. Food and Agriculture Organization of the United Nations and World Health Organization Expert Consultation Report, 2001;1–4.
2. Senok AC, Ismaeel AY, Botta GA. Probiotics:facts and myths. *Clin Microbiol Infect* 2005;11:958–966
3. Dietary Supplement Health and Education Act (DSHEA).42 USC 287C-11. 1994.
4. http://www.usprobiotics.org.
5. Lourens-Hattingh A, Viljoen BC. Yogurt as probiotic carrier food. *International Dairy Journal* 200;11:1–17.
6. Lavermicocca P. Highlights o new food research. *Digestive and Liver Disease* 2006;38:S295–S299
7. Mattila-Sandholm T, Myllärinen P, Crittenden R, Mogensen G, Fondén R, Saarela M. Technological challenges for future probiotic foods, *International Dairy Journal* 2002;12:173–182
8. Luckow T, Delahunty C. Which juice is 'healthier'? A consumer study of probiotic non-dairy juice drinks. *Food Quality and Preference* 2004;15:751–759
9. Fukushima Y, Kawata Y, Hara H, Terada A, Mitsuoka T. Effect of a probiotic formula on intestinal immunoglobulin A production in healthy children. *International Journal of Food Microbiology* 1998;42:39–44.
10. Sanders ME, Veld JH. Bringing a probiotic-containing functional food to the market: microbiological, product, regulatory and labeling issues. *Antonie van Leeuwenhoek* 1999;76:293–315
11. Reid G, Sanders ME, Gaskins HR, Gibson GR, Mercenier A, Rastall R, Roberfroid M, Rowland I, Cherbut C, Klaenhammer TR. New scientific paradigms for probiotics and prebiotics. *Journal of Clinical Gastroenterology* 2003;37(2):105–118.

12. Burton JP, Chilcott CN, Moore CJ, Speiser G, Tagg JR. A preliminary study of the effect of probiotic *Streptococcus salivarius* K12 on oral malodour parameters. *Journal of Applied Microbiology* 2006;100:754–764.
13. Burton J, Chilcott C, Tagg J. The rationale and potential for the reduction of oral malodour using *Streptococcus salivarius* probiotics. *Oral Diseases* 2005;11:29–31.

22 The Application of Prebiotics and Synbiotics in Pediatrics

Laure Catherine Roger and Anne Liza McCartney

Key Points

- Prebiotics are undigested carbohydrates that selectively enhance the indigenous probiotic-type organisms (i.e. lactic acid bacteria).
- Synbiotics are combinations of both probiotics and prebiotics, aimed at providing a synergistic effect.
- Results to date are very promising and such dietary regimes merit further investigation, especially with a focus on clinical outcomes/biomarkers.

Key Words: Bifidobacteria, functional foods, infants, prebiotics, synbiotics.

INTRODUCTION

As has been discussed in the preceding chapters, there is a long history associating members of the gut microbiota with health and well being. Indeed, high levels of beneficial bacteria or probiotics (including bifidobacteria) have been correlated with lower risk of infections and diseases [1–6]. The premise of prebiotics is to selectively enhance the indigenous probiotic-type organisms (i.e. lactic acid bacteria) [7]. Much of the work on prebiotic supplementation in infants has focused on fortification of infant formulae, with an aim to stimulate a microbiota more resembling that seen in breast-fed infants (i.e. bifidobacterially predominated). Very few studies have been published to date on the application of prebiotics in clinical pediatrics. One such study examined the impact of a prebiotic mixture in constipated infants [8]. Another study investigated the use of prebiotics after antibiotic treatment for acute bronchitis [9]. Synbiotics are combinations of both probiotics and prebiotics, aimed at providing a synergistic effect [7]. As well as eliciting the individual benefits of the component probiotic(s) and prebiotic(s), synbiotics can improve the survival and/or activity of the probiotic(s). Synbiotic applications are a relatively recent area of interest, which has not been extensively studied to date. However, more papers have been published on the application of synbiotics in clinical pediatrics than for prebiotics alone. This chapter aims to critically assess the

From: *Nutrition and Health: Probiotics in Pediatric Medicine*
Edited by: S. Michail and P.M. Sherman © Humana Press, Totowa, NJ

reported effects of prebiotics and synbiotics in pediatrics and to speculate on the relative merits and potential of such functional foods.

DEFINITIONS

Probiotics are 'a live microbial food ingredient that is beneficial to health' [10], and have been discussed in detail in previous chapters. *Prebiotics* are defined as 'nondigestible food ingredient that beneficially affects the host by selectively stimulating the growth and/or activity of one or a limited number of bacteria in the colon, and thus improves host health' [7]. The lactic acid bacteria form the major axis of interest in prebiotic selectivity. Fructo-oligosaccharides (FOS) and galacto-oligosaccharides (GOS) are the most common prebiotics (especially in the European market), although a number of other compounds have been touted as potential prebiotics (e.g. isomalto-oligosaccharides, xylo-oligosaccharides, lactulose). More work is necessary to evaluate the prebiotic properties of such substances and to meet the current EU regulations for functional foods. *Synbiotics* are 'a mixture of probiotics and prebiotics that beneficially affects the host by improving the survival and implantation of live microbial dietary supplements in the GI tract, by selectively stimulating the growth and/or by activating the metabolism of one or a limited number of health-promoting bacteria, and thus improving host welfare' [7].

APPLICATION OF FUNCTIONAL FOODS IN INFANTS

The use of prebiotics or synbiotics in early childhood may afford modulation of the developing microbiota and thus be employed to actively direct microbial ecology in the human infant. This is particularly interesting in light of increasing data associating certain bacteria with the onset of disease (including ulcerative colitis, colorectal cancer and Crohn's disease) [11]. Furthermore, certain patterns of colonization have been associated with necrotizing enterocolitis (frequently observed in pre-term infants) [12, 13] and autism [14, 15]. Functional foods (probiotics, prebiotics, or synbiotics) could provide useful tools to addressing such dysbiosis of the microbiota and, therefore, potentially impact infant health and/or quality of life. The longitudinal impact of supplementation during infancy is also of interest (for example, does the bacterial succession in early life form part of the blueprint for colonic health in latter life?), but is much more difficult to unravel.

PREBIOTICS IN PEDIATRICS

The greater proportion of studies investigating the use of prebiotics in infants relate to enhancing the bifidobacterial component of the microbiota in formula-fed infants. This has largely evolved from the observed predominance of bifidobacteria in the faecal microbiota of breast-fed infants, and their generally perceived improved health compared to their formula-fed counterparts [16]. Interest in the role of human milk oligosaccharides (HMO) in the microbiota composition of breast-fed infants has led to two theories; (i) that HMO are natural prebiotics which stimulate a bifidogenic effect, and (ii) that HMO are protective bioactive compounds which inhibit enteric pathogens and/

or their toxins [17]. Irrespective of their mechanism of action, the association of bifido-bacterial predominance with improved general health and well being (seen in breast-fed infants) has resulted in endeavours of the infant food industry to mimic this microbio-logical composition in formula-fed infants. Commercially available prebiotics, which are either extracted from natural sources (such as chicory or other plant materials) [18] or enzymatically synthesised from natural sugars [19], have thus been investigated for their potential use towards this end (Table 22.1).

Initial studies using FOS (1, 2 or 3 g/day doses) showed no significant impact on the bifidobacterial component of the infant microbiota [20]. Increased stool frequency was, however, observed in the 3 g/day group. More recently, a number of studies have reported a positive impact of FOS fortification on infants. Euler et al. [21] examined supplementation of formula with two FOS doses during a 5 weeks period. Fifty-eight healthy infants (aged 2–6 weeks old) were enrolled, 28 received 1.5 g/L FOS and the remaining 30 received 3 g/L FOS. Fourteen breast-fed infants (of the same age) were recruited as a control cohort.

Bifidobacterial levels were significantly higher following 1.5 g/L FOS supplementation ($9.1 \pm 1.33 \log_{10}$) compared to both the 3 g/L FOS group ($8.6 \pm 1.17 \log_{10}$) and breast-fed group ($8.0 \pm 1.37 \log_{10}$). However, initial bifidobacterial levels were slightly higher in the 1.5 g/L FOS group (8.2 ± 1.45, 8.8 ± 1.51 and $8.6 \pm 1.14 \log_{10}$ for breast-fed, 1.5 g/L FOS and 3 g/L FOS groups, respectively). Moreover, counts of bacteroides, enterococci and clostridia did not differ from the baseline counts during the supplementation, indicating selectivity of the prebiotic. Seven days after the end of supplementation, no statistical differences were found amongst the bacterial counts of the different feeding groups; however, the bifidobacteria were still higher in the 1.5 g/L FOS group. Importantly, the higher FOS dose was seen to increase adverse effects (such as flatulence and spitting up) compared to 1.5 g/L FOS [21].

Another study followed the effects of FOS (2 g/day for 6 weeks) on ten healthy infants (7–19 months old) [22]. Levels of bifidobacteria were slightly higher after supplementation, but no statistical significance was observed. However, FOS supplementation resulted in decreased clostridia ($P < 0.05$) and staphylococci levels. No adverse effects were seen in this study. Indeed, levels of flatulence, diarrhoea, fever and antibiotics treatment were significantly lower in the test group compared to the control group. The power of this study is limited due to the small cohort ($n = 20$) and use of cultivation methods for microbiological assessments [22].

Brunser et al. [9] investigated the effects of a mixture of oligofructose (short-chain FOS) and inulin (long-chain FOS) on the bacterial populations of infants following 7 days amoxicillin treatment (for acute bronchitis). It is generally considered that longer-chain prebiotics are more persistent throughout the colon (whilst oligofructose fermented in the proximal colon) and thus employing a mixture was aimed to stimulate a bifidogenic effect throughout the colon. Bifidobacteria were significantly higher after 7 days FOS supplementation compared to the standard formula group (partly due to a reduction in bifidobacteria in the control group). No other statistically significant differences were seen between the two feeding groups, although lactobacilli levels were higher in the FOS-fed group [9]. This study showed that supplementing the diet of amoxicillin-treated infants post-antibiotic therapy effectively maintained the bifidobacterial population. It would be interesting to examine the potential of prebiotic adjuvants

Table 22.1
Human feeding studies investigating the application of prebiotics in pediatrics

Reference	Subjects	Test product	Overall findings
Guesry et al. (20)[a]	7 to 20-day-old infants (n = 13 control, n = 11 1 g/day, n = 11 2 g/day, n = 12 3 g/day)	FOS (1 g/day, 2 g/day or 3 g/day) for 2 weeks	No change in bifidobacteria; increased stool frequency in 3 g/day group
Moro et al. (26)[b]	4 to 10-day-old infants (n = 33 placebo, n = 30 0.4 g/100 mL, n = 27 0.8 g/100 mL)	G9F1 (0.4 g/100 mL or 0.8 g/100 mL) for 4 weeks	Dose-related bifidogenic effect (higher counts with increasing prebiotic); increased lacto-bacilli after prebiotic; dose-related impact on stool consistency; fecal pH lowered in 0.8 g/100 mL group, compared to baseline
Boehm et al. (27)[b]	4 to 12-day-old pre-term infants (n = 12 breast-fed, n = 15 control, n = 15 test formula)	G9F1 (1 g/100 mL) for 4 weeks	Significantly increased bifidobacterial counts compared to control formula; harder stools in the control formula group
Knol et al. (48)[c]	4 to 12-week-old infants (n = 16 breast-fed, n = 18 control, n = 16 test formula)	G9F1 (0.8 g/100 mL) for 6 weeks	Increased bifidobacteria (% total), compared to both baseline and control formula
Schmelzle et al. (35)[c]	2 to 12-day-old infants (n = 57 control, n = 54 test formula); bacteriology was performed on subset (n = 28 control, n = 26 test formula)	G9F1 (0.8 g/100 mL) supplemented with high β-palmitic acid and partially hydrolyzed whey protein for 12 weeks	Significantly increased bifidobacterial counts and predominance (% total) compared to baseline and control formula; total bacterial counts significantly higher in control group compared to baseline; softer stools in test formula group
Xiao-ming et al. (25)[b]	Term infants (n = 26 breast-fed, n = 52 control, n = 69 test formula, n = 124 mixed fed)	GOS (0.24 g/dL) for 6 months	Significantly higher bifidobacteria and lacto-bacilli counts in test and breast-fed groups compared to control (at 3 and 6 months); acetic acid and stool frequency were significantly higher, and faecal pH significantly lower, in test and breast-fed groups

Bakker-Zierikzee et al. (32)[c]	Newborn infants (n = 34 breast-fed, n = 19 control, n = 19 probiotic (B. animalis; 6 × 10⁹ CFU/100 mL), n = 19 prebiotic formula)	G9F1 (6 g/L) for 16 weeks	No significant differences in %bifidobacteria or total SCFA between feeding groups; higher %acetate and lower %propionate, %butyrate and %iC4-5 SCFA compared to control and probiotic formula groups; significantly lower fecal pH than control formula (after 5 days) and probiotic formula (after week 8)
Euler et al. (21)[b]	2 to 6-week-old infants (n = 14 breast-fed, n = 28 1.5 g/L, n = 30 3 g/L)	FOS (1.5 g/L or 3 g/L) for 5 weeks; no control formula	Significantly higher bifidobacteria in 1.5 g/L FOS group, compared to breast-fed group
Fanaro et al. (36)[b]	Term infants (n = 15 control, n = 16 POS, n = 15 G9F1+POS)	POS (0.2 g/dL) with or without G9F1 (0.6 g/dL)	Significantly more bifidobacteria and lactobacilli, and significantly higher stool frequency with G9F1+POS formula, compared to control and POS formulae; significantly harder stools and higher fecal pH for control formula, compared to both test formulae
Haarman & Knol (30)[c,d]	3-month-old infants (n = 10 breast-fed, n = 10 control, n = 10 test formula)	G9F1 (8 g/L) for 6 weeks	Significant increase in bifidobacteria (% total) during G9F1 feeding, compared to baseline; breast-fed and G9F1-fed groups had significantly higher bifidobacteria (% total) at end of study, compared to control formula; G9F1 stimulated bifidobacterial species profile similar to breast-fed group
Knol et al. (28)[c]	7 to 8-week-old infants (n = 19 breast-fed, n = 19 control, n = 15 test formula)	G9F1 (0.8 g/100 mL) for 6 weeks	Significantly increased bifidobacteria (% total) compared to control group; faceal pH significantly lower versus control formula; SCFA ratios affected
Bakker-Zierikzee et al. (32)	Newborn infants (n = 19 control, n = 19 prebiotic formula)	G9F1 (6 g/L) for 16 weeks	Faecal sIgA levels significantly higher compared to control groups

(continued)

Table 22.1
(continued)

Reference	Subjects	Test product	Overall findings
Brunser et al. (9)[c]	1 to 2-year-old infants (n = 66 control, n = 64 test formula)	FOS (4.5 g/L) for 7 days	Significantly higher bifidobacteria compared to control group
Haarmen et al. (31)[d]	3-month-old infants (n = 10 breast-fed, n = 10 control, n = 10 test formula)	G9F1 (8 g/L) for 6 weeks	Significant increase in lactobacilli predominance (% total) in breast-fed and test formula groups, compared to baseline; similar profile diversity to breast-fed group
Scholtens et al. (39)	4 to 6-month-old infants (n = 9 control, n = 11 test product)	G9F1 (4.5 g/day) for 6 weeks	Significant increase in bifidobacteria, compared to baseline
Bongers et al. (8)	3 to 20-week-old constipated infants (n = 38; crossover design trial)	G9F1 (8 g/L) supplemented with palmitic acid and partially hydrolyzed whey protein, for 3 weeks	No microbiological analysis; improved stool consistency, but not frequency, compared to control formula
Costalos et al. (29)[c]	Newborn infants (n = 70 control, n = 70 test formula)	G9F1 (4 g/L) for 12 weeks	Significantly lower clostridia and higher bifidobacterial levels (non significant) compared to control group; softer stools, lower fecal pH and greater stool frequency than the controls
Kapiki et al. (23)[b]	Healthy pre-term infants (n = 20 control, n = 36 test formula)	FOS (4 g/L) for 7 days	Significantly higher bifidobacteria and bacteroides than the control group; decreased Escherichia coli and enterococci; increased stool frequency
Kim et al. (24)[b]	12-week-old orphans (n = 14; crossover designed trial)	FOS (0.2 g/kg/day) for 3 weeks (base formula contained FOS and GOS 1.5 g/100 g powder)	Significantly higher bifidobacteria and lactobacilli than control formula (magnitude of bifidobacterial increase was related to initial levels); significantly heavier stools than control formula

Waligora-Dupriet et al. (22)[d]	7 to 19-month-old infants (n = 10 control, n = 10 test formula)	FOS (2 g/day) for 44 days	Slight increase in bifidobacteria; significant decrease in clostridia compared to control group; decreased flatulence, diarrhoea, vomiting, and fever than control group

Abbreviations: FOS, fructo-oligosaccharides; G9F1, 90% galacto-oligosaccharides+10% fructo-oligosaccharides; POS, acidic oligosaccharides derived from pectin hydrolysis

[a]Method of determining bifidobacterial levels not provided
[b]Cultivation assays employed
[c]Fish analysis used
[d]Real-time PCR used

to antibiotic therapy—with an aim to prevent or reduce the microbial dysbiosis associated with antibiotic administration, as opposed to stimulating recovery.

Two further studies have examined the effects of FOS supplementation on the infant microbiota [23, 24]. One week feeding of FOS (4 g/L) significantly increased bifidobacteria and bacteroides counts in healthy pre-term infants, compared to control formula [23]. Stool frequency was also increased by prebiotic supplementation, whilst *Escherichia coli* and enterococci levels were lower than in the control group. The second study involved a cross-over design with inulin supplementation (0.2 g/kg/day) of a base formula already containing FOS (oligofructose) and GOS (1.5 g/100 g powder). Inclusion of inulin significantly increased bifidobacterial and lactobacilli counts, the magnitude of increment correlating with initial levels (i.e. higher increases seen in infants with lower starting levels) [24]. However, the cultivation protocol employed in this study is not ideal, with faecal homogenates frozen prior to cultivation work. Inulin supplementation also resulted in heavier stool weights; though, again, the methodology afforded inaccuracies (namely, weight of soiled nappy minus weight of clean nappy; no consideration of urine content or stool consistency [wet weight]).

GOS containing infant formulae are commercially available in Japan, and have been for a number of years; yet, few studies have been published on the effects of GOS supplementation in infants [16]. Xiao-ming and colleagues [25] examined whether feeding formula supplemented with 0.24 g/dL GOS elicited similar microbiological and fermentation profiles to those seen in breast-fed infants. After 3 months of feeding, the cultivable bifidobacteria and lactobacilli levels were significantly higher in the breast-fed and GOS-fed groups, compared to the control formula group. Whilst similar counts were seen for the breast-fed and GOS-fed groups, there was greater inter-individual variation within the GOS-fed group. At 6 months of age the bifidobacterial and lactobacilli levels remained significantly lower in the control group. Faecal pH was significantly lower, and SCFA levels significantly higher, in GOS-fed and breast-fed groups at both time points [25].

Under the premise of better mimicking the oligosaccharide composition of human milk, numerous studies have investigated a GOS:FOS combination (G9F1; comprising 90% GOS and 10% FOS). As previously reviewed [17], the majority of prebiotic supplementation studies focused on G9F1. These studies showed that G9F1 was well tolerated by infants and induced a microbiota that was dominated by bifidobacteria [26–28]. Furthermore, stool consistency, pH and SCFA levels were more similar to those seen in breast-fed infants following G9F1 supplementation, compared to the control formula.

A recent G9F1 feeding study in healthy newborns corroborated the findings of earlier studies in relation to stool characteristics (frequency, consistency and faecal pH)—although the bifidobacterial levels were not significantly different between the G9F1-fed infants and the control group [29]. Interestingly, the clostridial counts were significantly lower following G9F1 ingestion, compared to controls.

Prebiotic feeding studies have generally focused on the tolerance and well being of infants, as well as monitoring a few interesting or predominant bacterial populations. However, very few studies have examined the diversity or dynamics within these populations. This is a little short sighted, as simply stimulating similar levels or predominance of bifidobacteria to that seen in breast-fed infants may not correlate with conferring health benefits. The species diversity may be critical to clinical/health outcome. It is, therefore, also important to investigate the effects of supplementation at species level. To date, one prebiotic feeding study has examined the effects of probiotic supplementation on the species diversity of certain members of the faecal microbiota using real-time PCR (rtPCR) [30, 31].

Haarman and colleagues [30, 31] examined the impact of 6 weeks G9F1 supplementation on the bifidobacterial and lactobacilli populations of healthy infants. The control group had higher levels of *Bifidobacterium catenulatum* at the end of the study, whilst lower levels of *B. adolescentis* were observed in the G9F1-fed and breast-fed groups [30]. This study showed that G9F1 elicited similar levels and diversity of bifidobacteria as breast-feeding. However, only 50% of the bifidobacterial population was detected using this array of *Bifidobacterium* species-specific primers, indicating that further diversity may exist. Alternatively, this may reflect the limitations of the technique (rtPCR being prone to either over- or under-estimation, especially in bacterial populations with non-homologous copy number of the target gene/sequence between species/strains). G9F1 also generated significantly higher levels of lactobacilli compared to the control formula [31]. *L. acidophilus*, *L. paracasei* and *L. casei* were the predominant species in both the G9F1-fed and breast-fed groups. While the control group had more *L. delbrueckii*.

Bakker-Zierikzee et al. [32] examined the effects of 1 month G9F1 (6 g/L) feeding on immunoglobulin IgA in neonates. Significantly more secretory IgA (sIgA) was observed following G9F1 supplementation, compared to the control group. As sIgA are involved in mucosal immunity and are crucial for proper immune development of the GI tract and infant well being [33, 34], such stimulation by prebiotic supplementation is very interesting. Furthermore, sIgA are resistant to preteolytic degradation in the GI tract, and can aggregate pathogenic bacteria and block attachment to the mucosal membrane [4]. As such, dietary modulation of endogenous IgA levels could be a useful catalyst for maturation and development of the infant immune system.

A few studies have investigated the impact of G9F1 supplementation together with other additions. The first two incorporated β-palmitic acid and partially hydrolyzed whey proteins in the G9F1 fortified formulae [8, 35]. In the first study, bifidobacteria were significantly increased compared to baseline and control formula (both in terms of numerics and predominance [% total]) [35]. The test formula also led to significantly softer stools, compared to the control formula. Total bacterial levels were significantly less in the test group than the control group. The study by Bongers et al. [8] examined stool characteristics of constipated infants during a cross-over study with G9F1, palmitic acid and partially hydrolyzed whey proteins. Constipation is a common symptom of formula-fed infants. Consequently, fortified formulae, which may alleviate constipation, are of great interest (both to the industry and parents). Supplementation was shown to improve stool consistency (softer stools than the control formula) but not frequency [8]. Fanaro et al. [36], however, added acidic oligosaccharides derived from pectin hydrolysis (POS) to G9F1 containing formula (G9F1+POS); as a control, they also used standard formula supplemented with POS. They showed significantly more bifidobacteria and lactobacilli, together with significantly greater stool frequency in the G9F1+POS-fed group. The placebo group (who received maltodextrin supplemented formula) had significantly harder stools and higher faecal pH compared to both POS and G9F1+POS groups (36). However, the lactobacilli data and stool frequency data were merely referred to in the manuscript and not provided for the reader. A more concerning issue was the storage of faecal samples at -80°C prior to the cultivation work. Cultivation work should be performed on fresh samples, which are transferred to the laboratory and processed as soon as possible after collection, to avoid biasing due to storage conditions (oxygen content, freezing and thawing, ice crystals). Not all bacteria survive freezing as well as others and/or resuscitate from freezing at the same rate as other organisms. As such, the accuracy and reproducibility of such a research strategy is questionable – especially if inconsistent storage times are used for different samples.

A limited number of studies have been published in regard to the application of prebiotic supplemented cereals or weaning products [37–39]. Duggan and colleagues [37] demonstrated improved stool characteristics in Peruvian infants fed FOS-supplemented infant cereal, compared to control cereal. At the same time, Moore et al. [38] reported that FOS-supplemented cereals were well tolerated in weaning infants and led to more regular and softer stools than the control cereal. The recent study by Scholtens and co-workers [39] showed that G9F1-supplemented weaning products were well tolerated (during a 6 weeks feeding study) and elicited a significant increase in bifidobacteria compared to baseline levels.

SYNBIOTICS IN PEDIATRICS

Most pediatric studies using synbiotic products have either involved case studies or clinical cohorts. One recent study, however, examined the effects of a G9F1 synbiotic (G9F1 mixed with *B. longum* [10^7 CFU]) in healthy infants [40]; although no microbiological analysis was performed. The synbiotic was well tolerated and stool frequency was significantly increased after 4 months compared to the control group. No other significant differences were seen between the two groups, in relation to stool characteristics or weight gain (Table 22.2).

Between 2001 and 2003, a Japanese research group presented two case studies where synbiotic feeding (*B. breve* Yakult and *L. casei* Shirota [1×10^9] with GOS [3 g/day]) demonstrated clinical improvement [41, 42]. The first case study comprised ~ 2 years synbiotic feeding of a young girl suffering from short-bowel syndrome [41]. The child's nutritional status improved during the course of synbiotic treatment. At baseline, the child's faecal microbiota was classified as 'abnormal' with low bifidobacterial levels (6.9 $\log_{10}$ CFU/g faeces), high *E. coli* and *Candida* counts (9.20 and 9.36 $\log_{10}$ CFU/g faeces, respectively) and lactobacilli non-detectable by the culture system used. Synbiotic therapy not only enhanced the levels of the administered probiotics in the child, but also indigenous species of *Bifidobacterium* and *Lactobacillus*. Furthermore, *E. coli* and *Candida* colonization decreased dramatically during synbiotic treatment. Overall, the girl's nutritional, health status and faecal microbiota improved over the 2 years [41]. The second case study involved a 9-month-old girl with laryngotracheoesophageal cleft (type IV) and life-threatening weight problems [42]. After 10 months synbiotic treatment she had gained weight and her health was clinically improved. A third case study using the same synbiotic showed improved stool appearance and increased faecal anaerobe:aerobe ratio after ~ 4 months synbiotic feeding [43]. This case study involved a 3-month-old boy suffering from multiple-resistant *Staphylococcus aureus* (MRSA) and enterocolitis. MRSA is a concern as it is becoming harder to eradicate with antibiotics and alternative means of clearance are of particular interest. In this instance, synbiotic administration

Table 22.2
Human feeding studies investigating the application of synbiotics in pediatrics

Reference	Subjects	Test product	Overall findings
Kanamori et al. (41)[a]	4-year-old girl suffering from short-bowel syndrome	*Bifidobacterium breve* and *Lactobacillus casei* (1×10^9) with GOS (3 g/day) for ~ 2 years	Nutritional state improved; *Escherichia coli* and *Candida* colonization dramatically decreased; bifidobacteria and lactobacilli levels proliferated throughout
Kanamori et al. (42)[a]	9-month-old girl with laryngotracheoesophageal cleft (type IV) and life-threatening weight problems	*B. breve* and *L. casei* (1×10^9) with GOS (3 g/day) for 10 months	Improvement of illness; weight gain; faecal recovery of administered probiotics; increased faecal SCFA levels
Kanamori et al. (43)[a]	3-month-old boy with MRSA and enterocolitis	*L. casei* with GOS (3 g/day); followed by *B. breve* for ~ 4 months	Improved stool appearance; increased % faecal anaerobes
Kanamori et al. (44)[a]	2 to 10-year-old children suffering from short-bowel syndrome and repetitive enterocolitis ($n = 6$)	*B. breve* and *L. casei* (1×10^9) with GOS (3 g/day) for 1 year	Weight gain; improved intestinal microbiota; faecal recovery of administered probiotics
Gotteland et al. (45)	5 to 12-year-old children colonised with *Helicobacter pylori* ($n = 45$ antibiotics; $n = 46$ *L. acidophilus* (10^9 lyophilised bacteria); $n = 50$ synbiotic)	*Saccharomyces boulardii* (250 mg lyophilised bacteria/day) with inulin (5 g/day) for 8 weeks	12% *H. pylori* eradication; antibiotics more effective treatment (66% eradication); significant difference in the $\delta^{13}CO_2$ over base-line values before and after treatments in synbiotic group, but not probiotic group
Passeron et al. (46)	Children >2 years old with signs of atopic dermatitis ($n = 24$ lactulose and potato starch; $n = 24$ synbiotic)	*L. rhamnosus* Lcr35 (1.2×10^9 CFU) with lactulose and potato starch for 3 months	No microbiological analysis, significant improvement of atopic dermatitis signs in both groups; no significant difference between prebiotic and synbiotic groups

(continued)

Table 22.2
(continued)

Reference	Subjects	Test product	Overall findings
Kukkonen et al. (47)[a]	Pregnant women with high risk of neonates having allergic disease and their newborns (n = 464 control; n = 461 synbiotic)	2 strains of *L. rhamnosus*, *B. breve* and *Propionibacterium freudenreichii* ssp. *shermanii* with GOS (0.8 g/day) for 6 months	No overall preventative effect on allergic disease; significant decrease in atopic eczema; higher bifidobacterial and lactobacilli levels compared to placebo
Puccio et al. (40)	Healthy newborns (n = 55 control; n = 42 synbiotic)	*B. longum* with G9F1 (4 g/L) for ~ 4 months	No microbiological analysis; significantly increased stool frequency compared to control group; no significant differences in weight gain and stool characteristics

Abbreviations: GOS, galacto-oligosaccharides; G9F1, 90% galacto-oligosaccharides+10% fructo-oligosaccharides.

[a]Cultivation assays employed

was included as an adjuvant to antibiotic treatment. Stool appearance (i.e. colour) improved and increased predominance of anaerobes was seen after 4 months of antibiotic plus synbiotic therapy. Indeed, the stool appearance seen post-therapy resembled that of a healthy 3-month-old infant [43].

The same research group also followed a cohort of six children suffering from short-bowel syndrome and repetitive enterocolitis (age range 2–10 years) [44]. The same synbiotic was administered to this cohort of pediatric patients for 1 year and elicited improved faecal microbiota, weight gain and overall improvement in general health and well being.

More recently a randomised open study investigated the impact of *Saccharomyces boulardii* with inulin synbiotic (*S. boulardii*+InFOS) and probiotic treatment (*L. acidophilus*) in *Helicobacter pylori* positive children (aged 5–12 years; $n = 50$ and $n = 46$, respectively) [45]. A control group, treated with antibiotics (lanzoprazole, amoxicillin and clarythromycin), was also included ($n = 45$). Conventional *H. pylori* treatment (i.e. antibiotics) provided the best eradication rate of the study groups (66%), compared to 12% for the *S. boulardii*+InFOS group and 6.5% for the probiotic group. Interestingly, spontaneous clearance was not seen for any of the 81 untreated asymptomatic (*H. pylori* positive) children. Differences in the $\delta^{13}CO_2$ over baseline values before and after treatment were statistically significant in the *S. boulardii*+InFOS group, but not the probiotic group [45]. Antibiotic therapy was the superior clinical treatment regime, but it would be particularly interesting to investigate the combination of antibiotics and synbiotics in pediatric *H. pylori* eradication in light of this data.

The use of probiotics in atopic dermatitis and other allergic diseases in pediatrics has been a topic of particular interest, with positive results for certain probiotic preparations (potentially strain specific effects). One study has investigated the application of either 'prebiotic' (lactulose and potato starch; LacPS) or synbiotic (*L. rhamnosus* Lcr35 [1.2×10^9 CFU] with LacPS) (46). No control group was included in the study and microbiological analysis was not performed. The main outcomes monitored were signs of clinical improvement (e.g. SCORAD scores) and use of ointments. Both prebiotic and synbiotic treatments significantly improved SCORAD scores compared to baseline. Addition of probiotic to prebiotics did not significantly alter the clinical outcome [46]. A second study recruited pregnant women with high risk of having neonates with allergic disease [47]. Prior to giving birth, the pregnant women ingested either synbiotic (2 strains of *L. rhamnosus*, *B. breve* and *Propionibacterium freudenreichii* ssp. *shermanii* with GOS (0.8 g/day); $n = 461$) or placebo control ($n = 464$). After birth, formula-fed neonates received either synbiotic or control formula for 6 months; whilst the lactating mothers of breast-fed infants continued to consume the product (synbiotic or placebo). Synbiotic administration elicited a significant decrease in atopic eczema compared to the control group; however, there was no difference in overall allergic disease between the two groups. Bifidobacterial and lactobacilli levels were significantly higher in the synbiotic group [47].

The major criticism (scientifically at least) of the work on synbiotics is the lack of appropriate controls. The scientific community generally considers that evaluation of synbiotic effect necessitates demonstration of the effects elicited by each component (i.e. probiotics and prebiotics alone). Only then can the combination be truly evaluated. However, it remains to be determined whether such all-encompassing studies are required—especially if a clinical improvement or benefit is observed. Of course the mechanism of effect is of academic interest, as is the potential expansion of our understanding of the clinical state that such knowledge may afford.

SUMMARY AND CONCLUSION

The majority of prebiotic and synbiotic studies have concentrated on FOS and/or GOS. However, there is an increasing list of potential prebiotics, and research groups continue in their endeavours to identify and/or develop novel prebiotics (including so-called 'designer' prebiotics, which may have multiple functions—beyond that of selective fermentation by beneficial bacteria). A great deal of interest and scientific investment has been directed at the G9F1 prebiotic mixture, with multiple feeding studies demonstrating the bifidogenic effect of supplementation. However, only one synbiotic study has incorporated this prebiotic mixture to date. This is expected to change during the next decade. Indeed, the application of synbiotics in pediatrics is very much a 'watch this space' topic (as to a certain degree is the application of prebiotics in pediatrics, especially clinically). The results to date are very promising and such dietary regimes certainly merit further investigation, especially with a focus on clinical outcomes/biomarkers. The potential of synbiotic combinations to improve survival, implantation and/or activity of probiotics bodes well for extending the clinical applications of these beneficial strains in pediatric medicine.

REFERENCES

1. Lopez-Alarcon M, Villalpando S, Fajardo A. Breast-feeding lowers the frequency and duration of acute respiratory infection and diarrhea in infants under six months of age. *J Nutr* 1997;127:436–443.
2. Wilson AC, Forsyth JS, Greene SA, Irvine L, Hau C, Howie PW. Relation of infant diet to childhood health: seven year follow up of cohort of children in Dundee infant feeding study. *Br Med J* 1998;316:21–25.
3. Harmsen HJM, Wildeboer-Veloo AC, Raangs GC, Wagendorp AA, Klijn N, Bindels JG, Welling GW. Analysis of intestinal flora development in breast-fed and formula-fed infants by using molecular identification and detection methods. *J Pediatr Gastroenterol Nutr* 2000;30:61–67.
4. Wold AE, Adlerberth I. Breast feeding and the intestinal microflora of the infant –implications for protection against infectious diseases. *Adv Exp Med Biol* 2000;478:77–93.
5. Hoppu U, Kalliomaki M, Laiho K, Isolauri E. Breast milk--immunomodulatory signals against allergic diseases. *Allergy* 2001;56(Suppl 67):23–26.
6. Howie PW. Protective effect of breastfeeding against infection in the first and second six months of life. *Adv Exp Med Biol* 2002;503:141–147.
7. Gibson GR, Roberfroid MB. Dietary modulation of the human colonic microbiota: introducing the concept of prebiotics. *J Nutr* 1995;125:1401–1412.
8. Bongers MEJ, de Lorijn F, Reitsma JB, Groeneweg M, Taminiau JAJM, Benninga MA. The clinical effect of a new infant formula in term infants with constipation: a double-blind, randomized cross-over trial. Nutr J 2007;6:8 (http://www.nutritionj.com/content/6/1/8).
9. Brunser O, Gotteland M, Cruchet S, Figueroa G, Garrido D, Steenhout P. Effect of a milk formula with prebiotics on the intestinal microbiota of infants after an antibiotic treatment. *Pediatr Res* 2006;59:451–456.
10. Salminen S, Bouley C, Boutron-Ruault M-C, Cummings JH, Franck A, Gibson GR, Isolauri E, Moreau M-C, Roberfroid M, Rowland R. Functional food science and gastrointestinal physiology and function. *Br J Nutr* 1998;80(Suppl 1):S147–S171.

11. Guarner F, Malagelada JR. Gut flora in health and disease. *Lancet* 2003;361:512–519.
12. Millar MR, Linton CJ, Cade A, Glancy D, Hall M, Jalal H. Application of 16S rRNA gene PCR to study bowel microflora of preterm infants with and without necrotizing enterocolitis. *J Clin Microbiol* 1996;34:2506–2510.
13. Hoy CM, Wood CM, Hawkey PM, Puntis JW. Duodenal microflora in very-low-birth-weight neonates and relation to necrotizing enterocolitis. *J Clin Microbiol* 2000;38:4539–4547.
14. Song Y, Liu C, Finegold SY. Real-time PCR quantification of clostridia in feces of autistic children. *Appl Environ Microbiol* 2004;70:6459–6465.
15. Parracho MRT, Bingham MO, Gibson GR, McCartney AL. Differences between the gut microflora of children with autistic spectrum disorders and that of healthy children. *J Med Micro* 2005;54:987–991.
16. Ghisolfi J. Dietary fibre and prebiotics in infant formulas. *Proc Nutr Soc* 2003;62:183–185.
17. Roger LC, McCartney AL. Prebiotics and the infant microbiota. In: Tannock GW, (ed) Probiotics & Prebiotics: Scientific Aspects. Norfolk: Caister Academic Press, 2005:195–216.
18. Delzenne NM. Oligosaccharides: state of the art. *Proc Nutr Soc* 2003;62:177–182.
19. Goulas AK, Cooper JM, Grandison GS, Rastall RA. Synthesis of isomaltooligosaccharides and oligodextrans in a recycle membrane bioreactor by the combined use of dextransucrase and dextranase. *Biotechnol Bioeng* 2004;88:778–787.
20. Guesry PR. Important progress in infant nutrition. Arch Pediatr 2000;7(Suppl 2):197s–199s.
21. Euler AR, Mitchell DK, Kline R, Pickering LK. Prebiotic effect of fructo-oligosaccharide supplemented term infant formula at two concentrations compared with unsupplemented formula and human milk. *J Pediatr Gastroenterol Nutr* 2005;40:157–164.
22. Waligora-Dupriet AJ, Campeotto F, Nicolis I, Bonet A, Soulaines P, Dupont C, Butel MJ. Effect of oligofructose supplementation on gut microflora and well-being in young children attending a day care centre. *Int J Food Microbiol* 2007;113:108–113.
23. Kapiki A, Costalos C, Oikonomidou C, Triantafullidou A, Loukatou E, Pertrohilou V. The effect of a fructo-oligosaccharide supplemented formula on gut flora of preterm infants. *Early Hum Dev* 2007;83:335–339.
24. Kim SH, Lee da H, Meyer D. Supplementation of baby formula with native inulin has a prebiotic effect in formula-fed babies. *Asia Pac J Clin Nutr* 2007;16:172–177.
25. Xiao-ming B, Xiao-yu Z, Wei-hua Z, Wen-liang Y, Wei P, Wei-li Z, Sheng-mei W, van Beusekom CM, Schaafsma A. Supplementation of milk formula with galacto-oligosaccharides improves intestinal micro-flora and fermentation in term infants. *Chin Med J* 2004;117:927–931.
26. Moro G, Minoli I, Mosca M, Fanaro S, Jelinek J, Stahl B, Boehm G. Dosage-related bifidogenic effects of galacto- and fructooligosaccharides in formula-fed term infants. *J Pediatr Gastroenterol Nutr* 2002;34:291–295.
27. Boehm G, Lidestri M, Casetta P, Jelinek J, Negretti F, Stahl B, Marini, A . Supplementation of a bovine milk formula with an oligosaccharide mixture increases counts of faecal bifidobacteria in preterm infants. *Arch Dis Child Fetal Neonatal Ed* 2002;86:F178–F181.
28. Knol J, Scholtens P, Kafka C, Steenbakkers J, Groß S, Helm K, Klarczvk M, Schöpfer H, Böckler H-M, Wells J. Colon microflora in infants fed formula with galacto- and fructo-oligosacchardes: more like breast-fed infants. *J Pediatr Gastroenterol Nutr* 2005;40:36–42.
29. Costalos C, Kapiki A, Apostolou M, Papathoma E. The effect of a prebiotic supplemented formula on growth and stool microbiology of term infants. Early Hum Dev 2007;Apr10 [Epub ahead of print]. (doi:10.1016/j.earlhumdev.2007.03.001).
30. Haarman M, Knol J. Quantitative real-time PCR assays to identify and quantify fecal *Bifidobacterium* species in infants receiving a prebiotic infant formula. *Appl Environ Microbiol* 2005;71:2318–2324.
31. Haarman M, Knol J. Quantitative real-time PCR analysis of fecal *Lactobacillus* species in infants receiving a prebiotic infant formula. *Appl Environ Microbiol* 2006;72:2359–2365.
32. Bakker-Zierikzee AM, Tol EA, Kroes H, Alles MS, Kok FJ, Bindels JG. Faecal SIgA secretion in infants fed on pre- or probiotic infant formula. *Pediatr Allergy Immunol* 2006;17:134–140.
33. Field CJ. The immunological components of human milk and their effect on immune development in infants. *J Nutr* 2005;135:1–4.
34. Lonnerdal B. Nutritional and physiologic significance of human milk proteins. *Am J Clin Nutr* 2003;77:1537S–1543S.

35. Schmelzle H, Wirth S, Skopnik H, Radke M, Knol J, Bockler HM, Bronstrup A, Wells J, Fusch C. Randomized double-blind study of the nutritional efficacy and bifidogenicity of a new infant formula containing partially hydrolyzed protein, a high beta-palmitic acid level, and nondigestible oligosaccharides. *J Pediatr Gastroenterol Nutr* 2003;36:343–351.

36. Fanaro S, Jelinek J, Stahl B, Boehm G, Kock R, Vigi V. Acidic oligosaccharides from pectin hydrolysate as a new component for infant formulae: effect on intestinal flora, stool characteristics, and pH. *J Pediatr Gastroenterol Nutr* 2005;44:186–190.

37. Duggan C, Penny ME, Hibberd P, Gil A, Huapaya A, Cooper A, Coletta F, Emenhiser C, Kleinman RE. Oligofructose-supplemented infant cereal: 2 randomized, blinded, community-based trials in Peruvian infants. *Am J Clin Nutr* 2003;77:937–942.

38. Moore N, Chao C, Yang LP, Storm H, Oliva-Hemker M, Saavedra JM. Effects of fructo-oligosaccharide-supplemented infant cereal: a double-blind, randomized trial. *Br J Nutr* 2003;90:581–587.

39. Scholtens PA, Alles MS, Bindels JG, van der Linde EG, Tolboom JJ, Knol J. Bifidogenic effects of solid weaning foods with added prebiotic oligosaccharides: a randomised controlled clinical trial. *J Pediatr Gastroenterol Nutr* 2006;42:553–559.

40. Puccio G, Cajozzo C, Meli F, Rochat F, Grathwohl D, Steenhout P. Clinical evaluation of a new starter formula for infants containing live *Bifidobacterium longum* BL999 and prebiotics. *Nutrition* 2007;23:1–8.

41. Kanamori Y, Hashizume K, Sugiyama M, Mortomi M, Yuki N. Combination therapy with *Bifidobacterium breve*, *Lactobacillus casei*, and galactooligosaccharides dramatically improved the intestinal function in a girl with short bowel syndrome. *Digestive Dis Sci* 2001;46:2010–2016.

42. Kanamori Y, Hashizume K, Sugiyama M, Mortomi M, Yuki N, Tanaka, R. A novel synbiotic therapy dramatically improved the intestinal function of a pediatric patient with laryngotracheo-esophageal cleft (LTEC) in the intensive care unit. *Clin Nutr* 2002;21:527–530.

43. Kanamori Y, Hashizume K, Kitano Y, Tanaka Y, Morotomi M, Yuki N, Tanaka, R. Anaerobic dominant flora was reconstructed by synbiotics in an infant with MRSA enteritis. *Pediatr Int* 2003;45:359–362.

44. Kanamori Y, Sugiyama M, Hashizume K, Yuki N, Morotomi M, Tanaka R. Experience of long-term synbiotic therapy in seven short bowel patients with refractory enteroclitis. *J Ped Sur* 2004;39:1686–1692.

45. Gotteland M, Poliak L, Cruchet S, Brunser O. Effect of regular ingestion of Saccharomyces boulardii plus inulin or Lactobacillus acidophilus LB in children colonized by Helicobacter pylori. *Acta Paediatr* 2005;94:1747–1751.

46. Passeron T, Lacour JP, Fontas E, Ortonne JP. Prebiotics and synbiotics: two promising approaches for the treatment of atopic dermatitis in children above 2 years. *Allergy* 2006;61:431–437.

47. Kukkonen K, Savilahti E, Haahtela T, Juntunen-Backman K, Korpela R, Poussa T, Tuure T, Kuitunen M. Probiotics and prebiotic galacto-oligosaccharides in the prevention of allergic diseases: a randomized, double-blind, placebo-controlled trial. *J Allergy Clin Immunol* 2007;119:192–198.

48. Knol J, Steenbakkers GMA, van der Linde EGM, Groß S, Helm K, Klarczvk M, Schöpfer H, Kafka C. Bifidobacterial species that are present in breast-fed infants are stimulated in formula-fed infants by changing to a formula containing prebiotics. *J Pediatr Gastroenterol Nutr* 2002;34:477.

23 The Future of Probiotics

Eamonn MM Quigley

Key Points

- While animal models have demonstrated efficacy for killed bacteria, or even bacterial products or components, this strategy has not, as yet, been explored or validated in man.
- Not all probiotics are the same and extrapolations from one to another should be resisted at all times.
- Critical examinations of the actual constituents of commercially available probiotic preparations have revealed worrying deviations from those included in the product label.
- Few probiotic preparations have shown the actual concentration of the probiotic product at the desired site of action.
- Several probiotic questions that remain unanswered are discussed in this chapter.

Key Words: Future, probiotic, quality.

INTRODUCTION

The reader may be excused for hesitating when confronted by a piece that purports to address the future of an issue or a concept that has been around for almost 100 years; surely the future of such an entity is not in question and certainly, you will say, its course should by now be clearly set? Yet, so capricious has been the story of probiotics over this century that it has been only in very recent years that the true potential of this field has come to be appreciated and a few glimpses of the future fleetingly snatched. Before we embark on that most risky and, some would say, doomed, of tasks, namely, predicting the future, let us take stock, firstly, of where we are and, secondly, of the issues that still confront us. Perhaps, if we can crystallize the latter, the future may take care of itself.

From: *Nutrition and Health: Probiotics in Pediatric Medicine*
Edited by: S. Michail and P.M. Sherman © Humana Press, Totowa, NJ

PROBIOTICS 2007; PROGRESS AND MANY PITFALLS

The concept of probiotics has been with us since the observations of Metchnikoff among Bulgarian peasants in the first decade of the last century. For much of the intervening time, however, the concept has languished in the realm of "alternative" or "natural" medicine and scarcely attracted the interest of either science or conventional medicine. Several factors have, of late, conspired to dramatically change the profile of probiotics and the probiotic concept. These include rapid progress, now aided by evolving molecular techniques, in our appreciation of the vital role of the enteric flora (microbiota) in health and disease; the application of modern science to the study of probiotics per se, resulting in the accurate classification of individual probiotic organisms coupled with detailed descriptions of their genetic, microbiological and immunological properties; extensive in vivo and in vitro studies of the impact of various probiotics on a variety of biological systems and, finally, and most recently, well conducted clinical trials of probiotics in specific clinical scenarios in man and domestic animals.

Despite all of this progress several problems persist in relation to these areas, which continue to sully the image of probiotics. It is important at this stage to reflect on the most widely accepted (FAO/WHO) definition of a probiotic, which is as follows:

"Live microorganisms which when administered in adequate amounts confer a health benefit on the host" [1].

Two issues deserve special emphasis: the focus on "live" organisms and the insistence on conferring "a health benefit on the host". Firstly, while it is readily acknowledged that studies in a number of animal models have demonstrated efficacy for killed bacteria, or even bacterial products or components [2–4, in generating a number of anti-inflammatory and anti-infective effects, this strategy has not, as yet, been explored or validated in man. Secondly, it is obvious from the latter part of this definition that clinical claims in man, be they in the augmentation of health or in the treatment of disease, must be supported by credible clinical trial data. Currently, probiotics are not regulated as drugs and have been able to come on to the market as food supplements or other designations, which have allowed them, to a greater or lesser extent, to make a variety of "health" claims in the absence of supporting data. This is changing and will change even more rapidly as new regulations appear in Europe and North America to govern this area. At present the consumer is not being served, not only by the aforementioned issues relating to "health" claims, but also by major problems with quality control. Firstly, it is not unusual for the benefits of a given species or organism to be touted based on evidence derived from studies involving other organisms and species, despite the fact that detailed studies have demonstrated that, in terms of a probiotic property, be it immune modulation [5–8] or anti-bacterial activity [6, 9, 10], there are tremendous differences between different lactobacilli and bifidobacteria, not to mind between lactobacilli and bifidobacteria, for example. No two probiotics are the same and extrapolations from one to another should be resisted at all times. Secondly, an individual who is about to consume a given probiotic preparation should know exactly what he or she is about to take: is it live, what is it's concentration, will the organism survive as it makes contact with acid, bile and digestive enzymes as it transits the gut and what will be the actual concentration of the organism at it's desired site of action? Few probiotic preparations have been characterized and formulated with sufficient rigor to allow the manufacturer to provide answers to these critical questions. Of further concern, critical examinations of the actual constituents of commercially available probiotic preparations have revealed worrying deviations from those included in the product label [11–15].

Nevertheless, evidence for efficacy for specific probiotics in certain clinical conditions continues to accumulate. Most notable have been studies in diarrheal illnesses. Several studies have reported that probiotics may be effective in shortening the duration of acute diarrheal illnesses in children, such as that related to rotavirus infection [16]. Probiotics also appear to be effective in antibiotic-associated diarrhea [17–19], pouchitis [20,21] and, perhaps, some instances of inflammatory bowel disease [22,23]. More recently, several studies have evaluated probiotics in one of the most common gastroenterological ailments, irritable bowel syndrome (IBS); while several preparations have demonstrated benefits in terms of individual IBS-related symptoms [24], only one, *Bifidobacterium infantis* 35625, has produced consistent global benefit in IBS [8, 25].

THE FUTURE OF PROBIOTICS

Rather than make wild speculations regarding the future, or even risking modest predictions, I will now attempt to identify those areas where, to my mind, the greatest challenges persist and the most important questions remain unanswered.

Quality Control and Regulation

If the field of probiotics is to progress further and gain acceptance within the hallowed halls of science, quality control and appropriate regulation must occur. Inevitably, this will take place on a nation-by-nation basis but, however accomplished, must ensure that the consumer or the prescriber is sufficiently informed of the nature of any given product and assured of the accuracy of its label, including its shelf life, and the validity of health claims. It is incumbent on the medical and scientific communities to actively engage in these processes and to thereby ensure that new requirements and regulations in relation to quality control have scientific credibility and validity. This is a matter of great urgency; failure, may result in a gradual ebbing away of confidence in the entire area and the loss of valuable products because the public simply cannot differentiate them from impostors.

Probiotic Characterization

As individual probiotic organisms are subjected to genomic analysis [26], the stage is set for both the accurate definition of each individual organism and the identification, on the genome, of areas of interest in relation to a particular property or action. This must be the way forward for both the definition of individual organisms and the comparison of their individual characteristics. Parallel developments such as the, recently announced, National Institutes of Health (NIH) project to identify the human microbiome (http://nihroadmap.nih.gov/hmp/) will ultimately lead to the accurate description of the enteric flora and their metabolic properties and in so doing will facilitate a complete delineation of the interactions (good and bad) between bugs and the host. In so doing, considerable progress should be made in defining the basis for the beneficial actions of probiotic bacteria.

Mechanism of Action

While genomics and metabolomics may suggest certain roles for certain probiotics, these must, ultimately, be further elucidated in appropriate biological systems, including man. Indeed, a further component of the characterization of a probiotic must be the definition of it effects, if any, in a variety of contexts. Does the organism exert anti-bacterial or anti-viral properties, what are its effects on immune responses? Again a standardized and validated approach to the interrogation of a given organism in relation to a particular use must be developed, where possible. Currently, the methodologies and test systems to be employed to assess the efficacy of an organism against, say *Clostridium difficile* are well characterized but how does one evaluate the potential impact of an organism in IBS, a disorder whose pathogenesis remains unknown? With regard to the latter, one can only do what the pharmaceutical industry has done for decades, test the organism in relation to putative pathophysiological mechanisms such as, in the case of IBS, dysmotility [27] or visceral hypersensitivity [4, 28, 29]. Proposals to use a probiotic in man must have a plausible scientific rationale, hype and appeals to "being natural" should no longer be sufficient.

Waking the Dead

As emphasized at the outset of this chapter, the current definition of probiotics insists on the inclusion of live organisms. This is appropriate given the persisting absence of any data to suggest efficacy for anything other than live organisms in man. This will undoubtedly change; bacteria are metabolically active organisms which produce a variety of molecules with biological activity [4, 29]. As already mentioned, bacterial DNA has been demonstrated to exert anti-inflammatory activity on certain systems [2, 3]; it seems reasonable to assume that other bacterial components, such as the cell wall or its outer coat, may prove effective in certain contexts. The whole area of bacterial components and bacterial products will be an exceptionally active one in the coming years. In clinical terms, this approach has already shown dividends through the isolation of probiotic products with specific anti-bacterial activities [30, 31]. There is much more to come.

More Trials

Performing clinical trials with probiotics is not easy. Quite apart from the aforementioned issues in relation to strain selection for a given indication, the clinical investigator is faced with significant obstacles in choosing formulation, dose and duration of study. Dose is, for the most part, a "black box" in this field, very few dose ranging studies have been attempted and extrapolations from animal studies must always remain mindful of the fact that weight for weight probiotic doses used in the mouse or the rat exceed by several logs those used in man. We must attempt to get our doses right! Here, however, we encounter the issue of formulation; what may be most acceptable to the patient (e.g. a once-a-day capsule) may not permit the inclusion of an optimal dose of the organism. These challenges must and will be met; our obligation then is to ensure the performance of clinical trials whose design is optimal for the given indication. Only then can we recommend probiotics to our patients.

Probiotics could, in the future, act as vehicles for the targeted delivery of therapeutic molecules to the gut. It has already been shown that probiotics can be genetically engineered to deliver interleukin (IL)-10 to the intestinal mucosa using an ingenious system which ensures that the organism will not survive outside of the host [32–34]. In similar studies, probiotics such as *Lactobacillus lactis* and a commensal species of *Escherichia coli* have been engineered to express egg albumin to reduce food allergy [35, 36], either Yersinia LcrV [37] or trefoil factors [38] to heal murine colitis and, a GM1 ganglioside receptor to ameliorate enterotoxin-induced diarrhea in a rabbit ileal ligated-loop model [39]. These exciting developments have the potential to move the field into a new era of "designer" probiotics whereby specific manipulations will be invoked in order to address a particular deficiency or disease state.

One great advantage that probiotics currently enjoy in the clinical arena, and in comparison to conventional pharmaceuticals, is that of safety. We must remain vigilant in this area and perform the same rigorous and extensive phase IV, post-marketing, surveys that have become the norm elsewhere. Here again genomic analysis will provide an important supportive role by identifying pathogenicity islands or features that suggest the potential for transference of antibiotic resistance [26].

New Horizons; Moving Beyond the Gut

For obvious reasons, including their source and the well-documented interactions between the microbiota and the gut, studies of probiotics have, to date, concentrated in large part on intestinal disorders. Hints to suggest efficacy for probiotics in disorders beyond the gut accumulate and include, for example, non-alcoholic fatty liver disease [40], arthritis [41], allergy [42] and even obesity [43]. The latter is in keeping with very recent and exciting data on the role of the gut flora in obesity [44]. As our understanding of microbiota-host interactions increases, new applications for probiotics will arise. As the true importance of the microbiota in human homeostasis comes to be recognized the therapeutic potential of probiotics can begin to be realized.

SUMMARY AND CONCLUSION

Having languished for years in the nether world of the "alternative", probiotics have enjoyed a very recent and very rapid acceleration in scientific investigation and clinical application. In some instances the latter has, regrettably, preceded the former, an approach that, coupled with continuing issues with quality control and regulation, continues to dog the credibility of this area. These hurdles can and will be overcome and will allow scientifically based and rigorously tested probiotic products to assume their rightful place in the therapeutic armamentarium. In the future, the arrival of a range of therapeutic products that includes not just live organisms (probiotics) but genetically engineered organisms as well as molecules elaborated by probiotics or even components of these organisms, will herald the advent of the era of pharmacobiotics.

REFERENCES

1. Joint FAO/WHO expert consultation on evaluation of health and nutritional properties of probiotics in food including powder milk with live lactic acid bacteria. October 2001.
2. Rachmilewitz D, Kayatura, Karmeli F, et-al.. Toll-like receptor 9 signaling mediates the anti-inflammatory effects of probiotics in murine experimental colitis. *Gastroenterology* 2004; 126: 520 – 8.
3. Jijon H, Backer J, Diaz H, Yeung H, Thiel D, McKagney C, De Simone C, Madsen K. DNA from probiotic bacteria modulates murine and human epithelial and immune function. *Gastroenterology* 2004;126:1358–1373.
4. Kamiya T, Wang L, Forsythe P, Goettsche G, Mao Y, Wang Y, Tougas G, Bienenstock J. Inhibitory effects of *Lactobacillus reuteri* on visceral pain induced by colorectal distension in Sprague-Dawley rats. *Gut* 2006;55:191–196.
5. McCarthy J, O'Mahony L, O'Callaghan L, Sheil B, Vaughan EE, Fitzsimons N, Fitzgibbon J, O'Sullivan GC, Kiely B, Collins JK, Shanahan F. Double blind, placebo controlled trial of two probiotic strains in interleukin 10 knockout mice and mechanistic link with cytokine balance. *Gut* 2003;52:975–980.
6. Madsen K, Cornish A, Soper P, McKaigney, C, Jijon H, Yachimel C, Doyle J, Jewell L, De Simone C. Probiotic bacteria enhance murine and human intestinal epithelial barrier function. *Gastroenterology* 2001; 121:580–91.
7. Hart AL, Lammers K, Brigidi P, Vitali B, Rizzello F, Gionchetti P, Campieri M, Kamm MA, Knight SC, Stagg AJ. Modulation of human dendritic cell phenotype and function by probiotic bacteria. *Gut* 2004;53:1602–1609.
8. O'Mahony L. McCarthy J, Kelly P, Shanahan F, Quigley EM. Lactobacillus and bifidobacterium in irritable bowel syndrome: symptom responses and relationship to cytokine profiles. *Gastroenterology* 2005; 128:541–51.
9. O'Mahony L, O'Callaghan L, McCarthy J, Shilling D, Scully P, Sibartie S, Kavanagh E, Kirwan WO, Redmond RP, Collins JK, Shanahan F. Differential cytokine response from dendritic cells to commensal and pathogenic bacteria in different lymphoid compartments in humans. *Am J Physiol.* 2006;290:G839–G845.
10. Jijon H, Backer J, Diaz H, Yeung H, Thiel D, McKagney C, De Simone C, Madsen K. DNA from probiotic bacteria modulates murine and human epithelial and immune function. *Gastroenterology* 2004;126:1358–1373.
11. Hamilton-Miller JM, Shah S, Winkler JT. Public health issues arising from microbiological and labelling quality of foods and supplements containing probiotic microorganisms. *Public Health Nutr.* 1999;2:223–9.
12. Coeuret V, Gueguen M, Vernoux JP. Numbers and strains of lactobacilli in some probiotic products. *Int J Food Microbiol.* 2004;97:147–56.
13. Szajewska H, Fordymacka A, Bardowski J, Gorecki RK, Mrukowicz JZ, Banaszkiewicz A. Microbiological and genetic analysis of probiotic products licensed for medicinal purposes. *Med Sci Monit.* 2004;10:BR346–50
14. Drisko J, Bischoff B, Giles C, Adelson M, Rao RV, McCallum R. Evaluation of five probiotic products for label claims by DNA extraction and polymerase chain reaction analysis. *Dig Dis Sci.* 2005;50:1113–1117.
15. Theunissen J, Britz TJ, Torriani S, Witthuhn RC. Identification of probiotic microorganisms in South African products using PCR-based DGGE analysis. *Int J Food Microbiol.* 2005;98:11–21.
16. Allen SJ, Okoko B, Martinez E, Gregorio G, Dans LF. Probiotics for treating infectious diarrhoea. *Cochrane Database Syst Rev.* 2004;(2):CD003048.
17. D'Souza AL, Rajkumar CH, Cooke J, et-al.. Probiotics in prevention of antibiotic associated diarrhea: meta-analysis. *BMJ* 2002;324:1361–6.
18. Szajewska H, Skorka A, Dylag M. Meta-analysis: Saccharomyces boulardii for treating acute diarrhoea in children. *Aliment Pharmacol Ther.* 2007;25:257–64.
19. de Vrese M, Marteau PR. Probiotics and prebiotics: effects on diarrhea. *J Nutr.* 2007;137(3 Suppl 2):803S–11S.
20. Gionchetti P, Rizzello F, Helwig U, Venturi A, Lammers KM, Brigidi P, Vitali B, Poggioli G, Miglioli M, Campieri M. Prophylaxis of pouchitis onset with probiotic therapy: a double-blind, placebo-controlled trial. *Gastroenterology* 2003;124:1202–9.
21. Mimura T, Rizzello F, Helwig U, Poggioli G, Schreiber S, Talbot IC, Nicholls RJ, Gionchetti P, Campieri M, Kamm MA. Once daily high dose probiotic therapy (VSL#3) for maintaining remission in recurrent or refractory pouchitis. *Gut* 2004;53:108–14.
22. Sheil B, Shanahan F, O'Mahony L. Probiotic effects on inflammatory bowel disease. *J Nutr.* 2007;137(3 Suppl 2):819S–24S.
23. Quigley EMM. Probiotics in the management of colonic disorders. *Curr Gatroenterol Rep* 2007;9:434–440.
24. Quigley EM, Flourie B. Probiotics and irritable bowel syndrome: a rationale for their use and an assessment of the evidence to date. *Neurogastroenterol Motil.* 2007;19:166–72.

25. Whorwell PJ, Altinger L, Morel J, Bond Y, Charbonneau D, O'Mahony L, Kiely B, Shanahan B, Quigley EM. Efficacy of an encapsulated probiotic *Bifidobacterium infantis* 35624 in women with irritable bowel syndrome. *Am J Gastroenterol.* 2006;101:326–33.

26. Claesson MJ, Li Y, Leahy S, Canchaya C, van Pijkeren JP, Cerdeno-Tarraga AM, Parkhill J, Flynn S, O'Sullivan GC, Collins JK, Higgins D, Shanahan F, Fitzgerald GF, van Sinderen D, O'Toole PW. Multireplicon genome architecture of Lactobacillus salivarius. *Proc Natl Acad Sci U S A* 2006; 103(17):6718–23.

27. Verdu EF, Bercik P, Bergonzelli GE, Huang XX, Blenerhasset P, Rochat F, Fiaux M, Mansourian R, Corthesy-Theulaz I, Collins SM. Lactobacillus paracasei normalizes muscle hypercontractiltiy in a murine model of postinfective gut dysfunction. *Gastroenterology* 20004;127:826–37.

28. Verdu EF, Bercik P, Verma-Gandhu M, Huang X-X, Blenerhasset P, Jackson W, Mao Y, Wang L, Rochat F, Collins SM. Specific probiotic therapy attenuates antibiotic induced visceral hypersensitivity in mice. *Gut* 2006;55:182–90.

29. Ait-Belgnaoui A, Han W, Lamine F, Eutamene H, Fioramonti J, Bueno L, Theodorou V. Lactobacillus farciminis treatment suppresses stress-induced visceral hypersensitivity: a possible action through interaction with epithelial cells cytoskeleton contraction. *Gut* 2006;55:1090–94.

30. Rea MC, Clayton E, O'Connor PM, Shanahan F, Kiely B, Ross RP, Hill C. Antimicrobial activity of lacticin 3,147 against clinical Clostridium difficile strains. *J Med Microbiol.* 2007;56(Pt 7):940–6.

31. Corr SC, Li Y, Riedel CU, O'Toole PW, Hill C, Gahan CG. Bacteriocin production as a mechanism for the antiinfective activity of Lactobacillus salivarius UCC118. *Proc Natl Acad Sci U S A.* 2007;104:7617–21.

32. Vandenbroucke K, Hans W, Van Huysse J, Neirynck S, Demetter P, Remaut E, Rottiers P, Steidler L. Active delivery of trefoil factors by genetically modified Lactococcus lactis prevents and heals acute colitis in mice. *Gastroenterology* 2004;127:502–13.

33. Braat H, Rottiers P, Hommes DW, Huyghebaert N, Remaut E, Remon JP, van Deventer SJ, Neirynck S, Peppelenbosch MP, Steidler L. A phase I trial with transgenic bacteria expressing interleukin-10 in Crohn's disease. *Clin Gastroenterol Hepatol.* 2006;4:754–9.

34. Frossard CP, Steidler L, Eigenmann PA. Oral administration of an IL-10-secreting Lactococcus lactis strain prevents food-induced IgE sensitization. *J Allergy Clin Immunol.* 2007;119:952–9.

35. Huibregtse IL, Snoeck V, de Creus A, Braat H, De Jong EC, Van Deventer SJ, Rottiers P. Induction of ovalbumin-specific tolerance by oral administration of *Lactococcus lactis* secreting ovalbumin. *Gastroenterology* 2007;133:517–28.

36. Maillard MH, Snapper SB. Teaching tolerance with a probiotic antigen delivery system. *Gastroenterology* 2007;133:706–9.

37. Foligne B, Dessein R, Marceau M, Poiret S, Chamaillard M, Pot B, Simonet M, Daniel C. Prevention and treatment of colitis with *Lactococcus lactis* secreting the immunomodulatory Yersinia LcrV protein. *Gastroenterology* 2007;133:862–74.

38. Vandenbroucke K, Hans W, Van Huysse J, Neirynck S, Demetter P, Remaut E, Rottiers P, Steidler L. Active delivery of trefoil factors by genetically modified *Lactococcus lactis* prevents and heals acute colitis in mice. *Gastroenterology* 2004;127:502–13.

39. Focareta A, Paton JC, Morona R, Cook J, Paton AW. A recombinant probiotic for treatment and prevention of cholera. *Gastroenterology* 2006;130:1688–95.

40. Li Z, Yang S, Lin H, et-al.. Probiotics and antibodies to TNF inhibit inflammatory activity and improve nonalcoholic fatty liver disease. *Hepatology* 2003;37:343–50.

41. Sheil B, McCarthy J, O'Mahony L, Bennett MW, Ryan P, Fitzgibbon JJ, Kiely B, Collins JK, Shanahan F. Is the mucosal route of administration essential for probiotic function? Subcutaneous administration is associated with attenuation of murine colitis and arthritis. *Gut* 2004;53:694–700.

42. Osborn D, Sinn J. Probiotics in infants for prevention of allergic disease and food hypersensitivity. *Cochrane Database Syst Rev.* 2007 Oct 17;4:CD006475.

43. Lee HY, Park JH, Seok SH, Baek MW, Kim DJ, Lee KE, Paek KS, Lee Y, Park JH. Human originated bacteria, Lactobacillus rhamnosus PL60, produce conjugated linoleic acid and show anti-obesity effects in diet-induced obese mice. *Biochim Biophys Acta.* 2006;1761:736–44.

44. Turnbaugh PJ, Ley RE, Mahowald MA, Magrini V, Mardis ER, Gordon JI. An obesity-associated gut microbiome with increased capacity for energy harvest. *Nature* 2006;444:1027–31.

Section F
Probiotic Future

24   The Quality Control of Probiotics in Food and Dietary Supplements

Sheryl H. Berman

Key Points

- Different properties of food probiotics and dietary supplements are discussed in this chapter.
- Guidelines for the manufacture of probiotics and the current state of federal regulation of probiotics in food products and dietary supplements are described.
- Good manufacturing guidelines are being put forth at least for dietary supplements.
- Guidelines and resources are provided to healthcare providers so that they may advise patients about probiotic products.

Key Words: Probiotics, products, quality, safety, supplements.

INTRODUCTION

When examining the safety of probiotics in food or dietary supplements, there are at least two perspectives to address for the health care professional. One perspective is determining what type of adverse events are seen with the use of probiotics. With that determination comes several questions. How common are these adverse events? Do these events influence or preclude the use of probiotics in adult or pediatric populations? What about specialized populations such as pregnant women, the elderly or immune compromised persons?

Before one can assess the adverse events associated with probiotic use, however, it is essential to know the properties of the product one is evaluating. Is that product viable, pure, and consistent with labeling as to microbe identification and quantities stated? In other words, are the reported adverse events due to the product itself, or lack of the product or contamination? These fundamental questions relate to the second important perspective of probiotic safety, quality control.

From: *Nutrition and Health: Probiotics in Pediatric Medicine*
Edited by: S. Michail and P.M. Sherman © Humana Press, Totowa, NJ

This chapter addresses the many quality control issues related to probiotics. What processes are involved in the quality control of probiotics? How does the quality control of probiotic foods differ from that of probiotic supplements? What are the pertinent federal regulations with respect to viability, purity, and accurate labeling? Are there recommendations for good manufacturing practices of probiotic foods and dietary supplements? Taking all of these questions together, guidelines and resources are provided to healthcare providers so that they may advise their patients about high quality probiotic products. Products that will, at the very least, do no harm and at best, enhance the health of patients.

PROBIOTICS IN DIFFERENT FORMS

Probiotics are available in two main forms; food and dietary supplements. Each is subject to different quality control processes and different regulations to monitor quality control. Several types of probiotic foods are available. The most common probiotic foods in the USA include dairy products such as yogurt, yogurt drinks, milk, cheese, and kefir. Other fermented foods, such as sauerkraut and kimchee, may include probiotic organisms in certain circumstances. Probiotics are also available as dietary supplements in the form of liquid, tablets, pearls, or capsules. Let us address quality control in food probiotics first.

PROBIOTICS IN FOODS

Many bacteria and yeasts are useful in the production of fermented food products. Often, the microbial organisms used to initiate fermentation in foods are referred to as "starter cultures" and not "probiotic cultures". Some companies may add "probiotic organisms" such as *Lactobacillus acidophilus* and *Bifidobacterium bifidum* to the "starter cultures". Although fermentation of the food is allowed to go to completion in a number of products, more often in the commercial manufacture of fermented foods, the fermentation process is stopped before the final step in the manufacturing process. Stopping the fermentation process increases the shelf life of the product by retarding spoilage. The most common process used to stop the fermentation process is pasteurization, which involves heating a food to a specific temperature for a specified time in order to stop microorganisms from growing.

Due to the heating associated with pasteurization, it is unlikely that live "starter cultures" or even "probiotic organisms" remain in the pasteurized final fermented food product. Some companies will add additional probiotic organisms to the food product after pasteurization. Although pasteurizing a food product is more the rule than the exception with most milk products, some companies may choose not to kill the original organisms via pasteurization. For example, most yogurts are not pasteurized after being "cultured". Whether a manufacturer chooses to stop the fermentation process prematurely or not, there must be "adequate numbers" of live microorganisms in the final food product. Furthermore, an "adequate number" of live microorganisms must be recognized "probiotic strains" of microorganisms. If both of these criteria are met, the food may be labeled as a "probiotic food".

QUALITY CONTROL OF PROBIOTICS IN FOOD

As of August 2007, there are no requirements for a minimal number of microorganisms in foods in order for those foods to be classified as "probiotic foods" in the USA. Nor is there agreement as to which microorganisms can be classified as "probiotic organisms" in "probiotic foods". Certain food associations have made recommendations for the number of organisms and/or the type of microorganisms in their food products, but these are recommendations, not requirements. For example, the National Yogurt Association recommends the minimal presence of 10^8 viable organisms per gram of a yogurt product at production. To encourage compliance among manufacturers and confidence from consumers, the National Yogurt Association will add a seal (Live Active Seal) to products containing this minimal count of microorganisms. The quantification of microorganisms within a product must be certified by independent microbiologists to qualify for the Live Active Seal. The National Yogurt Association however, does not specify whether these organisms are "probiotic organisms" or organisms such as *L. bulgaricus* and *Streptococcus thermophilus* that are used as "starter cultures" [1].

RECOMMENDED CRITERIA FOR EVALUATING FOOD PROBIOTICS

In October 2001, the World Health Organization and the Food and Agriculture Organization of the United Nations (WHO/FAO) held a meeting in Co'rdoba, Argentina to generate guidelines, recommend criteria and identify methodologies for use in evaluating probiotics in food [2, 3]. Meeting attendees adopted the definition of probiotics, 'Live microorganisms which when administered in adequate amounts confer a healthy benefit on the host' and defined the properties of probiotics to support this definition. According to the WHO/FAO, all food probiotics should possess the following properties:

1. Identification of the genus, species, and strain by reliable methodology: The gold standard for identification of genus, species and subspecies (strain) is nucleic acid hybridization. The particular strain should be deposited in an international culture collection such as the American Type Culture Collection (ATCC).
2. *In vitro* characterization of the organism: There are a number of tests that help characterize the properties of probiotic microorganisms. Several of these *in vitro* properties are directly correlated to human or *in vivo* properties. Suggested tests include bile acid resistance which helps predict the survivability in gastric acids, bile salt hydrolase activity which helps predict the formation of bile salts capable of inducing diarrhea [4] and adherence to mucus and epithelial cells which help predict the ability of the organisms to temporarily colonize the gastrointestinal and genitourinary tracts [5].
3. Safety assessment: Several concerns need to be addressed with regard to probiotic safety. Specifically, the side effects or adverse effects of the probiotic organisms, if any, and the association of these organisms with sepsis must be elucidated. The potential of these organisms to produce toxins or hemolysins that may bring harm to the person ingesting them should also be identified. Last, but not least, are the antibiotic resistance patterns of the organism and the ability of the organism to transfer these resistance genes to other gastrointestinal or genitourinary flora. This is essential to both individual and public health. *In vitro*, animal and phase one human studies should be used as complementary approaches to assess safety concerns.

4. Assessment of Efficacy: Phase two human trials, preferably double-blind placebo controlled, are recommended to assess efficacy of any particular probiotic species and strain. These phase two trials should be followed by phase three trials which compare probiotic treatments with standard, commonly used treatments for a specific health concern or pathology.

When *in vitro* properties, safety, and efficacy have been established for a particular species and strain of probiotic organism, the FAO/WHO suggests guidelines for the appropriate labeling of the food product containing that organism. The label should display the genus, species, strain, and the number of viable bacteria estimated at the end of shelf life. In addition, the shelf life and storage conditions should be specified for the product. Information for the consumer to contact the company is a final piece of recommended information that should be associated with the food product.

Probiotics in Dietary Supplements

As mentioned in section 1.1, probiotics are available as dietary supplements in capsules, tablets, pearls, and liquids. The range of probiotic species in dietary supplements is much more diverse than found in food. The primary genera seen in probiotic supplements include *Lactobacillus* and *Bifidobacterium* species. Lists of the different Lactobacilli and Bifidobacteria commonly used in supplements are provided in Tables 24.1 and 24.2. Many of the species found in probiotic dietary supplements are also found as normal microbial flora in the human intestinal or genitourinary tracts

Table 24.1
Lactobacilli commonly used in dietary supplements

Lactobacillus species	Recognized as gastro-intestinal flora	Recognized as Genitourinary flora	Not recognized as GI or GU flora
L. acidophilus	X		X
L. brevis	X		
L. bulgaricus			X
L. casei	X		
L. cellobiosus			X
L. crispatus		X	
L. curvatus			X
L. delbrueckii			X
L. fermentum	X		
L. gallinarum			X
L. gasseri		X	
L. iners			X
L. jensenii		X	
L. johnsonii			X
L. plantarum	X		
L. reuterii			X
L. rhamnosus			X
L. salivarius			X
L. sporogenes			X
L. vaginalis		X	

Table 24.2
Bifidobacteria commonly used in dietary supplements

Bifidobacterium species	Recognized as gastro-intestinal Flora	Not recognized as gastrointestinal flora
B. adolescentis		X
B. animalis		X
B.bifidum	X	
B. brevis		X
B. infantis	X	
B. lactis	X	
B. longum	X	
B. thermophilum		X

(see Tables 24.1 and 24.2). Bacterial genera other than *Lactobacillus* and *Bifidobacterim* are also used in probiotic dietary supplements and they include *Bacillus, Streptococcus, Enterococcus,* and *Escherichia* (*E. coli*). *Sachromyces boulardii* (baker's yeast) and *S. cervesiae* (brewer's yeast) are nearly genetically identical yeasts also used as probiotic organisms.

PREBIOTICS, DELAYED RELEASE OR ENTERIC COATING OF SUPPLEMENTS

In addition to the multitude of probiotic strains available in dietary supplements, the delivery of these products is quite variable. For example, some manufacturers may 'enteric coat' their product or have gastrointestinal disintegration delayed in a 'time-release formula'. The purpose of enteric coating or a delayed release formula is to protect the probiotic bacteria from degradation by gastric acids and digestive enzymes. In addition, numerous products may contain "prebiotics" such as fructo-oligosacchardies (FOS) or inulin. Prebiotics are substances that can function as food sources for probiotic organisms, particularly those of the Bifidobacteria genus [6, 7]. As there have been few, well-controlled studies comparing these special formulations with supplements that do not have them, we cannot scientifically critique these formulations. At this time, there is no compelling scientific evidence that the presence of enteric coating, a time-release formula or prebiotics increase the antibacterial, immune, or other physiological proper-ties of probiotic organisms in dietary supplements or foods.

REGULATION OF PROBIOTIC DIETARY SUPPLEMENTS BY THE FDA

The Food and Drug Administration controls the regulation of food, prescription drugs, over the counter (OTC) drugs and dietary supplements in the USA. In 1994, the Dietary Supplement Health and Education Act (DSHEA) was passed by Congress. This act amended previous statutes that regulated dietary supplements. It created a variety of specific provisions for the regulation of dietary supplements. These provi-sions included the definition of a dietary supplement, dietary supplement product safety, nutritional statements and claims, ingredient and nutritional labeling, the ability to establish good manufacturing procedures and practices, and the classification of "new" dietary ingredients.

PROVISIONS OF DSHEA 1994

The Dietary Supplement Health and Education Act (DSHEA) defined dietary supplements as "a vitamin, mineral, or herb in pill, capsule, or liquid form that supplements the diet but is not represented as a sole meal" [8, 9]. The act puts the "burden of proof" for safety on the manufacturers of the dietary supplements. Although some individuals may liken this to the "fox guarding the hen house", this system of safety self-regulation has historically been in use by the food industry for many years. DSHEA 1994 helped classify dietary supplements as resembling food more than pharmaceuticals. In addition, DSHEA 1994 specifies that literature about the dietary supplement must be displayed separately from the product, may not contain false or misleading information and does not promote a particular product.

Some individuals and consumer groups consider the most important aspect of DSHEA to be its provisions for dietary supplement labeling. The ability to claim prevention, treatment, or cure for a particular pathology or disease is strictly forbidden under DSHEA 1994 [10]. Label statements that address general "well being" or the effect of the dietary supplement on "structure and function" of the body are allowed as long as they are truthful and have the following disclaimer "This statement has not been evaluated by the Food and Drug Administration. This product is not intended to diagnose, treat, cure, or prevent any disease." In addition, the dietary supplement label must contain nutritional information such as the name and quantity of each ingredient and particular plant origin, if applicable.

Further provisions of DSHEA include the prohibition of ingredients that were not marketed before 1994 unless the ingredient was already in common use and with a history of safe use. Manufacturers proposing to use new ingredients in dietary supplements are required to notify the FDA 75 days before marketing the product. This notification must be accompanied by evidence that the ingredient "will reasonably be expected to be safe." More information regarding DSHEA 1994 can be attained by going to: http://www.healthy.net/public/legallg/fedregs/S784_ENR.HTM>http://www.cfsan.fda.gov/~dms/dietsupp.html

GOOD MANUFACTURING PRACTICES FOR DIETARY SUPPLEMENTS

The primary way to protect dietary supplement users is for good manufacturing practices (GMPs) to be established, practiced, and regulated. As discussed above, the Food and Drug Administration is not directly responsible for regulating the safety of dietary supplements. In addition, until June, 2007 the FDA did not require or recommend good manufacturing practices (GMPs) for the dietary supplement industry. In 1994, DSHEA ensured the ability of the FDA to establish GMPs for the supplement industry. Until recently, the FDA had not formally done so but, instead, relied upon the dietary supplement manufacturers themselves to establish these guidelines and recommendations.

Since 1994, many suggestions have been put forth to follow up on DSHEA with regard to good manufacturing practices [11,12]. In June 2007, 13 years after DSHEA 1994 and the deregulation of supplements by the federal government, good manufacturing practices for the dietary supplement industry were finally initiated by the FDA in the USA [13]. These good manufacturing practice guidelines provide for a gradual implementation that is dependent upon the size of the dietary supplement company (greater than 500 employees, less than 500 employees and less than 20 employees). However, GMPs will apply to all companies manufacturing dietary supplements by the year 2010 [13]. Prior to the establishment of GMPs in June, 2007, the National Sanitation Foundation (NSF), one of two auditing bodies in the USA. that "certifies" dietary supplement companies with regard to good manufacturing practices, launched its "One Step Ahead Program". This program, a web based service center, was developed to help manufacturers get ready for the new FDA GMP guidelines [14].

PROVISIONS OF THE FDA GOOD MANUFACTURING PRACTICES GUIDELINES

The new good manufacturing practice guidelines address several areas in the manufacture, packaging, labeling, and storage of dietary supplements. These include personnel, physical plant, equipment, record keeping and remediation practices. Manufacturers are required to evaluate the identity, purity, quantity, and composition of the dietary supplements using state of the art scientific practices. Within these practice guidelines, companies have the flexibility to change methods of evaluation as scientific protocols are improved [13].

Regardless of how soon the FDA implements its new GMPs, the USA is far behind many other countries in establishing good manufacturing practices for dietary supplements. Canada, Australia, the European Union and Japan have all established good manufacturing practices for dietary supplements and foods containing probiotics. These regulations vary greatly with the country but most address issues mentioned above in addition to enforcement of the regulations [15–22]. With the gradual implementation of GMPs by the FDA still to be accomplished, and the policing of these recommendations still unclear, the quality control and regulation of all dietary supplements in the USA still remains in the hands of the production companies.

GMPS AND SELF-REGULATION BY THE DIETARY SUPPLEMENT INDUSTRY

Consumer groups and patient advocacy groups are likely to applaud the FDA for establishing good manufacturing practices for companies manufacturing dietary supplements including probiotics. At this time, however, it is unclear how these recommendations will be followed by the dietary supplement industry. The FDA GMPs contain no guidelines for policing or evaluating companies for adherence to these practices. If the dietary supplement industry will continue to regulate their own quality control, one must ask what the companies are doing now with regard to quality control? Specifically, what are the processes involved in the manufacture of probiotic supplements and where should quality control processes be present? Are the companies that manufacture probiotics adequately monitoring the manufacture of these products? Is self-regulation working with regard to consumers and patients? The next section addresses these questions.

IS SELF-REGULATION OF PROBIOTIC SUPPLEMENTS WORKING?

In a word, no. At this time, self-regulation of probiotics by the manufacturers of dietary supplements in the USA is not keeping these products reliable or safe. Although a substantial number of companies already follow good manufacturing practices, data show problems with self-regulation in the probiotic dietary supplement industry overall. Numerous studies examining dietary supplements or food products have been conducted in which dietary supplements or food products are examined microbiologically for agreement with product labeling [23–31]. Studies have also examined the viability of microorganisms present, the colony count of organisms in the supplement and most importantly, the presence of contaminating microbes [26–31].

QUALITY CONTROL AND CONTAMINATION OF PROBIOTIC SUPPLEMENTS

Contamination of probiotic supplements deserves special mention because both the presence of contamination and the type of contamination are equally important where the health of a patient is concerned. Where do these microbial contaminants come from? Do they originate from the soil, the human gastrointestinal tract or human skin? What is the potential for a probiotic contaminant to cause disease in immune competent, immune suppressed or individuals with other serious medical conditions such as inflammatory bowel disease and cancer? Does this organism have the ability to pass on antibiotic resistance genes to other organisms? The results and conclusions of these studies have not been encouraging.

RESULTS OF QUALITY CONTROL STUDIES

Overall, these studies have found that the microbial identification of a significant proportion (approximately 20–25%] of products on the market do not match the labeling of these products [23–31]. There are three primary reasons for the mismatch between the label and identification of microorganisms. One is incorrect genetic identification. This does not imply problems with quality control but rather that the dietary supplement industry has not kept pace with the rapid improvements in genetic identification protocols. Subsequently, the renaming of a number of microorganisms, including probiotic organisms, has resulted in a high number of mismatches between genetic testing and product labeling. Most of these mismatches occur at the species level. The second and third reasons for mismatch between labeling and identification are due to deletions or additions of probiotic species. Both the absence of expected species or strains and the presence of unexpected species or strains are very problematic and are directly related to quality control.

First let us examine deletions. If something is on the label but is not viable or present in the product, this can be due to lack of addition of product in the first place or the death of the organism somewhere from manufacture until sampling. In a second scenario, the original organism may be detected via different methodologies but not be viable at the time of sampling.

With regard to additions, these are considered contaminants. It is likely that contamination occurred either in the manufacturing process or in the packaging process. Some contaminants are considered relatively harmless, some are considered "opportunistic" and some are considered "frank pathogens". These "harmless" contaminants may include probiotic organisms that were not efficiently separated from the original probiotic organism. Examples may include *Lactobacillus* or *Bifidobacterium* species other than what was listed on the label. Although probiotic organisms have been associated with sepsis and other infections [32–35], this is extremely rare and usually occurs in immune compromised individuals. Therefore, the addition of other "probiotic strains" is usually not detrimental to the health of consumers and patients.

Some contaminating organisms are considered opportunistic pathogens. These organisms are normally harmless in immune competent hosts, but have the potential for causing infection in immune compromised or immune suppressed persons. These organisms may originate from soil, such as *Bacillus subtilis* or from skin or intestinal tract such as *Staphylococcus aureus*, *Staphylococcus epidermidis*, or *Enterococcus* species (*Enterococcus faecium* and *E. faecalis*). Of these, *Enterococcus* species is worth special mention as it poses an additional risk. Although the organism is an opportunistic pathogen, it has the added risk of passing on resistance genes to multiple antibiotics to other microorganisms. Some *Enterococcus* species are among the most antibiotic resistant *Streptococcus* bacteria recognized [36, 37]. Other organisms well known as opportunistic or even "frank pathogens" to immune compromised persons include Gram-negative rods such as *Serratia marcescens*, *Escherichia coli*, *Klebsiella pneumoniae* and Pseudomonas species such as *Burkholderia cepacia* and *Pseudomonas aeruginosa*. All of these bacteria have been recovered from probiotic cultures [26, 30].

RECOMMENDATIONS FOR CLINICIANS

What recommendations can we make to healthcare professionals and their patients when choosing a probiotic that will be safe? The first and foremost step is to check the peer- reviewed literature and consumer websites. These resources provide clinicians and patients a way to check on the quality control of probiotic foods and supplements. Specifically, these resources indicate which brands have been tested for purity, viability, and efficacy with regard to immune support or specific health care problems. The most commonly used sites are listed in Table 24.3.

If a particular brand has not been reviewed, there are a few guidelines that have been published as a result of large-scale quality control studies. One is the use of refrigeration. Refrigeration should be assured during production, shipping, delivery, and storage. The presence of refrigeration in probiotic products is associated with decreased contamination and increased viability [38]. Even if the product does not require refrigeration, it is suggested that it be refrigerated once purchased. These are live microorganisms after all. The second is to purchase a probiotic supplement or food as close to its manufacturing date as possible. While many companies may not directly list the date of manufacture on the container, one can often determine this information from the lot

Table 24.3
Websites to investigate quality control of probiotics

Organization	Contact information	Comments
Consumer Labs	Consumerlab.com	Details results of quality control testing. Requires subscription.
National Sanitation Foundation	http://www.nsf.org/consumer	Information about dietary supplement manufacturer GMPs certification
National Products Association (formerly the National Nutritional Foods Association)	http://www.supplement-quality.com/testing/	Information about dietary supplement manufacturer GMPs certification
US Pharmacopeia	http://www.usp.org/ USPVerified/dietary-Supplements/	Details results of quality control testing.
National Library of Medicine Website	http://www.ncbi.nlm.nih. gov/sites/entrez?db = pubmed	Peer reviewed scientific papers on probiotics

number. Frequently, manufacture lot number are a combination of the day, month, and year of production. The third guideline is to use these supplements as quickly as possible. Even in a refrigerator, constant opening and closing of a bottle may add moisture to the contents of the bottle and moisture hastens decline of viability. A desiccant in the bottle is likely to help, but not totally prevent, the accumulation of moisture in the bottle. Another factor is cost. Although higher cost does not guarantee good quality and there are many good quality products at very reasonable prices ($0.25 a pill or less), there is a positive correlation between cost and viability [30]. Additionally, there is a positive correlation between cost and purity [30]. It is wise to check for the manufacturers' certification by one of two auditing and credentialing bodies in the USA (National Sanitation Foundation -NSF and National Nutrition Foods Association-NNFA). The primary problem with this recommendation is that the name of the original manufacturer may not be displayed on the final probiotic product.

ADDITIONAL RECOMMENDATIONS ON PRODUCT LABELING

The probiotic dietary supplement parameters discussed above may provide other useful information about the quality and efficacy of a particular product. Other things to look for on the probiotic supplement label include:

1. Listing of all genera, species, and strains (subspecies): Check the peer-reviewed literature for correlation of particular species or strains with efficacy. A positive clinical outcome may be associated with a particular strain or subspecies.
2. Specific properties of any strains like hydrogen peroxide (H_2O_2) production or adherence capabilities. See above discussion with regard to these properties.

3. Colony count: Although the optimal dose for probiotics is not known, recommended doses showing efficacy in scientific studies are in the 1–100 billion colony count per dose range. This usually translates to1–3 pills or capsules per day.

4. Quality control practices including independent laboratory assays for purity, viability, and colony count. This is evidence of good manufacturing practices.

5. The presence of fillers and other "inert" ingredients. Generally, minimal presence of fillers or inert ingredients is favorable and testing these inert ingredients for purity is highly recommended. This is another indication of following good manufacturing practices

6. The presence of a delayed release formula or the presence of enteric coating. Although there is no scientific evidence for improved quality with either property (see above), theoretically they may allow for greater survival and possibly provide equivalent clinical effect with lower microorganism numbers.

SUMMARY AND CONCLUSIONS

This chapter discusses the different properties of food probiotics and those found in dietary supplements. Included are the guidelines for the manufacture of probiotics and the current state of federal regulation of probiotics in food products and dietary supplements. Currently, it is encouraging that good manufacturing guidelines are being put forth at least for dietary supplements. However, the regulation of these practices remains to be determined. Until these good manufacturing practices are fully implemented and regulated, information for the clinicians and their patients is provided for assessing products that are on the market and choosing a probiotic that will have the best chance of promoting health.

REFERENCES

1. http://www.aboutyogurt.com/industryAndResources/pdfs/NYA-Seal-Program-Procedure.pdf.
2. Joint FAO/WHO Working Group Report on Drafting Guidelines for the Evaluation of Probiotics in Food. London, Ontario, Canada. 30 April and 2 May 2002.
3. FAO/WHO. Guidelines for the evaluation of probiotics in food. Food and Agriculture Organization of the United Nations and World Health Organization Working Group Report, 2002. http://www.fao.org/es/ESN/Probio/probio.htm
4. Donohue DC, Salminen S, Marteau P. Safety of Probiotic bacteria. In: S Salminen, A von Wright, (Eds), Lactic Acid Bacteria –Microbiology and Functional Aspects. New York: Marcel Dekker 1998:369–383.
5. Lee YK, Lim CY, Teng WL, Ouwehand AC, Tuomola EM, Salminen S. Quantitative approach in the study of adhesion of lactic acid bacteria to intestinal cells and their competition with enterobacteria. 2000; *Appl. Environ. Microbiol*, 66:3692–3697.
6. Biradar, SS, Patil, BM, Rasal, VP. Prebiotics for improved gut health. *Int. J. Nutr. Welln*. 2005; 2 (1).
7. Veereman-Wauters, G. Application of prebiotics in infant foods. *Br. J. Nutr.* 2005; 93:S57–S60.
8. http://www.fda.gov/opacom/laws/dshea.html
9. Full text of DSHEA at HealthWorld Online http://www.healthy.net/public/legal-lg/fedregs/S784_ENR. HTM > http://www.cfsan.fda.gov/~dms/dietsupp.html
10. http://www.cfsan.fda.gov/~dms/hclaims.html
11. Pineiro, M, and Stanton C. Probiotic bacteria: Legislative framework-requirements to evidence basis. *J. Nutr.* 2007; 137:850S–853S.

12. Reid G. The importance of guidelines in the development and application of probiotics. *Curr. Pharm. Design.* 2005; 11:11–15.

13. http://www.cfsan.fda.gov/~dms/supplmnt.html

14. http://www.nsf.org/business/newsroom/press_release.asp?p_id = 15466

15. http://www.hc-sc.gc.ca/dhp-mps/prodnatur/index_e.html

16. http://www.apvma.gov.au/qa/gmp_code_veterinary.pdf

17. http://www.foodstandards.gov.au/mediareleasespublications/mediareleases/mediareleases2005/fsanzseeksviewsonpro2909.cfm

18. http://canada.gc.ca/gazette/part1/ascII/g1–13551_e.txt

19. Australian Ministry of Health and Welfare. Notice: Guideline for Application and Evaluation of Nutritional Supplements. May 2001.

20. Australian Ministry of Health, Labor, Welfare, Notice on Treatment of "Nutritional Supplement" May 2001.

21. European Commision. Recommendation 97/618/EC (http://europa.eu.int/smartapi/cgi/sga_doc/smartapi!prod!CELEXnumdoc&Ig = EN&num-doc = 31997HO618&model = guichett).

22. European Commission.Regulation EC N 258/97 (http://europa.eu.int/smartapi/cgi/sga_doc?smartapi!celexapi!prod!CELEXnumdoc&Ig = EN&numdoc = 31997R0258&model = guichett).

23. Huys G., Vancanneyt M., D'Haene K, Vankerckhoven, V.,Goosens H., Swings J., Accuracy of species identity of commercial bacterial cultures intended for probiotic or nutritional use. *Res Microb.* 2006; 157:803–810.

24. Drisko J., Bischoff B., Giles, C., Adelson, M., Evaluation of five probiotic products for label claims by DNA extraction and polymerase chain reaction analysis digest. Dis. Sci. 2004; 50 (6): 1113–1117

25. Yeung, PS., Sanders, ME.,Kitts, CL.,Cano, R., Tong, PS., Species-specific identification of commercial probiotic strains. *J. Dairy Sci.* 2002; 85:1039–1051.

26. Hughes, VL and Hillier, SL. Microbiological characteristics of Lactobacillus products used for colonization of the vagina. Obstet. *Gynecol.* 1990; 75:244–248.

27. Zhong, W., Millsap, K., Bialkowska-Hobrzanska, H., and Reid, G. Differentiation of Lactobacillus species by molecular typing. *Appl. Environ. Microbiol.* 1998; 64:2418–2423.

28. Hamilton-Miller, JM., Shah, S., Smith, CT. "Probiotic" remedies are not what they seem. *Brit. Med. J.* 1996; 312:55–56.

29. Hamilton-Miller, JM., Shah, S., Winkler, JT. Public health issues arising from microbiological and labeling quality of foods and supplements containing probiotic organisms. *Pub. Health. Nutr.* 1999; 2:223–229.

30. Berman, SH, Spicer, D. Safety and reliability of Lactobacillus supplements in Seattle, Washington (a pilot study). Inter. J. Alter. Med. 2003; 1(2).

31. Schillinger, U., Isolation and Identification of lactobacilli from novel-type Probiotic and mild yoghurts and their stability during refrigerated storage. *Intern. J. Food Microbiol.* 1999; 47:79–87.

32. Saxelin M, Chuang NH, Chassy B, et al. Lactobacilli and bacteremia in southern Finland, 1989–1992. *Clin Infect Dis* 1996; 22:564–566.

33. MacGregor G, Smith AJ, Thakker B, et al. Yogurt biotherapy: contraindicated in immunosuppressed patients? *Postgrad Med J.* 2002; 78:366–367.

34. Land MH, Rouster-Stevens K, Woods CR, et al. Lactobacillus sepsis associated with probiotic therapy. *Pediatrics* 2005; 115:178–181.

35. Ha GY, Yang, CH, Kim, H, Chong, Y, Case of Sepsis Caused by Bifidobacterium longum *J. Clin. Microbiol.* 1999; 37:1227–1228.

36. Iwen, PC., Kelly, DM., Linder, J., Hinrichs SH., Dominguez EA., Rupp, ME., Patil, KD. Change in prevalence and antibiotic resistance of Enterococcus species isolated from blood cultures over an 8-year period. Antimicrob. *Agents Chemother.* 1997; 41(2):494–495.

37. Lund, B., Edlund, C., Barkholt, L., Nord, CE., Tvede, M., Poulsen, RL., Impact on human intestinal microflora of an Enterococcus faecium probiotic and vancomycin. *Scand. J. Infect. Dis.* 2000; 32:627–632.

38. Antunes, AC. Cazetto, TF., Bolini, HA., Viability of probiotic micro-organisms during storage, postacidification and sensory analysis of fat-free yogurts with added whey protein concentrate. *Intern. J. Dairy Techn.* 2005; 58(3):169–173. 2005

Index

Printed in the United States of America